RAPID INTERPRETATION OF ECGs IN EMERGENCY MEDICINE

A VISUAL GUIDE

Jennifer L. Martindale, MD

Harvard Affiliated Emergency Medicine Residency Program
Boston, Massachusetts

David F. M. Brown, MD

Vice Chair
Department of Emergency Medicine
Massachusetts General Hospital
Associate Professor
Division of Emergency Medicine
Harvard Medical School
Boston, Massachusetts

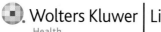. Wolters Kluwer | Lippincott Williams & Wilkins
Health

Philadelphia • Baltimore • New York • London
Buenos Aires • Hong Kong • Sydney • Tokyo

Senior Acquisitions Editor: Frances DeStefano
Product Director: Julia Seto
Production Manager: Alicia Jackson
Senior Manufacturing Manager: Benjamin Rivera
Senior Marketing Manager: Kimberly Schonberger
Design Coordinator: Stephen Druding
Production Service: SPi Global

Printed in China

Library of Congress Cataloging-in-Publication Data
Martindale, Jennifer L.
    Rapid interpretation of ECGs in emergency medicine : a visual guide / Jennifer L. Martindale, David F. M. Brown. — 1st ed.
        p. ; cm.
    Includes bibliographical references and index.
    ISBN 978-1-4511-2837-6 (pbk.)
    I. Brown, David F. M. II. Title.
    [DNLM: 1. Electrocardiography. 2. Emergencies.   WG 140]
    616.1'207547—dc23

2011045348

Care has been taken to confirm the accuracy of the information presented and to describe generally accepted practices. However, the authors, editors, and publisher are not responsible for errors or omissions or for any consequences from application of the information in this book and make no warranty, expressed or implied, with respect to the currency, completeness, or accuracy of the contents of the publication. Application of the information in a particular situation remains the professional responsibility of the practitioner.

The authors, editors, and publisher have exerted every effort to ensure that drug selection and dosage set forth in this text are in accordance with current recommendations and practice at the time of publication. However, in view of ongoing research, changes in government regulations, and the constant flow of information relating to drug therapy and drug reactions, the reader is urged to check the package insert for each drug for any change in indications and dosage and for added warnings and precautions. This is particularly important when the recommended agent is a new or infrequently employed drug.

Some drugs and medical devices presented in the publication have Food and Drug Administration (FDA) clearance for limited use in restricted research settings. It is the responsibility of the health care provider to ascertain the FDA status of each drug or device planned for use in their clinical practice.

To purchase additional copies of this book, call our customer service department at (800) 638-3030 or fax orders to (301) 223-2320. International customers should call (301) 223-2300.

Visit Lippincott Williams & Wilkins on the Internet: at LWW.com. Lippincott Williams & Wilkins customer service representatives are available from 8:30 am to 6 pm, EST.

RRS1202

RAPID INTERPRETATION OF ECGs IN EMERGENCY MEDICINE

A VISUAL GUIDE

WITH UTMOST GRATITUDE TO MY MOTHER, DEE, FOR MOVING
ME TO HELP OTHERS AND TO MY FATHER, PETER, FOR
ENCOURAGING ME TO EXPLORE. TO MY SISTER, CASSIDY, FOR
INSPIRING ME BY HER COURAGE, CREATIVITY, AND SUCCESS.
TO THE RESIDENTS AND FACULTY OF THE HARVARD
AFFILIATED EMERGENCY MEDICINE RESIDENCY PROGRAM,
FOR MAKING ME WANT TO BECOME A BETTER DOCTOR.

J.M.

DEDICATED TO THE RESIDENTS OF THE HARVARD AFFILIATED
EMERGENCY MEDICINE RESIDENCY, PAST, PRESENT, AND
FUTURE, WHO CONTINUE TO AMAZE AND INSPIRE ME.

D.F.M.B

PREFACE

Pattern recognition plays an essential role in the practice of medicine and making real-time diagnoses. The main objective of this book is to provide a visual tool that will help physicians and other emergency care providers quickly recognize important electrocardiogram (ECG) patterns. We believe that by the end of the book, the reader will have developed a mental repertoire of ECGs that represent medically significant conditions, including some that are potentially fatal.

We also believe that ECG interpretation can be demystified through the use of visual, easy-to-follow explanations. Our audience, therefore, is not only emergency physicians, but also physicians from other specialties; residents in emergency medicine, internal medicine, and family practice; physician assistants; nurse practitioners; and advanced medical students who want to become more competent in ECG interpretation without having to face the daunting task of relearning the math and physics of cardiac electrophysiology.

The format of the book is to first show an ECG in its native state to give the reader a chance to recognize and interpret salient features. The reader can then flip the page and look at the same ECG with abnormal patterns enlarged, highlighted in color, and described in brief text. This book is intentionally graphic and nontechnical. It is designed to help clinicians make visual diagnoses by pointing out abnormalities in a colorful and pictorial fashion.

We hope that in presenting this compilation of ECGs in a visually memorable way, we will help providers to recognize medical conditions requiring rapid diagnosis and management.

We would like to thank Keith A. Marill, MD and James K. Takayesu, MD, emergency medicine physicians at Massachusetts General Hospital, for their encouragement and helpful feedback. We would also like to thank all those who contributed ECGs to this collection.

CONTENTS

Preface   vi

1	Concept Review	1
2	Sinus Dysfunction	16
3	Bundle and Fascicular Blocks	27
4	AV Conduction Blocks	63
5	Premature Contractions	95
6	Abnormal QRS Morphology	117
7	Abnormal T Waves	161
8	QT Abnormalities and Electrolyte Disturbances	190
9	Voltage Abnormalities	227
10	Fast and Narrow	262
11	Fast and Wide	310
12	Ischemic Patterns	356
13	Paced Rhythms	430
14	Rapid Review	460

Appendix   471

Index   473

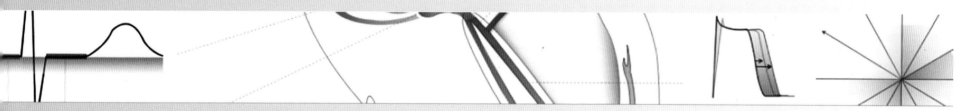

Action Potential—Myocardial Cell

The different phases of the action potential relate directly to the waveforms, intervals, and segments that constitute a cardiac cycle on the ECG. Each phase is distinguished by an alteration in cell membrane permeability to sodium, potassium, and calcium ions. A basic understanding of these phases and their major ion currents will help in learning the ECG features associated with conduction abnormalities, drug toxicities, and electrolyte disturbances.

The action potential of the myocardial cell is divided into five phases (phases 0–4). The first phase, phase 0, represents ventricular depolarization. Rapid depolarization depends on initial sodium entry that triggers the explosive influx of more sodium through fast-gated sodium channels. This phase takes the myocardial cell from its resting potential of –90 mV to a positive potential of 20 mV. The summation of this phase across the ventricular myocardium is represented on the ECG as the QRS wave.

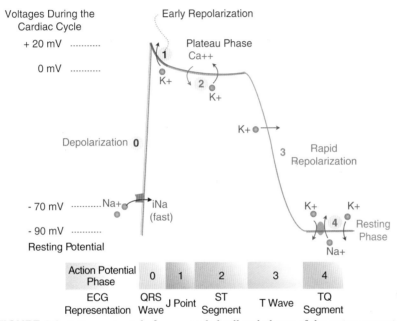

FIGURE 1.1 Action potential of a myocardial cell and phases of the action potential as they relate to ECG waves and segments.[1] The action potential also represents the cell membrane in this figure, with the area under the action potential representing intracellular space and the area above the action potential representing extracellular space.

Ventricular repolarization occurs during phases 1, 2, and 3. By phase 1, the fast sodium channels are closed (and inactivated), and the cell returns to a neutral potential by the opening of potassium channels that allow for the outward movement of potassium.

During phase 2, the neutral potential is maintained by balancing potassium efflux with the sustained entry of calcium ions. Calcium entry during this phase initiates the release of intracellular calcium stores necessary for sarcomere shortening and ventricular contraction. The ST segment corresponds to phase 2.

Phase 3 represents rapid repolarization to the negative resting potential by potassium ion efflux and the closure of calcium channels on the cell membrane. This phase corresponds to the T wave.

After the membrane returns to the resting potential, this potential is maintained during phase 4 by continued potassium efflux and the Na$^+$/K$^+$ ATPase pump (red oval). The ventricular myocardium is at its resting potential (phase 4) between the end of the T wave and the beginning of the next QRS wave (TQ segment).

Action Potential—Pacemaker Cell

Cardiac pacemaker cells are specialized to spontaneously depolarize and initiate action potentials. The action potential of pacemaker cells is divided into three phases (phases 0, 3, and 4). Spontaneous phase 4 depolarization (represented by an upsloping phase 4 in the action potential) distinguishes pacemaker cells from myocardial cells. During this phase, slow inward sodium current results in the gradual rise of the membrane potential toward its threshold potential. The current responsible for phase 4 depolarization is also known as the pacemaker current or funny current (I_f).

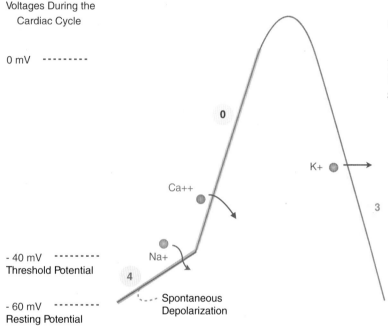

FIGURE 1.2 Action potential of a pacemaker cell. Lines of the action potential also represent the cell membrane of the pacemaker cell.

Once threshold potential is attained, calcium channels open to depolarize the cell during phase 0.

Repolarization occurs in phase 3 with the opening of potassium channels and closure of calcium channels. When the membrane potential returns to its resting potential, sodium channels immediately open again.

The slope of phase 4 is directly affected by sympathetic and parasympathetic tone. Sympathetic stimulation results in a steeper phase 4 and consequently a faster heart rate. Norepinephrine (NE) released from sympathetic nerves increases the membrane's permeability to sodium. Vagal tone decreases the slope of phase 4 and consequently, the heart rate. Acetylcholine (ACh) released by the vagus nerve increases the cell membrane's permeability to potassium while decreasing its permeability to sodium.[2]

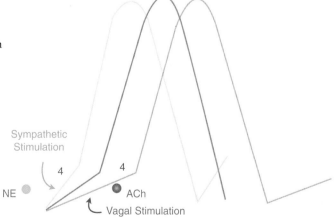

FIGURE 1.3 Effect of sympathetic and parasympathetic stimulation on phase 4 of the pacemaker action potential.

Refractory Periods

Once myocardial cells have entered phase 0 depolarization, the cells become refractory to the conduction of incoming impulses. This allows cells to recover from depolarization. The relative differences in refractory states depend on the state of the fast sodium channels. Refractory states are defined by the strength of impulse required for a myocardial cell to generate and propagate an action potential. Fig. 1.4 shows how these different refractory periods relate to phases of the action potential.[2] Refractory periods are especially relevant to ECG rhythms resulting from a reentry circuit and to antiarrhythmic drugs that prolong the duration of the action potential.

Effective Refractory Period

During phases 0 to 2 and part of phase 3, the myocardial cell is unable to propagate an action potential in response to a stimulus, regardless of the strength of that stimulus.

Relative Refractory Period

Before the cell has returned to its resting membrane potential of –90 mV, it may respond to a stronger-than-normal stimulus. This can occur during phase 3 of repolarization. The response to this stimulus is slower than normal.

Supranormal Period

A smaller-than-normal impulse can elicit a normal action potential.

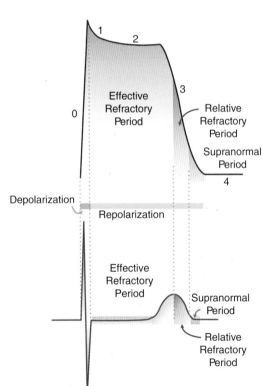

FIGURE 1.4 Refractory periods during different phases of the action potential and cardiac cycle on ECG.

Reentry Circuits

A reentrant circuit consists of two separate pathways that differ in refractory period duration. An impulse may simultaneously encounter a group of refractory cells and a group of cells ready to conduct. Conduction preferentially occurs down the pathway out of its refractory period.

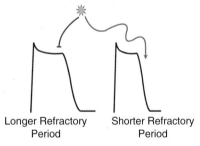

Longer Refractory Period   Shorter Refractory Period

FIGURE 1.5 Variable refractory periods play a key role in reentry. Drugs that prolong the action potential and effective refractory period are used to terminate reentrant circuits.

Class IA Antiarrhythmics

Quinidine, procainamide, and disopyramide prolong the effective refractory period by blocking the sodium channels responsible for rapid depolarization, thereby prolonging phase 0. This is represented on the ECG by QRS widening.

Class III Antiarrhythmics

Amiodarone, dofetilide, and ibutilide prolong the action potential duration by blocking the outward flow of potassium during phase 3. This increases the effective refractory period of cardiac myocytes. On the ECG, this is represented by QT prolongation.

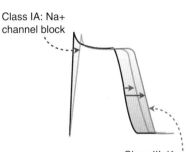

Class IA: Na+ channel block

Class III: K+ channel block

FIGURE 1.6 Effect of Na+ channel blockade and K+ channel blockade on action potential duration.

Conduction Anatomy

Normal conduction is essential to coordinated and efficient ventricular contraction. Impulses from the sinus node activate atrial myocardium and travel down internodal tracts to the AV node. After a brief delay at the AV node, simultaneous conduction down the right and left bundle branches allows for synchronous contraction of the right and left ventricles. Simultaneous conduction down the left anterior and posterior fascicles of the left bundle branch allows for coordinated contraction of the left ventricular free wall.

Action
Potential

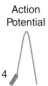

4

Sinus Node

The sinus node is located in the superior aspect of the right atrium near the superior vena cava and contains pacemaker cells with automaticity. The sinus node is the dominant pacemaker of the heart because its pacemaker cells are capable of reaching the threshold potential the fastest. This is reflected by a steep phase 4 of their action potential.

Internodal Pathways

AV Node

The AV node is located in the lower right atrium near the coronary sinus and septal leaflet of the tricuspid valve. The node can be divided into three regions based on their different electrophysiologic properties. The nodal region, shown in Fig. 1.8, is the middle segment and lacks automaticity. This part of the AV node contributes to conduction delay between the atria and ventricles. The atrial and nodo-His regions of the AV node contain pacemaker cells.[1]

Right Ventricle

Bundle of His

The Bundle of His, or common bundle, stems from the AV node before it bifurcates into the right and left bundle branches.

Left Bundle Branch

The left bundle branch is short and separates into *three* fascicles (only two are depicted here and throughout this book): the left anterior fascicle, the septal fascicle, and the left posterior fascicle. The role of the septal fascicle is less understood.

Left Posterior Fascicle

The left posterior fascicle activates the posterior and inferior segments of the left ventricle.

Left Anterior Fascicle

The left anterior fascicle activates the anterior and superior segments of the left ventricle.

Purkinje Fibers

The Purkinje fibers arise from the bundle branches and spread throughout the subendocardium. The endocardium is the first part of the cardiac muscle to become depolarized. Purkinje fibers also have automaticity. When other pacemakers fail to take over, the Purkinje fibers may fulfill the pacemaker role.

Right Bundle Branch

The right bundle branch travels alongside the left anterior fascicle down the interventricular septum.

FIGURE 1.7 Anatomy of the conduction system.

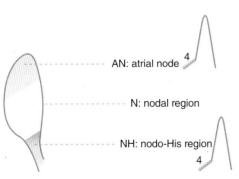

AN: atrial node   4

N: nodal region

NH: nodo-His region

4

FIGURE 1.8 Properties of the AV node

Retrograde Conduction Patterns

Basic teaching of conduction anatomy addresses anterograde conduction down normal pathways from the sinus node to the His-Purkinje system. Conduction can also occur in retrograde fashion (in a ventricular to atrial direction) through normal and bypass conduction pathways.

From Atrium to Sinus Node

A premature atrial impulse travels to both the AV node and sinus node (A). This impulse can depolarize the sinus node and effectively reset the pacemaker while it travels through the AV node and His-Purkinje system.

From AV Node to Atrium

Retrograde conduction can also occur from a focus or reentrant circuit within the AV node (B). Retrograde conduction from the AV node to atria can result in atrial depolarization. When not buried by a QRS wave, this can result in the appearance of a retrograde P wave on the ECG.

Concealed Retrograde Conduction

Retrograde conduction may reach the AV node but fail to penetrate and depolarize atrial tissue (C). By reaching the AV node, however, a retrograde impulse can render the AV node refractory to the next incoming atrial impulse. The next sinus P wave will be blocked and appear without an associated QRS complex.

From Ventricle to Atrium

Ventriculoatrial conduction can occur by retrograde conduction through normal conduction pathways or through a bypass tract (C and D).

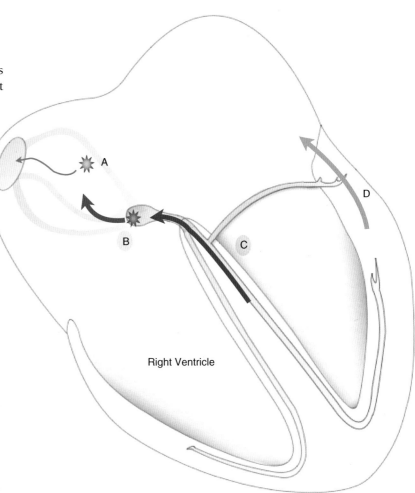

FIGURE 1.9 Retrograde conduction patterns.

Axis and the Frontal Leads

The ECG axis is a vector representation of the direction of current. Axis can be described for P, QRS, and T waves, but when unspecified, the term usually refers to the QRS axis (representing the direction of ventricular current and depolarization). There are several approaches for determining the QRS axis.

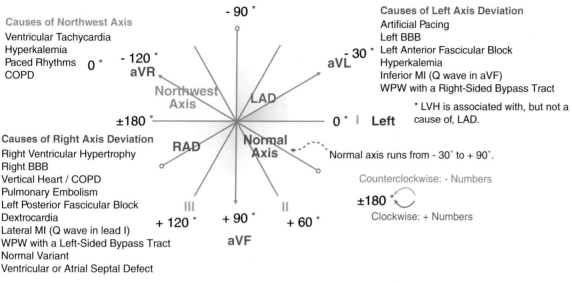

FIGURE 1.10 Frontal plane leads and the hexaxial reference system.

The Hexaxial Method

One approach to determining the QRS axis is to make use of isoelectric (equiphasic) QRS waves in limb leads. A lead with an isoelectric QRS wave is likely to be perpendicular to the axis, as the vector sum of such a wave (zero) reflects the absence of any current moving toward or away from that lead. The axis is then 90° clockwise or counterclockwise from the isoelectric lead (Fig. 1.11). The perpendicular lead with the positive QRS complex is the QRS axis (current is moving toward that lead). Each limb lead is perpendicular to another limb lead on the ECG.

The Quadrant Method

To get a quick sense of whether there is axis deviation, look at the QRS complexes in leads I and aVF, and simplify the hexaxial system into quadrants.

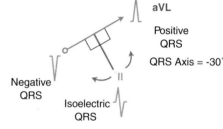

FIGURE 1.11 Perpendicular relationship between two leads used to determine axis.

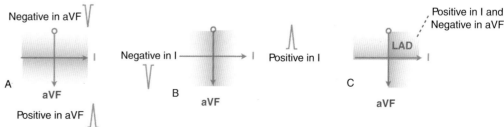

FIGURE 1.12 Use of I and aVF for axis determination. **A.** When the QRS wave in aVF is positive, the axis will be classified as either normal axis or right axis deviation. **B.** When the QRS wave is positive in I, the axis will be normal or deviated to the left. **C.** The combination of a negative QRS wave in aVF and a positive QRS wave in I indicates left axis deviation.

The Precordial Leads

Whereas the limb leads view the heart in the frontal plane, the precordial leads view it in the horizontal or transverse plane. Lead V1 is considered to be the window into the right ventricle. In general, leads V1 and V2 reflect the right ventricle and leads V5 and V6 reflect the left ventricle. The QRS complex becomes more positive progressing from V1 to V6.

Normally R waves are small in lead V1. Causes of tall R waves in this lead are listed below.[3]

Causes of a Tall R Wave in V1 (R > S)

Right Bundle Branch Block
Right Ventricular Hypertrophy
Hypertrophic Cardiomyopathy
Posterior MI
Paced Rhythm
Wolff-Parkinson-White Syndrome
Normal Variant (children/adolescents)
Duchenne Muscular Dystrophy
Dextrocardia

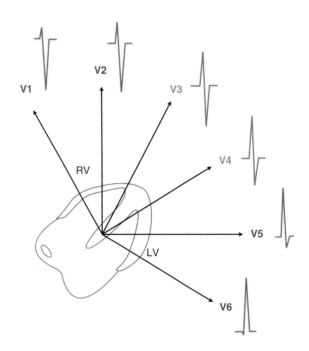

FIGURE 1.13 Normal relationship between precordial leads and the heart.

Lead Misplacement: An obvious aberration in the sequence of wave progression from V1-V6 is commonly due to incorrect lead placement.

Normally, the QRS complexes transition from being predominately negative to positive in leads V2-V4. When transition with isoelectric complexes occurs in V5 or V6 or the R wave amplitude is less than 3 mm in lead V3, the ECG is said to demonstrate "poor R-wave progression" or "loss of anterior forces." Causes of poor R-wave progression are listed below.[4]

Causes of Poor R-Wave Progression

Left Bundle Branch Block
Left Ventricular Hypertrophy
Anterior MI
Right Ventricular Hypertrophy/COPD

The QRS Wave

The morphology of the QRS wave is governed by the sequence of ventricular activation and the dominant vector force associated with each step. Normal ventricular depolarization can be simplified into two steps: depolarization of the septum followed by depolarization of the ventricular free walls. Because the Purkinje fibers are located just beneath the endocardium, activation of the ventricular walls spreads from endocardium to epicardium.

Septal Depolarization

The left aspect of the septum is the first part of the ventricles to depolarize. Normal septal depolarization occurs in a left-to-right direction. This results in the small septal R wave in the right precordial lead V1 and the small septal Q wave in V6.

Ventricular Depolarization

Depolarization of left and right ventricular free walls normally occurs simultaneously. The right-to-left depolarization in the larger and thicker left ventricle comprises the dominating vector force. The ECG interprets this depolarization as a right-to-left force even though depolarization in the right ventricle slightly opposes this force. This dominant vector accounts for the large S wave in V1 that transitions in V3/V4 to become the large R wave in the left precordial leads (V6) .

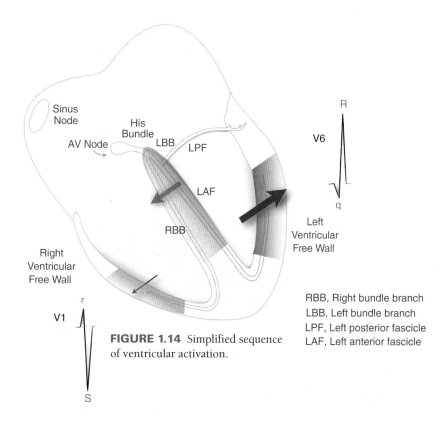

FIGURE 1.14 Simplified sequence of ventricular activation.

RBB, Right bundle branch
LBB, Left bundle branch
LPF, Left posterior fascicle
LAF, Left anterior fascicle

Rate

In regular rhythms, rate can easily be determined by dividing the number 300 by the number of large boxes in a single cardiac cycle (R-R interval). The number 300 is based on the fact that each large box represents 200 msec (0.2 sec or one fifth of a second). A minute is comprised of 300 of these large boxes.

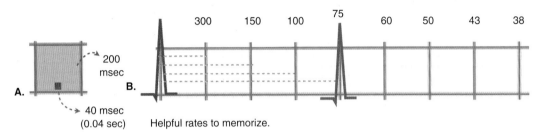

FIGURE 1.15 **A.** Duration of small and large boxes; **B.** Relationship between R–R distances and ventricular rates (bpm).

For irregular rhythms, a simple and fast way to approximate the rate is to count the number of cardiac cycles occurring in six seconds and to multiply this number by 10. Some ECG printouts include markers to indicate 3-second intervals. In those that don't, the number of cardiac cycles within 30 large boxes can be counted and multiplied by 10. In the rhythm below, there are six cardiac cycles; the approximated rhythm is 60 bpm .

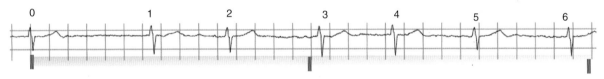

FIGURE 1.16 Calculating ventricular rate in atrial fibrillation using 6-second intervals.

Rhythm Nomenclature

Rhythm nomenclature can be confusing. The name of a rhythm is often based on origin and rate. Because the inherent automaticity differs among the sinus node, AV junction, and pacemaker cells in the ventricle, different rates are used for classifying escape and accelerated rhythms. The table below outlines rhythm classification based on different rates.

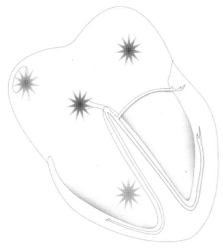

FIGURE 1.17 Locations of ectopic and pacemaker foci.

The AV junction includes the AV node and bundle of His. It is composed of pacemaker cells with an intrinsic rate of 40 to 60 bpm. Because the focus of this rhythm is proximal to the bifurcation of the bundle of His, both ventricles are activated synchronously and the QRS complex is narrow.

A ventricular escape rhythm is typically less than 40 bpm and produces wide QRS complexes.

TABLE 1.1 Classification of rhythms based on rates.

Sinus Node	Sinus Bradycardia	Normal Sinus Rhythm	Sinus Tachycardia
Typical Rate	<60 bpm	60–100 bpm	≥100 bpm

Atrial Foci	Wandering Atrial Pacemaker		Multifocal Atrial Tachycardia
Typical Rate	<100 bpm		≥100 bpm

AV Junction	Junctional Escape Rhythm	Accelerated Junctional Rhythm	Junctional Tachycardia
Typical Rate	<60 bpm	60–100 bpm	≥100 bpm

Ventricular Focus	Ventricular Escape Rhythm	Accelerated Ventricular Rhythm	Ventricular Tachycardia*
Typical Rate	<40 bpm	40–100 bpm	≥100 bpm

Some sources will define ventricular tachycardia when rates are greater than or equal to 120 bpm.

Waves, Intervals, and Segments

WAVES

P Wave: Atria are typically activated in a right-to-left direction as the electrical impulse spreads from the sinus node in the right atrium to the left atrium. The first half of the P wave therefore represents activation of the right atrium.

In normal sinus rhythm, P waves should be upright in the inferior leads (reflecting the superior to inferior direction of the impulse from sinus to AV node). The P wave in V1 is upright or biphasic.

QRS Wave: The QRS wave represents rapid ventricular depolarization and corresponds to phase 0 of the action potential. The QRS complex is widened by delay in the intraventricular conduction system and ventricular hypertrophy.

T Wave: The T wave corresponds to rapid repolarization (phase 3 of the action potential). Repolarization of the epicardium is followed by repolarization of the endocardium. The axis of the T wave should parallel that of the QRS wave when depolarization is normal.

U Wave: The U wave may be absent in the normal electrocardiogram. The source of the U wave is unclear but may represent His/Purkinje repolarization.

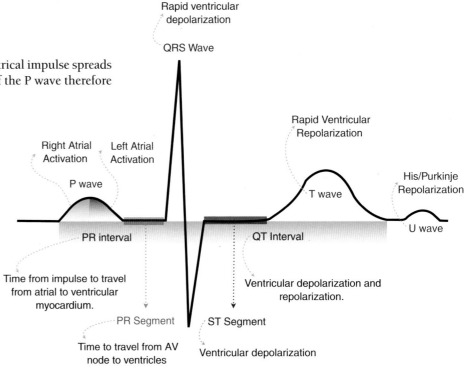

FIGURE 1.18 Electrocardiographic waves, intervals, and segments.

INTERVALS

PR Interval: The PR interval represents the time for an impulse to travel from the atria to the ventricles, including the time it takes to travel through the AV node and bundle of His. PR prolongation most often results from delayed conduction within the AV node. PR shortening classically occurs when an impulse travels from atrium to ventricle through an accessory pathway that bypasses the delay in conduction that occurs in the AV node.

QT Interval: The QT interval represents ventricular depolarization and repolarization, corresponding to phases 0 to 3 of the action potential and ventricular systole. QT prolongation often results from delay in repolarization.

R-R Interval: This corresponds to a complete cardiac cycle.

SEGMENTS

PR Segment: The time it takes for an impulse to travel from the AV node, through the His bundle, and to the ventricles is represented by the PR segment.

ST Segment: During phase 2 or plateau phase of the action potential, the influx of intracellular calcium and subsequent release of intracellular calcium stores allow for ventricular contraction. This phase is represented by the ST segment. Hypercalcemia results in a shortened ST segment; hypocalcemia results in a prolonged ST segment.

General Approach to ECG Interpretation

It helps to have a consistent and methodical approach to interpreting an ECG. With time and practice, this mental checklist can become second nature and completed rapidly. Certain ECG findings should prompt you to look for other ECG abnormalities and to ask relevant clinical questions (*in italics*).

Clinical History ECGs aren't produced in a vacuum; they come from patients with clinical histories and chief complaints. It helps to know if you are dealing with an elderly man with a history of angina complaining of chest pain or a middle-aged woman with lung cancer complaining of shortness of breath. These facts change your pretest probabilities of different clinical diagnoses (in the aforementioned examples, myocardial ischemia or cardiac tamponade, respectively) and thus your interpretation of different ECG morphologies and patterns.

Rate Your initial approach to rhythm analysis starts with defining the rate as normal, slow, or fast.

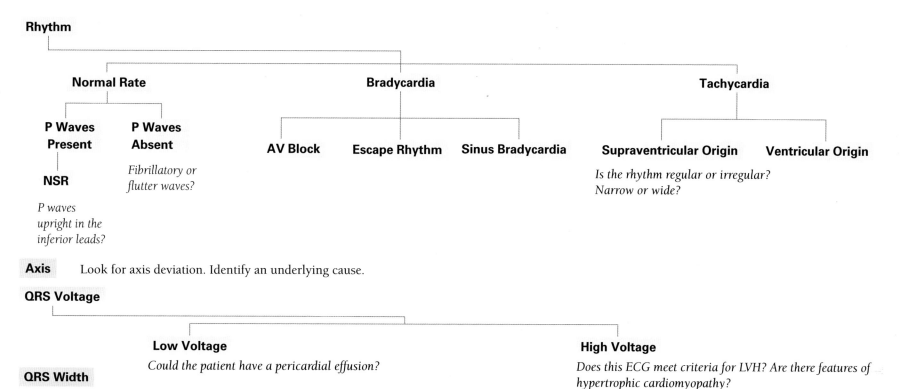

Rhythm

- **Normal Rate**
  - **P Waves Present**
    - **NSR**
    - *P waves upright in the inferior leads?*
  - **P Waves Absent**
    - *Fibrillatory or flutter waves?*
- **Bradycardia**
  - **AV Block**
  - **Escape Rhythm**
  - **Sinus Bradycardia**
- **Tachycardia**
  - **Supraventricular Origin**
    - *Is the rhythm regular or irregular? Narrow or wide?*
  - **Ventricular Origin**

Axis Look for axis deviation. Identify an underlying cause.

QRS Voltage

- **Low Voltage**
  - *Could the patient have a pericardial effusion?*
- **High Voltage**
  - *Does this ECG meet criteria for LVH? Are there features of hypertrophic cardiomyopathy?*

QRS Width

Wide QRS Complexes QRS complexes wider than 120 msec are abnormal. Look for an underlying cause.

Are criteria for RBBB or LBBB met?
Is there LVH?
Any reason to suspect hyperkalemia?
Are there visible pacer artifacts?
Any reason to suspect TCA or cocaine toxicity?

Intervals

PR Interval   A short PR interval may indicate an accessory pathway. A prolonged PR interval could indicate increased parasympathetic tone or AV nodal disease.

QT Interval   Look for QTc prolongation. If QTc prolongation is significant, look for underlying acquired causes and obtain a family history.

Signs of Ischemia

ST Segment   Look for ST depression or elevation in an anatomical lead distribution. Look for reciprocal changes.

T waves   T wave inversion in leads other than aVR is abnormal. Look for biphasic and inverted T waves.

Pathologic Q Waves   Look for pathologic Q waves in an anatomical lead distribution.

Wave Morphologies

P Waves   *Is the P wave morphology consistent within each lead? Is there evidence of right or left atrial enlargement?*

QRS Waves   *Are there delta waves? Are the QRS complexes suggestive of an incomplete bundle branch block?*

T Waves   *Are T waves peaked? Biphasic? Notched and possibly fused with U waves?*

U Waves   *Are there large U waves (near the same amplitude as preceding T waves)?*

Compare with Prior ECG   Valuable information can be gained from comparing current with prior ECGs.

References

1. Baltazar R. Basic Anatomy and Electrophysiology. *Basic and Bedside Electrocardiography*. Philadelphia, PA: Wolters Kluwer/Lippincott Williams & Wilkins; 2009:1–8.
2. Mohrman DE HL. Characteristics of Cardiac Muscle Cells. *Cardiovascular Physiology*. 7th ed. McGraw-Hill Professional; 2010.
3. Mirvis DaG, A. Electrocardiography. In: Bonow RM, D; Zipes, D; Libby P, ed. *Braunwald's Heart Disease: A Textbook of Cardiovascular Medicine*. 9th ed. Philadelphia, PA: Elsevier; 2011.
4. Zema MJ, Kligfield P. ECG poor R-wave progression: review and synthesis. *Arch Intern Med* 1982;142(6):1145–1148.

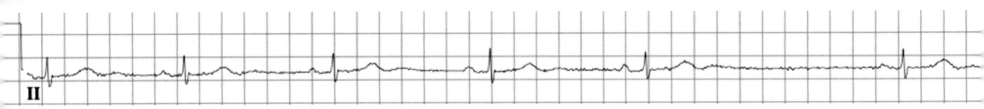

II

Sinus Arrhythmia

Sinus arrhythmia occurs in young and healthy individuals and is *not* a form of sinus node dysfunction. Sinus arrhythmia is characterized by variation in cardiac cycle length. Variation in cycle length is defined as a 120-msec or 10% change between the shortest and longest cycles.[1] Usually, the P wave morphology is invariable, and the PR interval is constant.

Sinus arrhythmia can cause light-headedness and syncope if pauses between sinus beats are long enough.

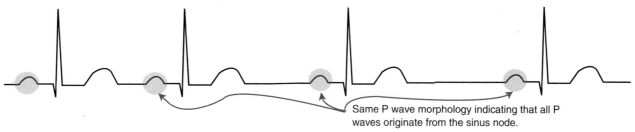

Same P wave morphology indicating that all P waves originate from the sinus node.

FIGURE 2.1 ECG appearance of sinus arrhythmia.

Sinus arrhythmia is classified into respiratory and nonrespiratory types.

Respiratory Sinus Arrhythmia   Inhibition of vagal tone during inspiration causes shortening of cardiac cycle length. On expiration, the cycle lengthens.

Nonrespiratory Sinus Arrhythmia   Phasic variation in cycle length is unrelated to the respiratory cycle. This may occur in patients who are taking digitalis.

Wandering Atrial Pacemaker

This is considered a variant of sinus arrhythmia in which the dominant pacemaker gradually wanders from the sinus node to a latent pacemaker in the atrium or AV junction. This is considered normal physiology.

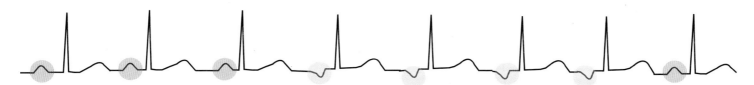

FIGURE 2.2 ECG appearance of a wandering atrial pacemaker. Changes in P wave morphology and cycle length are typically more gradual than what is depicted here.

As the cardiac cycle lengthens, the PR interval shortens and the P wave changes morphology to become negative. As the cardiac cycle shortens, the sinus node takes over again, and the sinus P wave reappears.

Different Types of Sinus Node Dysfunction

Sinus node dysfunction is common and primarily affects the elderly population. There are numerous reversible and irreversible causes. Irreversible causes of symptomatic sinus node dysfunction are often treated with permanent pacemakers.

Sinus Arrest In sinus arrest, the sinus node fails to spontaneously fire and produce an impulse. This results in a pause (absent P-QRS-T). The pause can be terminated by an escape beat. The escape beat occurs at a random time, resulting in a pause that is *not* a multiple of the preceding P-P interval. Technically a pause requires at least a two-second period during which sinus node activity (P waves) is absent.

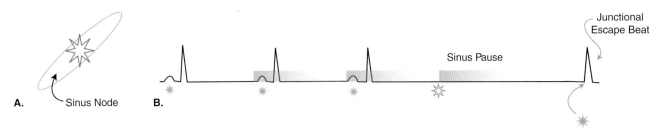

FIGURE 2.3 **A.** Failure to generate a sinus impulse. **B.** ECG appearance of sinus arrest/pause. *Blue stars* indicate sinus-generated impulses. The *white star* indicates failure of the sinus node to generate an impulse. The *pink star* indicates an impulse generated by the AV junction.

The sinus node may consistently fail to fulfill its role as pacemaker. Ventricular activation then comes from pacemaker cells in the AV junction or ventricles. The resultant rhythm is typically a junctional or ventricular escape rhythm.

Junctional Escape Rhythm The QRS complexes in a junctional escape rhythm are narrow. The rate is typically 40 to 60 bpm. P waves may be absent or appear inverted as retrograde P waves before or after QRS complexes.

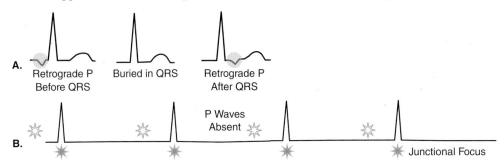

FIGURE 2.4 **A.** Different appearances of junctional escape beats. **B.** ECG appearance of persistent sinus arrest with junctional escape rhythm. *Purple stars* indicate impulses generated by pacemaker cells in the AV node. *White stars* indicate failure of the sinus node to fire.

Ventricular Escape Rhythm The QRS complexes of a ventricular escape rhythm are wide. The rate is typically 20 to 40 bpm.

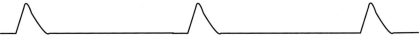

FIGURE 2.5 ECG appearance of a ventricular escape rhythm.

Sinoatrial Exit Block

The sinus node may generate an impulse, but this impulse may fail to propagate to the atria and appear on the ECG as a dropped P-QRS-T complex.

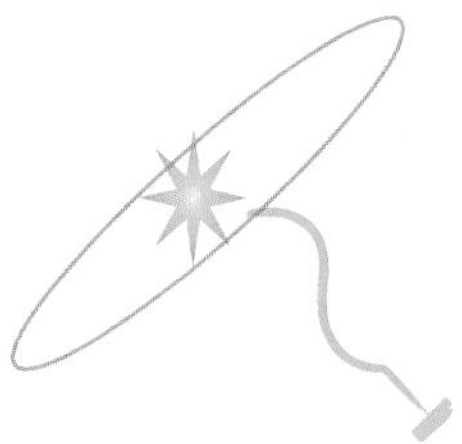

Causes   Increased vagal tone, medications, myocardial infarction, fibrosis, and myocarditis can cause SA exit block.[1]

Subtypes   Like conduction block classification in the AV node, sinoatrial block can be classified into first, second (types I and II), and third degree block.

First Degree SA Block   The time from the sinus impulse to exit to the atrium is prolonged. Because the sinus impulse itself is not represented on the ECG, there is no way to diagnose this electrocardiographically.

Second Degree SA Block

Type I   A progressive prolongation of sinoatrial conduction is represented by a shortening of the P-P interval prior to a pause. The duration of the pause is less than twice the duration of the shortest cycle length. The cycle following the pause is longer than that preceding the pause. Persistent type 1 second degree AV block can appear as grouped beating. This rhythm may be difficult to distinguish from sinus arrhythmia.

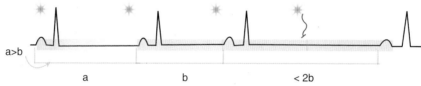

FIGURE 2.7 ECG appearance of type 1 second degree sinoatrial block.

Type 2   The duration of sinoatrial conduction is constant (P-P intervals are constant) prior to the pause. Unlike the pause secondary to sinus arrest, the pause generated by type 2 second degree sinoatrial block *is* a multiple of the preceding P-P interval.

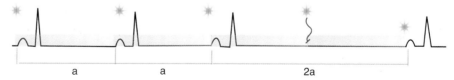

FIGURE 2.8 ECG appearance of type 2 second degree sinoatrial block.

Third Degree SA Block   P waves are absent. There is no way to differentiate third degree SA block from sinus arrest on the ECG.

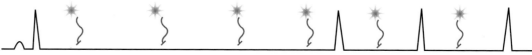

FIGURE 2.9 ECG appearance of third degree sinoatrial block is indistinguishable from that of sinus arrest.

FIGURE 2.6 Failure of sinus impulse to propagate secondary to sinoatrial block.

Inappropriate Bradycardia

Marked sinus bradycardia in a patient other than the well-conditioned athlete may be the result of sinus node dysfunction. Heart rates less than 50 bpm in an awake and active patient may result in symptoms of poor perfusion. Patients with normal resting heart rates that fail to appropriately increase with activity and exertion may have chronotropic incompetence. Chronotropic incompetence has been defined as a failure to achieve 70% to 80% of maximal heart rate at peak exercise.[2]

Tachycardia–Bradycardia Syndrome

Rhythms generated by ectopic foci (including atrial fibrillation, atrial flutter, and atrial tachycardia) may become the dominant rhythm when the sinus node fails to function. Sinus node dysfunction becomes evident when these dominant rhythms self-terminate and a long pause follows because the sinus node is unable to take over the pacemaker role. This pause either terminates in an escape impulse or results in asystole.

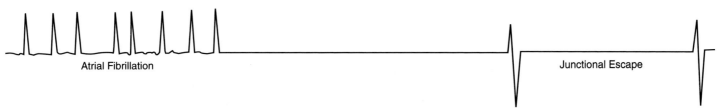

Atrial Fibrillation   Junctional Escape

FIGURE 2.10 ECG appearance of tachycardia–bradycardia syndrome. Atrial fibrillation followed by a pause recovered by a junctional escape.

Sick Sinus Syndrome

Sick sinus syndrome applies to different patterns of intrinsic sinus node dysfunction. Fibrofatty infiltration of nodal and surrounding tissue is thought to be the common pathway leading to sick sinus syndrome. Symptomatic patients may undergo placement of a permanent pacemaker.

Table 2.1 Several ECG patterns classified as sick sinus syndrome.

Inappropriate sinus bradycardia

Sinus arrest or exit block

Alternation between atrial tachyarrhythmias and slow atrial rates (tachy-brady syndrome)

Atrial Fibrillation with slow ventricular response

ECG 2.1a

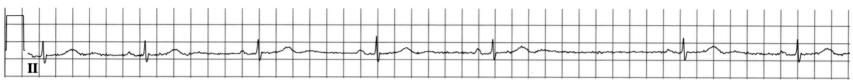

ECG 2.2a

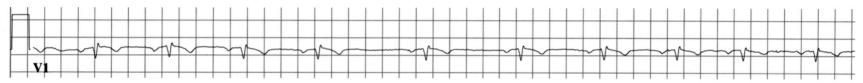

ECG 2.3a A 53-year-old asymptomatic male was referred from a clinic where he was found to have hyperkalemia (K = 6.4 mg/dL) and bradycardia.

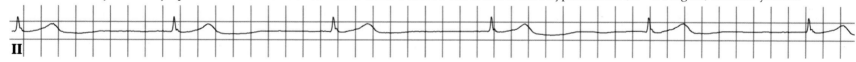

ECG 2.4a An 89-year-old woman complains of light-headedness with walking.

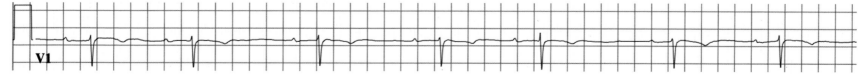

ECG 2.1b

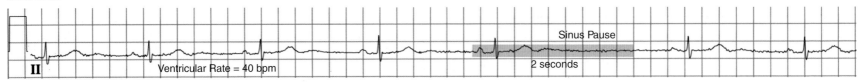

Sinus pauses can be an indication of underlying sick sinus syndrome.

Sinus Bradycardia with a 2.4-Second Sinus Pause

ECG 2.2b

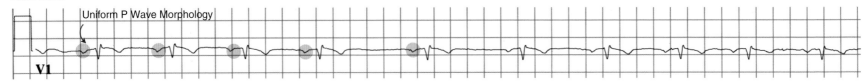

The uniform P waves followed by narrow QRS complexes indicate that despite the irregularity of the rhythm, its origin is the sinus node. If there were variability in the P wave morphology, the rhythm would be wandering atrial pacemaker.

Sinus Arrhythmia

ECG 2.3b   A 53-year-old asymptomatic male was referred from a clinic where he was found to have hyperkalemia (K = 6.4 mg/dL) and bradycardia.

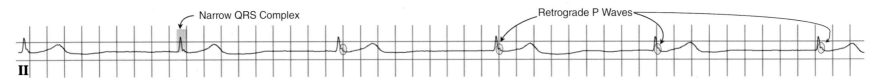

Hyperkalemia can cause bradyarrhythmias including junctional bradycardia.

Junctional Bradycardia

The underlying cause of this rhythm may be sinus arrest or sinoatrial exit block (third degree).

ECG 2.4b   An 89-year-old woman complains of light-headedness with walking.

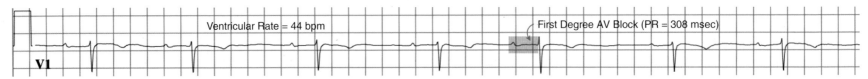

This patient was diagnosed with chronotropic incompetence.

Sinus Bradycardia with First Degree AV Block

ECG 2.5a   A 95-year-old female with a history of persistent atrial fibrillation complains of weakness and fatigue.

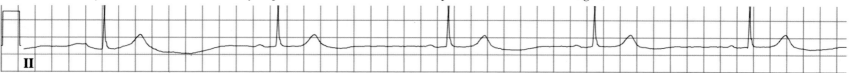

ECG 2.5b   A 69-year-old woman with a history of atrial fibrillation presents with syncope.

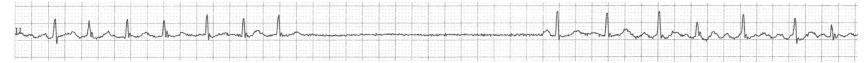

ECG 2.6

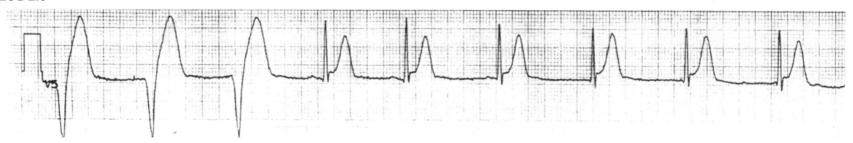

ECG 2.5a A 95-year-old female with a history of persistent atrial fibrillation complains of weakness and fatigue.

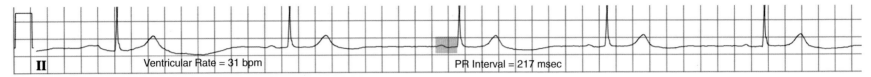

Sinus Bradycardia with First Degree AV Block

Bradycardia that is this marked is abnormal, even in a younger patient who is in a resting state. After this patient was admitted, she was observed to have a 6-second pause on telemetry and intermittent periods of atrial fibrillation with ventricular rates in the 100s. She was diagnosed with tachycardia–bradycardia syndrome and underwent placement of a permanent pacemaker.

ECG 2.5b A 69-year-old woman with a history of atrial fibrillation presents with syncope.

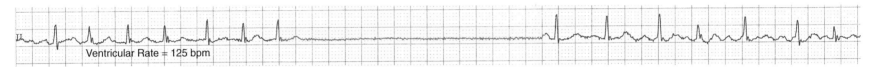

**Atrial Fibrillation with Rapid Ventricular
Response; 3-Second Sinus Pause**

Rapid atrial fibrillation followed by sinus pauses can occur in tachycardia-bradycardia syndrome.

ECG 2.6

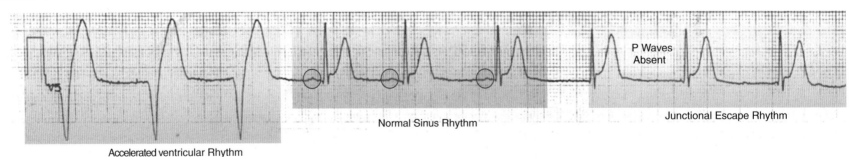

**Accelerated Idioventricular Rhythm; Normal
Sinus Rhythm; Sinus Arrest with Junctional Escape**

Three different rhythms were recorded from the same 12-lead ECG in the setting of a large anterolateral myocardial infarction.

References

1. Olgin JaZD. In: Bonow R, Zipes D, Libby P, ed. *Braunwald's Heart Disease: A Textbook of Cardiovascular Medicine.* 9th ed. Philadelphia, PA: Elsevier; 2011:771–824.
2. Katritsis D, Camm AJ. Chronotropic incompetence: a proposal for definition and diagnosis. *Br Heart J* 1993;70(5):400–402.

CHAPTER 3

Bundle and Fascicular Blocks

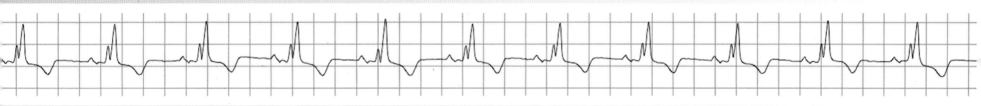

Right Bundle Branch Block

1. Septal Depolarization In the presence of a right bundle branch block (RBBB), septal depolarization occurs in a normal left-to-right pattern (*orange arrow*) but for a longer duration than normal.

The initial deflection is therefore positive in right-sided leads (V1) and negative in left-sided leads (V6).

2. Left Ventricular Activation The left ventricle is activated first in a right-to-left pattern (*blue arrow*) via the functional left bundle branch and distal Purkinje fibers.

This major leftward force accounts for the negative deflection sometimes present in V1 and the positive deflection in V6.

3. Right Ventricular Activation

The right ventricle is activated last by myocardial spread (*dotted red arrow*) from the left ventricle. This delayed activation is no longer opposed by left ventricular depolarization forces and accounts for the R' wave in V1 and a terminal wide S wave in V6 (Fig. 3.1A–C).

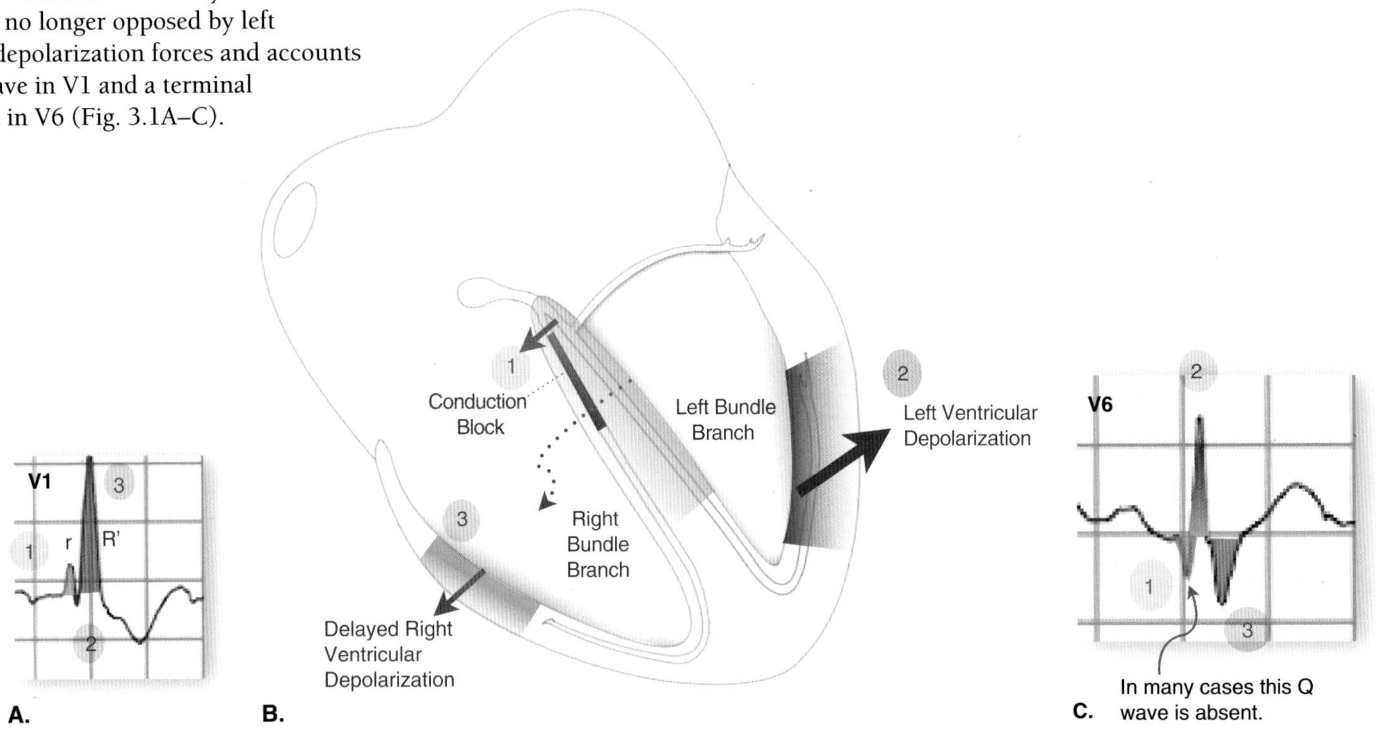

FIGURE 3.1 A. Appearance of RBBB in V1. B. Pattern of ventricular activation in RBBB. C. Appearance of RBBB in V6.

Right Bundle Branch Block

Criteria for RBBB[1]
1. QRS > 120 msec in adults
2. Right lead morphology: rSR', rsR', RR'; notched single R in V1 or V2
3. Left lead morphology: Terminal S wave in V6 and I; S wave of greater duration than R wave
4. R peak time greater than 50 msec in V1 and normal in leads V5 and V6

Different Possible QRS Morphologies in V1 (Fig. 3.2)

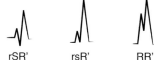

rSR'   rsR'   RR'

FIGURE 3.2 Some of the Morphologies of RBBB in lead V1.

Discordance

The ST segments and T waves in RBBB are discordant with (in the opposite direction of) the terminal portion of the QRS complex. These changes represent repolarization abnormalities secondary to abnormal depolarization (Fig. 3.3).

Suspect abnormal pathology (i.e., ischemia) if ST segments and T waves are concordant with the terminal portion of the QRS complex.

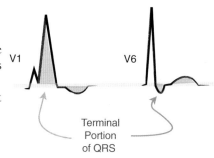

FIGURE 3.3 Diagram of appropriate discordance in RBBB.

Incomplete RBBB

Delay rather than complete block. QRS < 120 msec (Fig. 3.4).

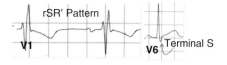

FIGURE 3.4 Leads V1 and V6 in an ECG demonstrating incomplete RBBB.

Causes of RBBB

RBBB can be a normal finding in healthy people. Pathologic causes to consider include severe pulmonary hypertension and pulmonary embolism. Other causes include acute myocardial ischemia, infiltrative diseases, valve disorders, and iatrogenesis (right heart catheterization, septal ablation).

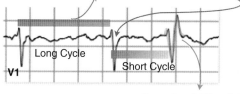

FIGURE 3.5 Ashman Phenomenon. RBBB morphology appears when a short cardiac cycle follows a long cycle.

Causes of RBBB Pattern

Ashman Phenomenon

The refractory period of the right bundle branch is inherently longer than that of the left bundle branch. Supraventricular rhythms conducted rapidly or irregularly (atrial fibrillation, atrial tachycardia) or beats conducted prematurely may simultaneously encounter a right bundle branch still in its refractory period and a left bundle branch ready to conduct (Fig. 3.5).

Ventricular Tachycardia from a Left Ventricular Focus

Ventricular conduction emanating from an ectopic focus in the left ventricle spreads from myocardial cell to myocardial cell to the right ventricle. This results in delayed right ventricular conduction represented on the ECG by wide positive QRS complexes in V1 and wide negative QRS complexes in V6.

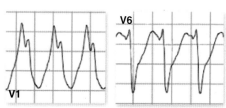

FIGURE 3.6 RBBB morphology in VT from a left ventricular focus.

Left Bundle Branch Block

1. Aberrant Septal Depolarization   The septum is depolarized abnormally from right to left and is delayed. The initial deflection is thus positive in lead V6 and negative in lead V1. This eliminates the normal septal Q waves in left-sided leads.

2. Ventricular Depolarization   Ventricular depolarization also proceeds in a right-to-left direction. The combination of right-to-left septal and ventricular depolarization creates wide monophasic complexes (QS in V1 and R wave in V6, I, and aVL) (Fig. 3.7A–C).

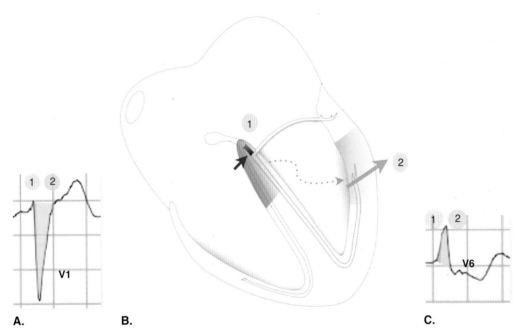

FIGURE 3.7 **A.** Appearance of LBBB in V1. **B.** Pattern of ventricular activation in left bundle branch block. **C.** Appearance of LBBB in V6.

Left Bundle Branch Block

Criteria for LBBB[2]
1. QRS > 120 msec in adults
2. Right-sided morphology: QS or rS in V1, V2
3. Left-sided morphology: monophasic, slurred, or notched R wave in V5, V6, and I, aVL
4. Absent septal Q wave in left precordial leads (Fig. 3.9)

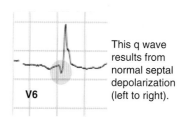

This q wave results from normal septal depolarization (left to right).

FIGURE 3.9 Septal Q wave.

Location
LBBB can result from proximal block in the left bundle before it divides into fascicles (pre-devisional) or from simultaneous conduction block in the left anterior and posterior fascicles (post-divisional).

Discordance
The ST segments and T waves in LBBB are discordant with (in the opposite direction of) the terminal portion of the QRS complex. These changes represent repolarization abnormalities secondary to abnormal depolarization and are more pronounced than in RBBB (Fig. 3.10).

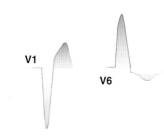

FIGURE 3.10 Discordance in LBBB.

Incomplete LBBB
Delay rather than complete block. QRS < 120 msec (Fig. 3.11).

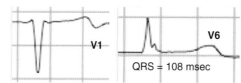

QRS = 108 msec

FIGURE 3.11 Incomplete LBBB.

Causes of LBBB
While LBBB can rarely occur in asymptomatic individuals free of cardiovascular disease, this block usually indicates underlying cardiac pathology. Common causes include degenerative disease of the conduction system, hypertension, coronary artery disease, aortic stenosis, myocarditis, and cardiomyopathy.[3]

Complicates Other Diagnoses

Ischemic Changes
Abnormal ST and T waves in LBBB can both mimic and mask ischemic changes in acute myocardial infarction. ECG stress test results in patients with LBBB are difficult to interpret. See page 372 for further description of ischemic changes in patients with LBBB.

Left Ventricular Hypertrophy
LVH and LBBB are often coexisting conditions. LBBB can be mistaken for LVH. Unopposed right-to-left ventricular spread of current increases the amplitude of the QRS complex. Both LBBB and LVH can cause ST- and T wave discordance from repolarization abnormalities. One way to differentiate LVH and LBBB is by looking for the presence of small septal Q waves in left-sided precordial leads. These will be absent in LBBB.

Clinical Significance
LBBB can result in varying degrees of intraventricular and interventricular dysynchrony and wall motion abnormalities. These wall motion abnormalities interfere with interpretation of echo stress test results. Sequential rather than simultaneous activation of the ventricles from LBBB can compromise effective contraction. Cardiac contractility becomes more compromised with greater delays in left ventricular conduction (i.e., wider QRS complexes).

Cardiac Resynchronization Therapy
Patients with symptomatic heart failure and BBB may benefit from cardiac resynchronization therapy (CRT). CRT entails placement of a biventricular pacemaker that stimulates the right and left ventricles simultaneously.

Left Bundle Branch Block Pattern

Other Causes of a LBBB Pattern

Ventricular Pacing

Ventricular pacing leads are embedded in the apex of the right ventricle. Ventricular activation is initiated by the tip of this lead when there is capture and ventricular activation proceeds from right to left.

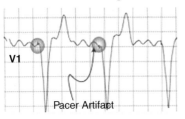
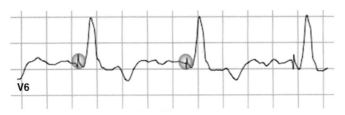

A.

Right-Sided Bypass Tract

A right-sided atrioventricular (AV) bypass tract that conducts in an anterograde fashion allows for early right ventricular activation. Ventricular activation then spreads in a right-to-left fashion away from the right ventricle.

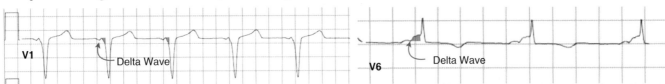

B.

Right Ventricular Outflow Tachycardia

Ventricular tachycardia emanating from a focus in the right ventricle will produce a wide-complex tachycardia with LBBB morphology.

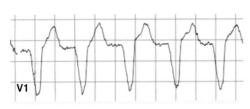
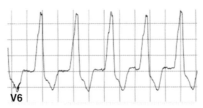

C.

FIGURE 3.8 Leads V1 and V6 in **A.** ventricular paced rhythm, **B.** ventricular pre-excitation down a right-sided bypass tract and **C.** right ventricular outflow tachycardia.

Left Anterior Fascicular Block

The left bundle branch splits into three fascicles: the left anterior fascicle (LAF), the left posterior fascicle (LPF), and the septal fascicle. The importance of the septal fascicle is uncertain, and it has no defining ECG characteristics. The anterior and posterior fascicles are the main fascicles that contribute to ventricular activation. Both fascicles normally activate the free wall of the left ventricle simultaneously. When a block occurs in either fascicle, both the QRS morphology and axis change. Left anterior fascicular block results in left axis deviation.

When the LAF is blocked, the left ventricular free wall is activated from the left posterior fascicle. Conduction is first directed inferiorly and posteriorly down the LPF before spreading in a delayed fashion to the anterior and superior portions of the left ventricle (Fig. 3.12).

Leads II, III, aVF   [rS] The initial deflection of the QRS wave is positive (R wave) as the left posterior fascicle is directed toward these leads. Activation of the left ventricle then spreads superiorly and to the left, away from II, III, and aVF, producing prominent S waves in these leads.

Leads I, aVL   [qR] Initial depolarization of the left ventricle is directed away from I and aVL, producing a Q wave in these leads. As activation then spreads superiorly and leftward, an R wave is produced in I and aVL (Fig. 3.13; Table 3.2).

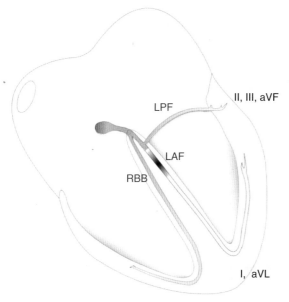

FIGURE 3.12 Diagram of left anterior fascicular block.

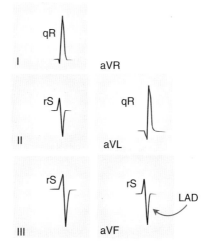

FIGURE 3.13 Limb lead ECG appearance of left anterior fascicular block.

LAF Location		Related Causes of LAFB
Runs down the septum alongside the left ventricular outflow tract	→	Hypertension Aortic valve disease Spontaneous closure of VSD
LAF Blood Supply		
Septal perforators coming off left anterior descending artery	→	Anterior MI

Table 3.1 Categorized causes of LAFB.

Table 3.2 Criteria for LAFB[4]
Left axis deviation
rS in inferior leads (II, III, aVF)
qR in lateral limb leads (I and aVL)
Delayed intrinsicoid deflection (time to peak R) in aVL
QRS < 120 msec (unless coexisting RBBB)

Left Posterior Fascicular Block

Left posterior fascicular block is the least common of the intraventricular conduction blocks and is an uncommon cause of right axis deviation. In left posterior fascicular block, the LAF first activates the anterior and superior portions of the left ventricle. Conduction to the inferior and posterior portions of the left ventricle supplied by the posterior fascicle is delayed.

Leads II, III, aVF   [qR] Initial conduction is directed away from these leads, and q waves are inscribed. As conduction proceeds toward these leads, positive QRS deflections follow.

Leads I, aVL   [rS] Conduction down the anterior fascicle toward these leads is normal. The QRS complex starts with a small R wave. As conduction then travels inferiorly, S waves are inscribed (Figs. 3.14–3.15).

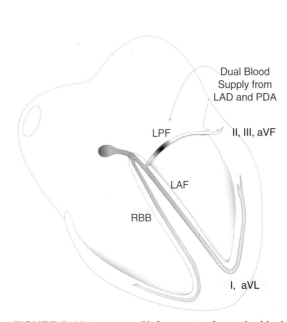

FIGURE 3.14 Diagram of left posterior fascicular block.

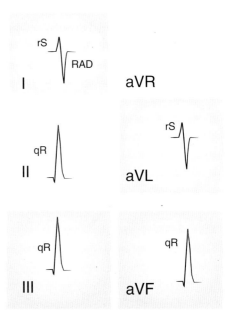

FIGURE 3.15 ECG limb lead appearance of left posterior fascicular block.

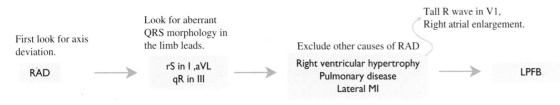

FIGURE 3.16 Approach to diagnosing left posterior fascicular block.[5]

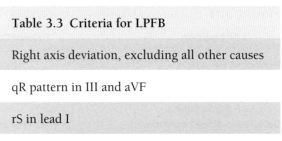

Table 3.3 Criteria for LPFB
Right axis deviation, excluding all other causes
qR pattern in III and aVF
rS in lead I
QRS < 120 msec (unless coexisting RBBB)

Bifascicular Block

Conduction pathways distal to the AV node can be thought of in terms of three fascicles, the right bundle branch, the left anterior fascicle and the left posterior fascicle. Bifascicular block generally refers to LAFB or LPFB in the presence of RBBB.

		ECG Findings
RBBB + LAFB	The most common type of bifascicular block is simultaneous block of the right bundle branch and LAF. RBBB and LAFB occur in combination for anatomical reasons. The LAF runs adjacent to the right bundle branch as it courses down the ventricular septum. Both are supplied by the LAD. In patients with acute LAD occlusion (anteroseptal MI), both RBBB and LAFB may be present. When there is simultaneous block of the RBB and LAF, conduction of the ventricles occurs solely through the left posterior fascicle (Fig. 3.17A).	RBBB + LAD + rS in II, III, aVF + qR in I, aVL
RBBB + LPFB	Since the LPF is the least vulnerable to conduction disease, concomitant conduction block in the right bundle branch and LPF signifies extensive conduction disease. First and second degree AV block frequently accompanies this combination of bifascicular block and can progress to complete heart block (Fig. 3.17B).	RBBB + RAD + rS in I, aVL + qR in II, III, aVF
LAFB + LPFB	Left bundle branch block can be considered a type of bifascicular block if there is simultaneous block of the anterior and posterior fascicles. The ECG does not allow one to infer whether the left bundle branch block occurs at the bundle or fascicular level (Fig. 3.17C).	LBBB

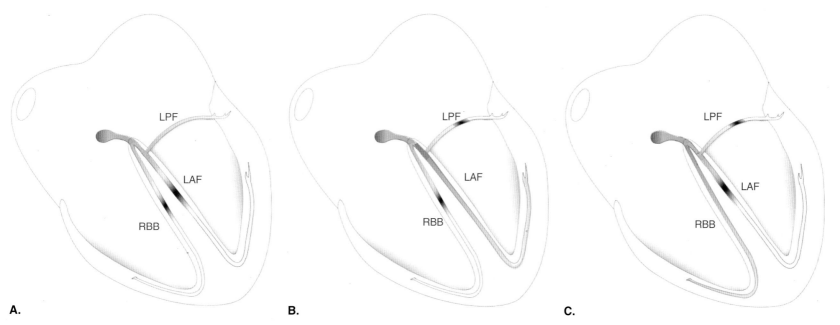

FIGURE 3.17 Diagram of different types of fascicular block. **A.** RBBB + LAFB. **B.** RBBB + LPFB. **C.** LAFB + LPFB.

Trifascicular Block

Trifascicular block indicates that some type of conduction delay is present in the right bundle branch as well as in the left bundle branch or both left anterior and posterior fascicles. Ventricular activation spreads from the fascicle with the smallest degree of conduction delay. Trifascicular blocks can deteriorate into complete AV block with ventricular escape rhythms. It is important to recognize trifascicular block so that a permanent pacemaker can be placed before ventricular activation depends on ventricular escape. ECG findings can be classified as definite or possible trifascicular block.[6]

Definite Trifascicular Block

Alternating Bundle Branch block

Evidence of LBBB and RBBB recorded at different times in the same patient indicates that conduction disease is present in all three fascicles (Fig. 3.18A).

RBBB + Alternating Fascicular block

This is rare. Precordial leads will demonstrate a fixed RBBB. Frontal leads will show alternating axis as left anterior fascicular block alternates with left posterior fascicular block (Fig. 3.18B).

RBBB or LBBB + Second Degree (Mobitz II) AV Block

Mobitz type II blocks usually occur below the AV node in the His-Purkinje system. In Mobitz II block, there is a fixed block in one of the bundle branches and intermittent block in the other branch. Dropped QRS complexes occur when there is simultaneous block in both bundle branches. Bifascicular block with 2:1 AV block is almost always a Mobitz II block and indicative of trifascicular block (Fig. 3.18C).

Possible Trifascicular Block

(Block might be proximal to the fascicles).

Bifascicular Block + First or Second Degree AV block (type I)

First or second degree block can occur proximal to the His bifurcation or represent conduction delay or block in the fascicle not involved in the bifascicular block (Fig. 3.18D).

Complete AV Block with Ventricular Escape

Complete heart block in a patient with prior evidence of bifascicular block is likely a manifestation of impaired conduction down the third fascicle (E1 in Fig. 3.18). Complete heart block is not necessarily a manifestation of trifascicular disease. Block may occur proximal to the bundle branches and a subsidiary pacemaker in the bundle of His may fail to take over (E2 in Fig. 3.18).

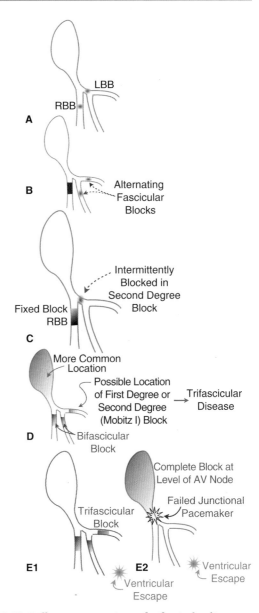

FIGURE 3.18 Different presentations of trifascicular disease. **A.** Alternating bundle branch block; **B.** Alternating fascicular block; **C.** Bundle branch block and Mobitz II block; **D.** Bifascicular Block and Mobitz I or first degree AV block **E1.** Block in all three fascicles with ventricular escape; **E2.** AV nodal block with failed junctional pacemaker.

ECG 3.1a

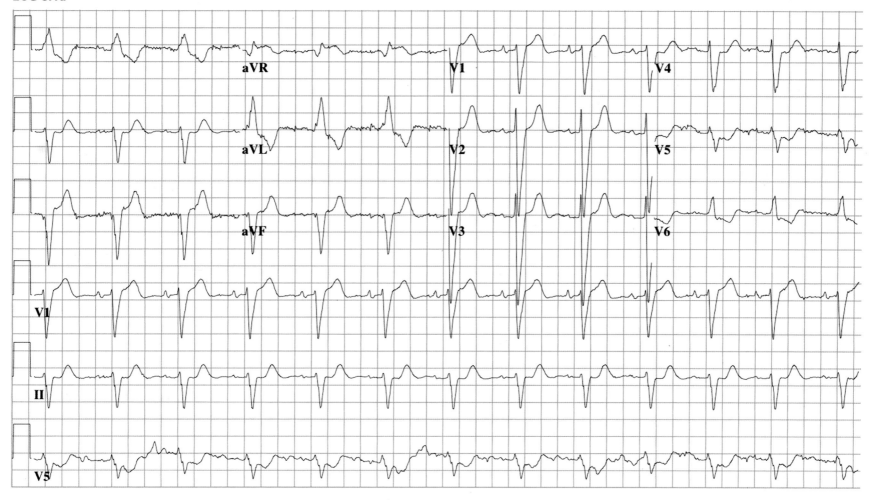

ECG 3.1b

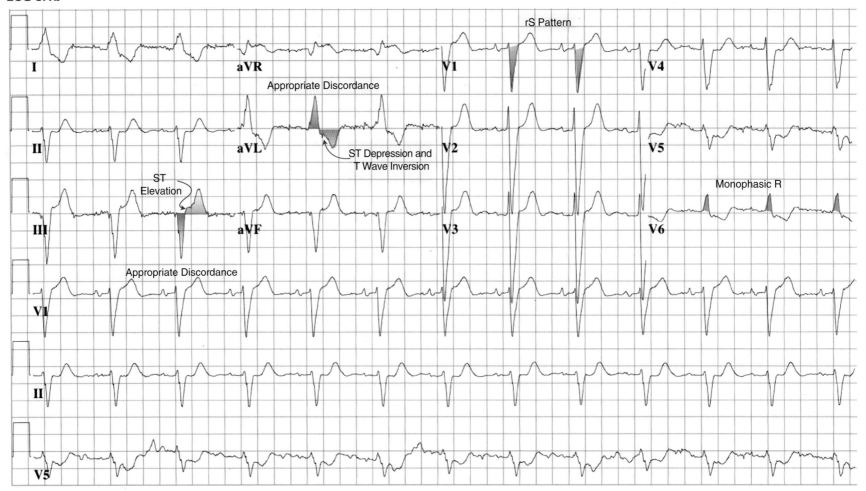

Left Bundle Branch Block

ECG 3.2a

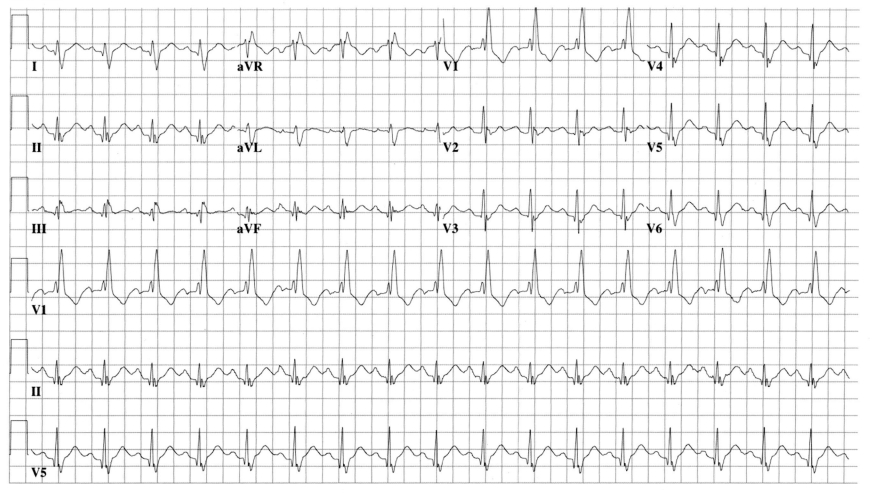

ECG 3.2b

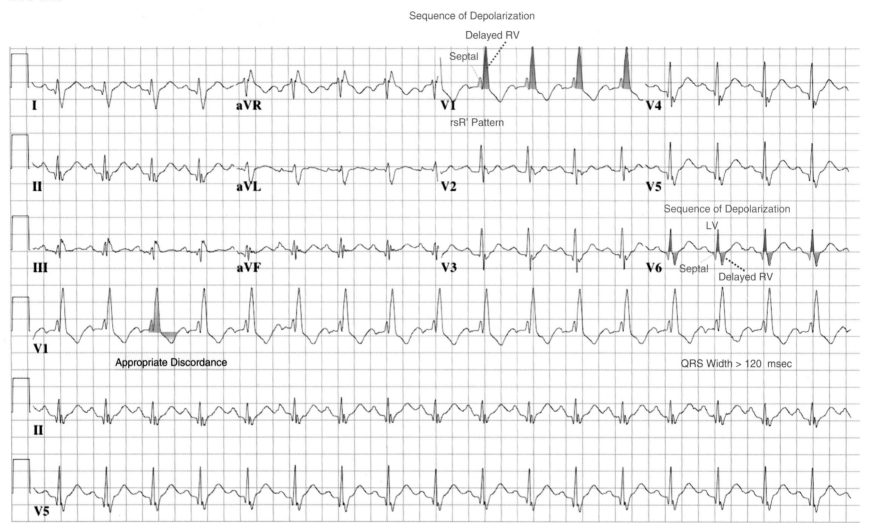

Right Bundle Branch Block

ECG 3.3a

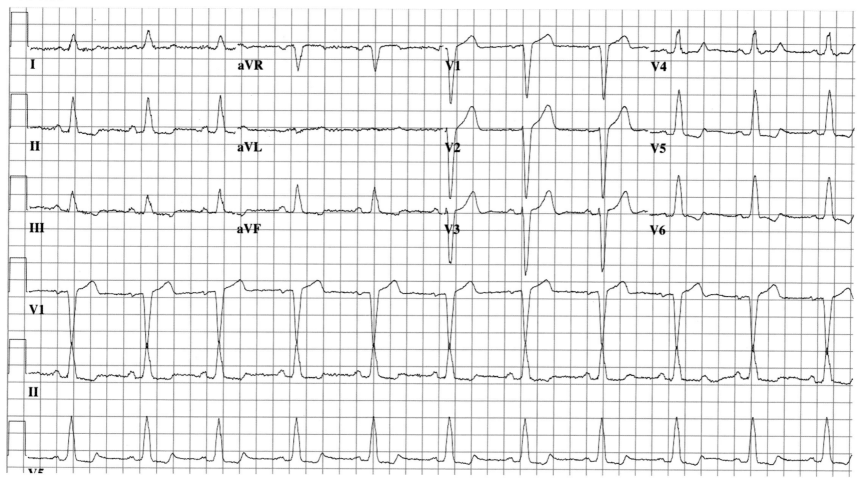

ECG 3.3b

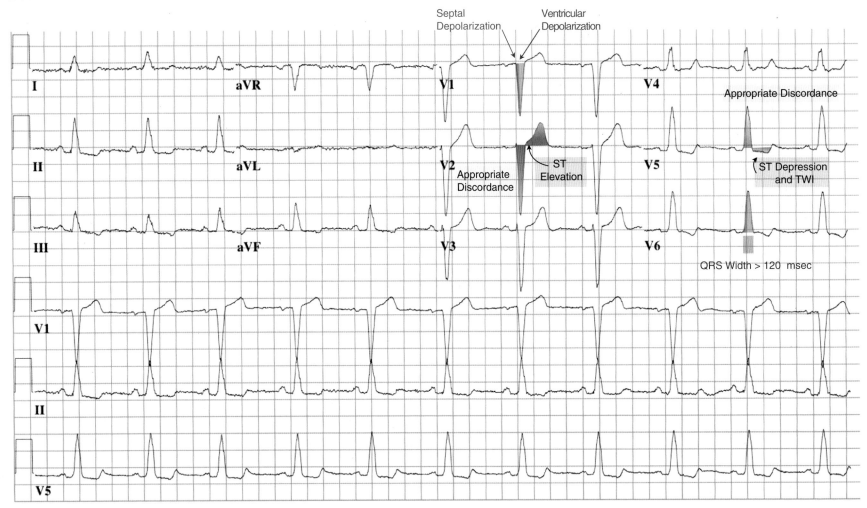

Left Bundle Branch Block

ECG 3.4a

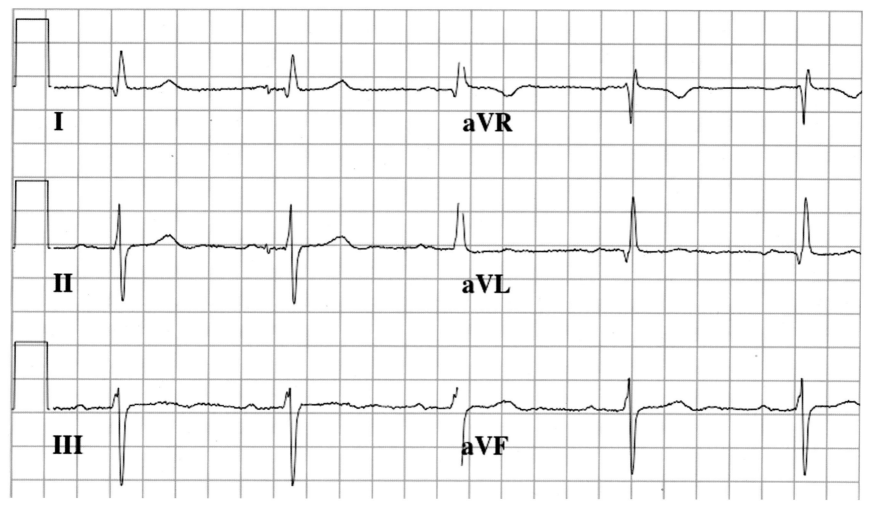

ECG 3.4b

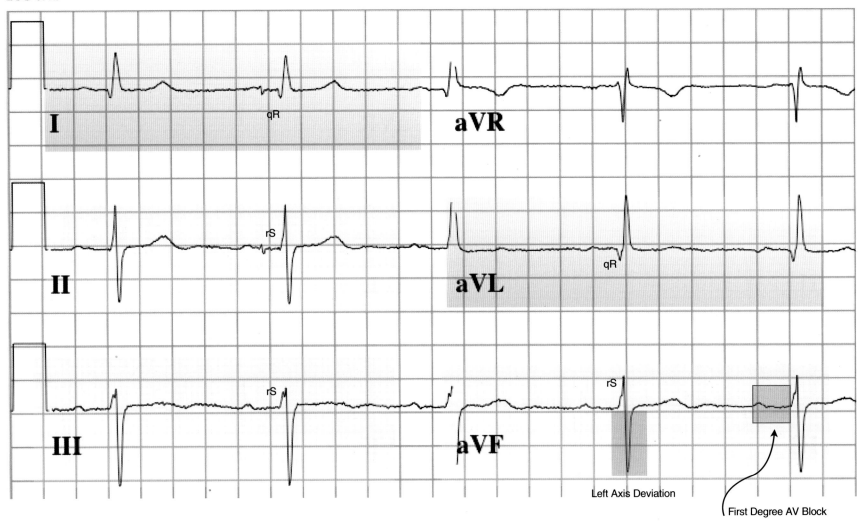

I

qR

aVR

II

rS

aVL

qR

III

rS

aVF

rS

Left Axis Deviation

First Degree AV Block

Left Anterior Fascicular Block

ECG 3.5a

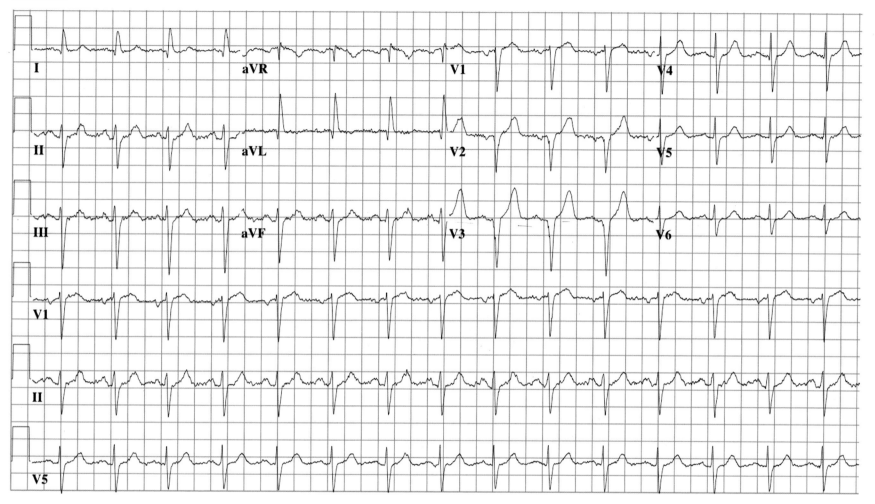

ECG 3.5b

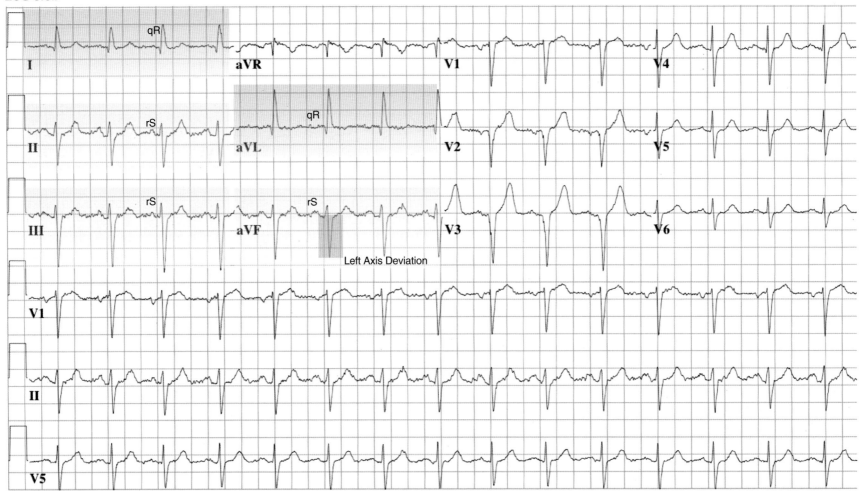

Left Anterior Fascicular Block

ECG 3.6a

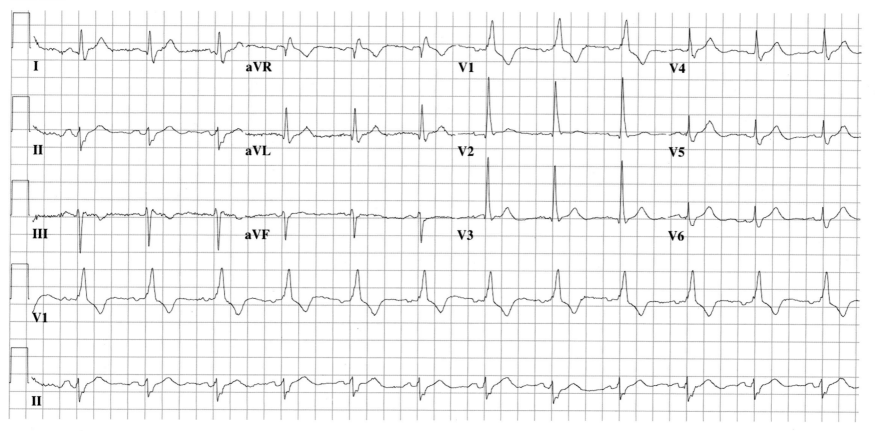

ECG 3.6b

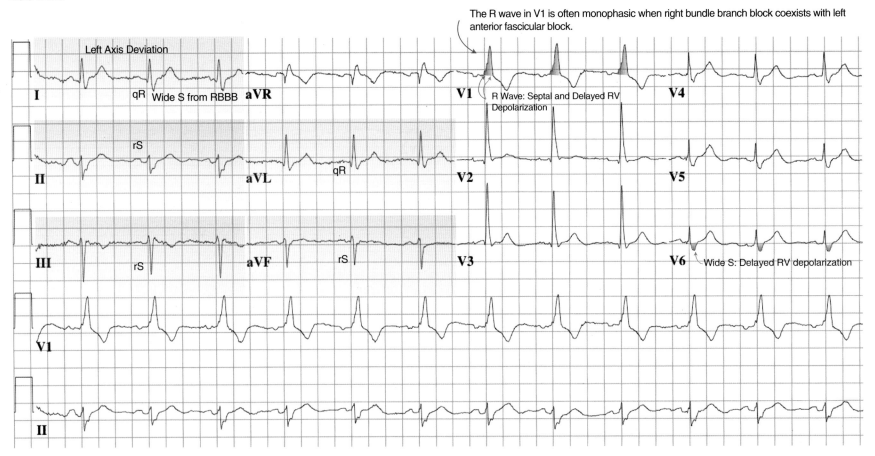

The R wave in V1 is often monophasic when right bundle branch block coexists with left anterior fascicular block.

Left Axis Deviation

I — qR Wide S from RBBB aVR

V1 — R Wave: Septal and Delayed RV Depolarization V4

II — rS aVL qR V2 V5

III — rS aVF rS V3 V6 — Wide S: Delayed RV depolarization

V1

II

Bifascicular Block: LAFB + RBBB

ECG 3.7a

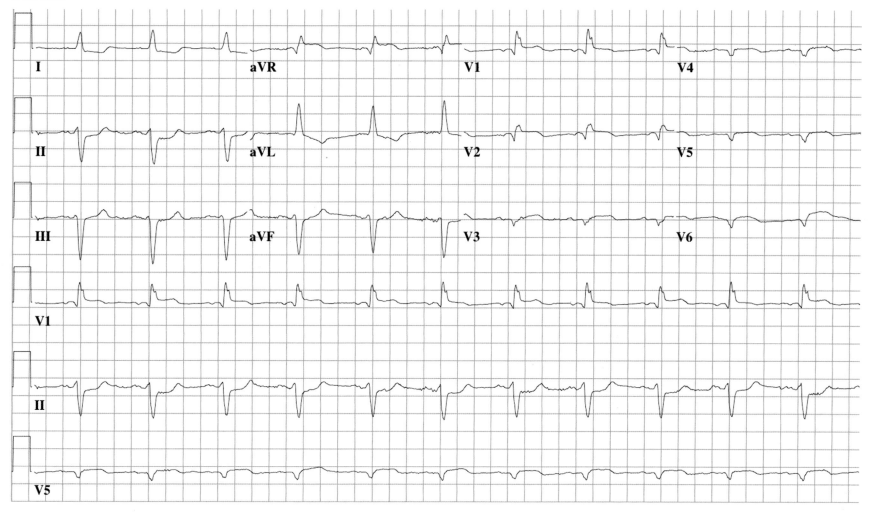

ECG 3.7b

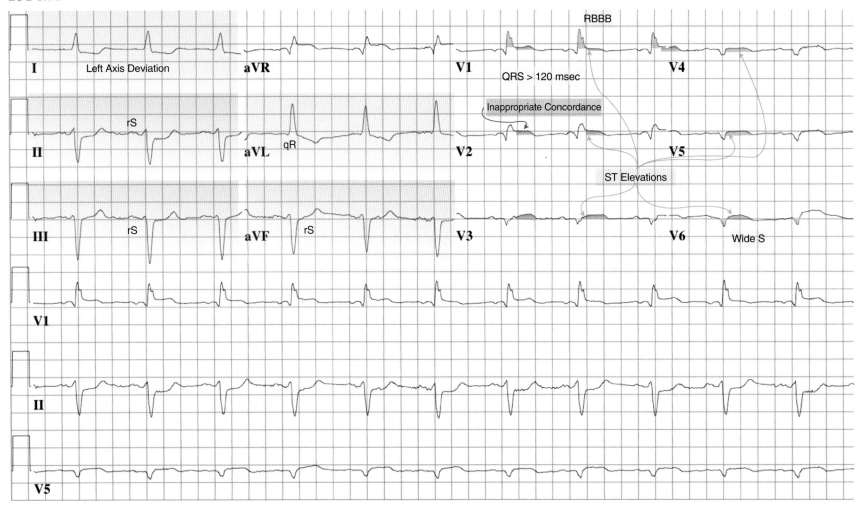

Bifascicular Block: LAFB and RBBB;
Anterior ST Elevation MI

Note the ST elevations across the precordial leads, indicating acute anterior myocardial infarction.
Bifascicular block may progress to complete heart block in the context of an anterior MI.

ECG 3.8a

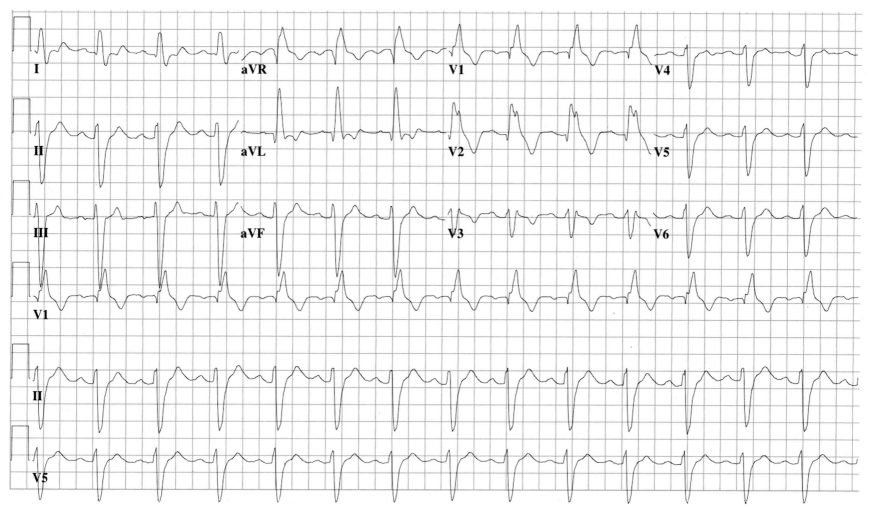

ECG 3.8b

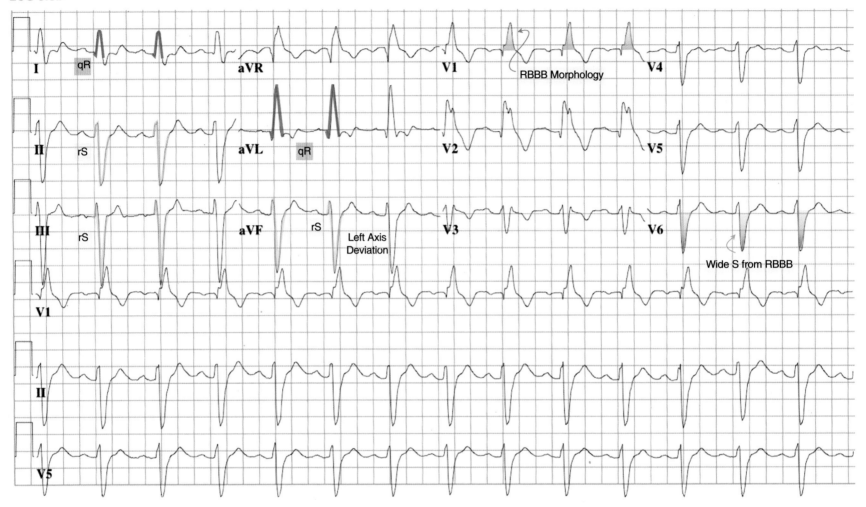

Bifascicular Block: LAFB + RBBB

ECG 3.9a

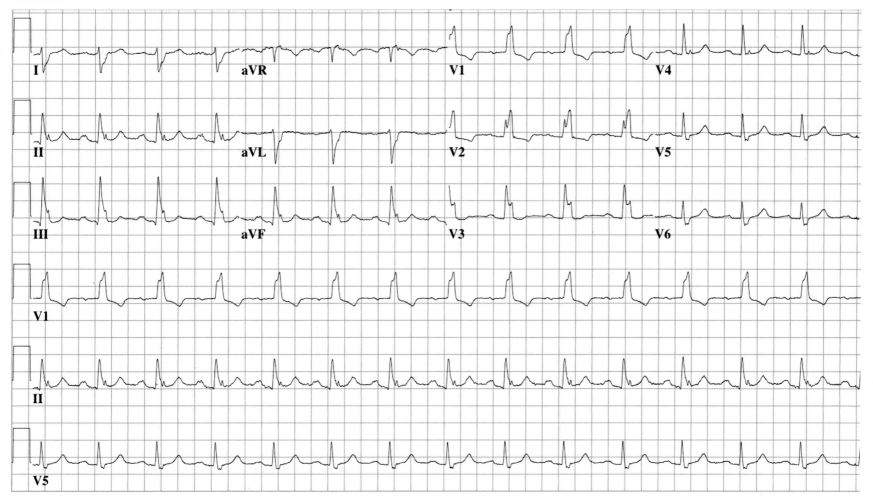

ECG 3.9b

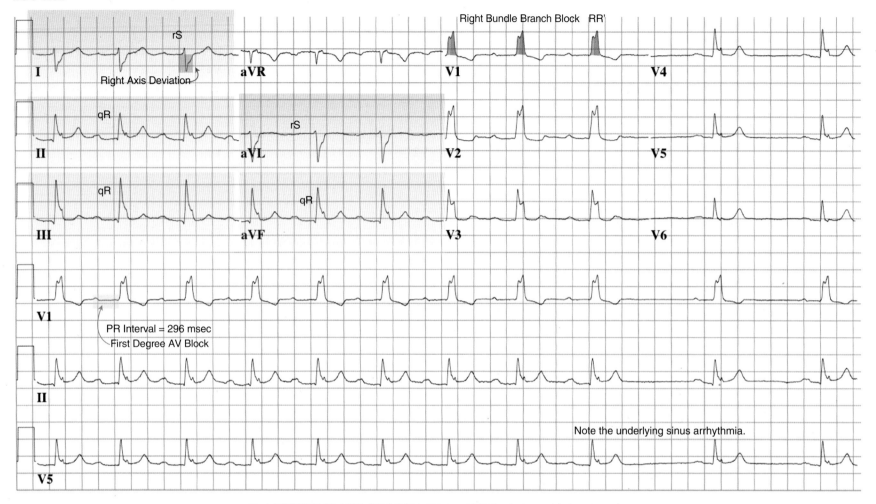

Possible Trifascicular Block: RBBB + LPFB + First Degree AV Block

ECG 3.10a

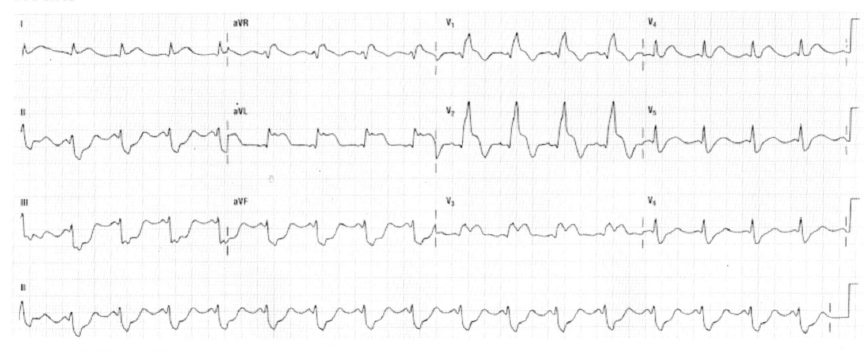

Image courtesy of Josh Kosowsky, MD

ECG 3.10b

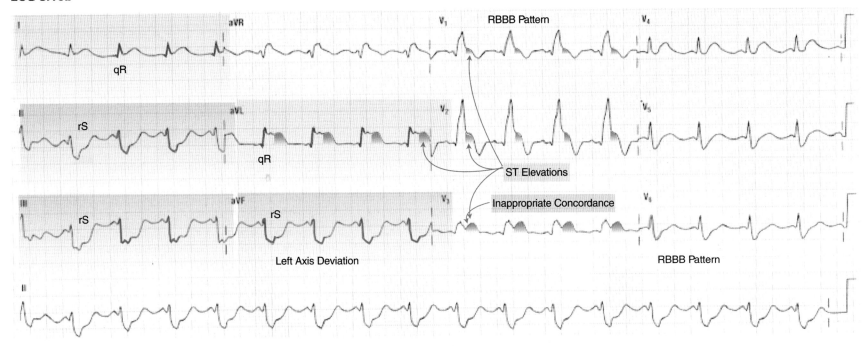

Bifascicular Block: RBBB + LAFB ; Anterior ST Elevation MI

The risk of new bifascicular block progressing to complete heart block in the setting of acute myocardial infarction is high. Acquired bifascicular block is more commonly associated with anterior myocardial infarction than with inferior infarctions.

ECG 3.11a

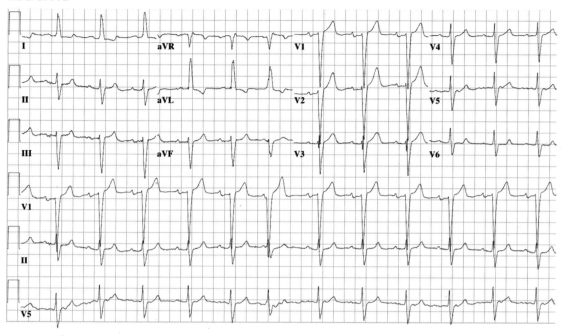

ECG 3.12a Same patient 6 months later…

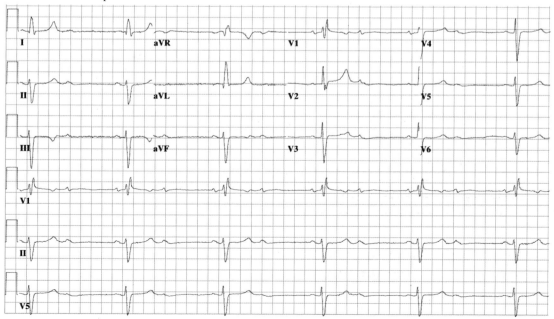

ECG 3.11b

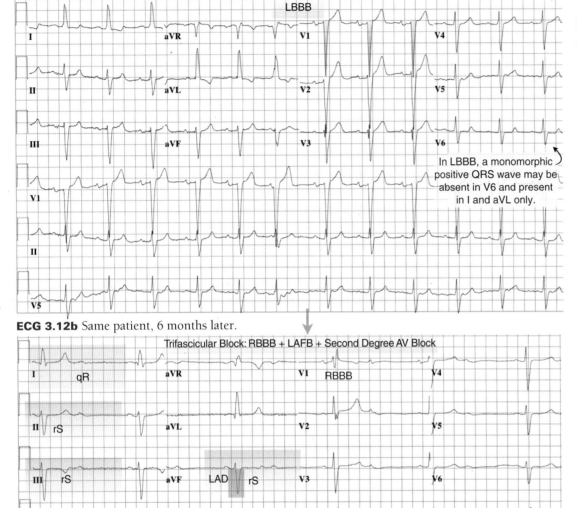

LBBB

In LBBB, a monomorphic positive QRS wave may be absent in V6 and present in I and aVL only.

ECG 3.12b Same patient, 6 months later.

Trifascicular Block: RBBB + LAFB + Second Degree AV Block

qR

rS

rS

LAD   rS

RBBB

2nd Degree 2:1 AV Block

Nonconducted P wave

This patient underwent pacemaker placement shortly after this ECG.

This patient initially presented with an ECG demonstrating left bundle branch block. Six months later, his ECG demonstrated fixed conduction block in the right bundle branch and LAF. Alternation of left bundle branch block to right bundle branch block meets criteria for definite trifascicular block.

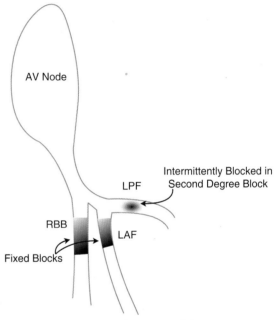

AV Node

Intermittently Blocked in Second Degree Block

LPF

RBB

LAF

Fixed Blocks

FIGURE 3.19 Presumed anatomy of this patient's conduction disease based on ECG 3.12b.

The second ECG alone suggests possible trifascicular disease. It demonstrates fixed blocks involving the right bundle branch and LAF. Intermittently dropped QRS complexes in this ECG (second degree block) most likely represent impulses blocked at the remaining left posterior fascicle (Fig. 3.19).

ECG 3.12c

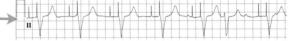

II

ECG 3.13a A 75-year-old male with coronary artery disease comes to the ED after having two syncopal episodes.

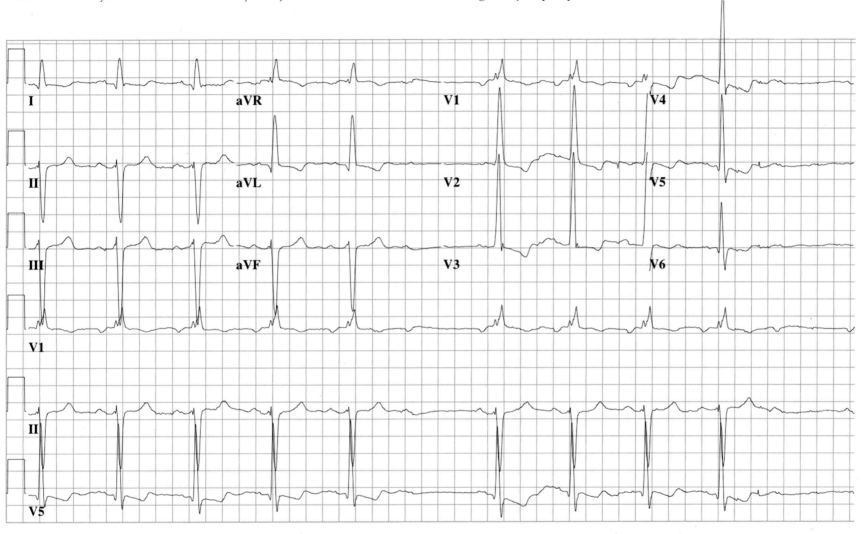

ECG 3.13b A 75-year-old male with coronary artery disease comes to the ED after having two syncopal episodes.

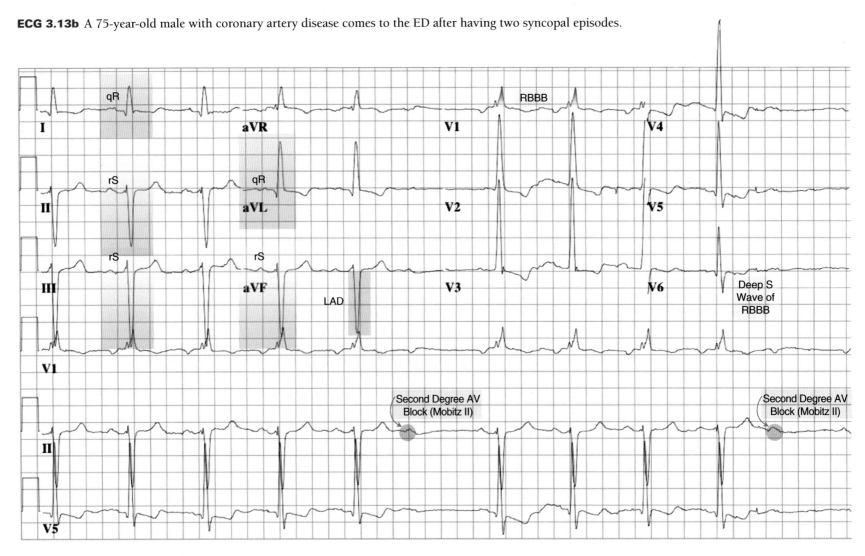

Trifascicular Block:
RBBB + LAFB + Second Degree AV Block (Mobitz II)

Rhythm strips obtained in the emergency department later demonstrated complete heart block. This patient underwent placement of a pacemaker the day following hospital admission.

References

1. Surawicz B, Childers R, Deal BJ, et al. AHA/ACCF/HRS recommendations for the standardization and interpretation of the electrocardiogram: part III: intraventricular conduction disturbances: a scientific statement from the American Heart Association Electrocardiography and Arrhythmias Committee, Council on Clinical Cardiology; the American College of Cardiology Foundation; and the Heart Rhythm Society. Endorsed by the International Society for Computerized Electrocardiology. *J Am Coll Cardiol* 2009;53:976–981.
2. Wagner G. Intraventricular conduction abnormalities. In: Wagner G, ed. *Marriott's Practical Electrocardiography*. Philadelphia, PA: Lippincott Williams & Wilkins; 2008:97–124.
3. Schneider JF, Thomas HE Jr, McNamara PM, et al. Clinical-electrocardiographic correlates of newly acquired left bundle branch block: the Framingham Study. *Am J Cardiol* 1985;55:1332–1338.
4. Elizari MV, Acunzo RS, Ferreiro M. Hemiblocks revisited. *Circulation* 2007;115:1154–1163.
5. Garcia D, Mattu A, Holstege CP, et al. Intraventricular conduction abnormality—an electrocardiographic algorithm for rapid detection and diagnosis. *Am J Emerg Med* 2009;27:492–502.
6. Baltazar R. ed. *Basic and Bedside Electrocardiography*. Philadelphia, PA: Wolters Kluwer/Lippincott Williams & Wilkins; 2009:138–147.

CHAPTER 4

AV Conduction Blocks

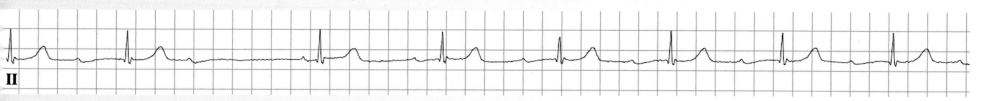

II

First Degree AV Block

First degree AV block is a delay in conduction, not a true block. First degree block represents conduction delay somewhere between the sinus node and ventricles. It most often occurs at the site of the AV node when a sinus impulse encounters a part of the AV node with a prolonged refractory period. The delay may also be located within the atria or bundle of His.

Causes

Increased Parasympathetic Tone	First degree block can be a normal finding in patients with increased parasympathetic (vagal) tone. Causes of increased vagal tone include sleeping, vomiting, coughing, and severe pain. Sinus bradycardia coexistent with first degree block is a clue that the cause of the first degree block is increased parasympathetic tone.
AV Nodal Blocking Agents	Beta-blockers, calcium channel blockers, digitalis
Ischemia	Can especially be seen with inferior wall MI.
Infiltrative Diseases	
Myocarditis	
Congenital Structural Heart Disease	Ebstein anomaly of the tricuspid valve, endocardial cushion defects

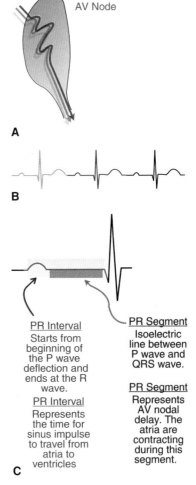

A

B

C

FIGURE 4.1 A. Diagram of first degree AV block; **B.** ECG appearance of first degree block. **C.** PR interval compared with PR segment.

PR Interval
Starts from beginning of the P wave deflection and ends at the R wave.

PR Interval
Represents the time for sinus impulse to travel from atria to ventricles

PR Segment
Isoelectric line between P wave and QRS wave.

PR Segment
Represents AV nodal delay. The atria are contracting during this segment.

ECG Features

All P waves are conducted in first degree block (each P wave is followed by a QRS complex). The PR interval is prolonged, lasting more than 200 milliseconds.

Pitfalls in Diagnosis

The duration of the PR interval can be as long as 1 second.[1] In extremely prolonged PR intervals, the P wave may be mistaken entirely for or become obscured by a T wave. When P waves are completely obscured by T waves, the rhythm may be mistakenly identified as a junctional bradycardia. (Fig. 4.2)

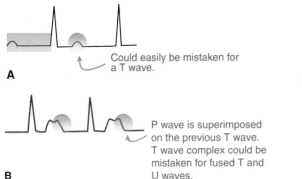

A

Could easily be mistaken for a T wave.

B

P wave is superimposed on the previous T wave. T wave complex could be mistaken for fused T and U waves.

FIGURE 4.2 A. P wave appears in place of T wave. **B.** P wave fused with T wave.

Second Degree AV Block: Mobitz I

Mobitz I block (also called Wenckebach block) usually occurs in the AV node. It rarely progresses to complete heart block. This type of block is often *reversible*.

Mechanism   In Mobitz I block, each successive atrial impulse finds the AV node in an earlier phase of the refractory period and takes longer to reach the ventricles.[2] When an impulse finds the AV node in its absolute refractory period, it becomes blocked (Fig. 4.3A,B).

Causes   Mobitz I block may be a normal physiologic finding in healthy individuals with enhanced vagal tone. Beta-blockers, calcium channel blockers, and digitalis are extrinsic reversible causes. The acute phase of an inferior MI may cause block at the level of the AV node. Inflammation and degenerative disease of the conduction system are other common causes.

ECG Features

Lengthening of PR Intervals   Mobitz I is characterized by progression of PR interval length followed by nonconducted P waves. The greatest increase in conduction time occurs between the first and second beats (Fig. 4.3C). The absolute increase in conduction time decreases with each subsequent beat in a Wenckebach cycle.[1]

A PR interval may shorten and lengthen before the nonconducted beat. A few beats preceding the nonconducted P wave may show no change in PR interval duration.[3]

Variable R-R Intervals   The R-R interval immediately following a pause is longest, and progressively shortens with each subsequent cardiac cycle within a Wenckebach group.

PR Shortest After the Block   The PR interval is predictably the shortest after the block. Sometimes this is the only way to tell that the second degree block is Mobitz I. Progressive prolongation of the PR interval can be very subtle.

Subtle Lengthening of PR Intervals

Shortest PR Interval

FIGURE 4.4 ECG appearance of Mobitz I second degree block with only slight lengthening of PR intervals preceding a blocked impulse.

Grouped Beating   Blocked P waves can separate QRS complexes into groups. QRS complexes tend to appear in pairs, as the most common atrial to ventricular conduction ratio is 3:2.

Location   Mobitz classification is based on ECG patterns, not the anatomical location of the block.

AV Nodal   Type I block is almost always at the level of the AV node. QRS complexes are typically narrow.

Infranodal   Not all Mobitz I blocks occur at the AV node. They can also occur at the level of the His-Purkinje system. Wider QRS complexes typically accompany infranodal Mobitz I block.

Pitfalls   A common pitfall is to mistake blocked premature atrial complexes (PACs) for second degree AV block. PACs occur earlier than would be suspected of a sinus beat, and their associated P waves often have a different morphology than that of the sinus P wave.

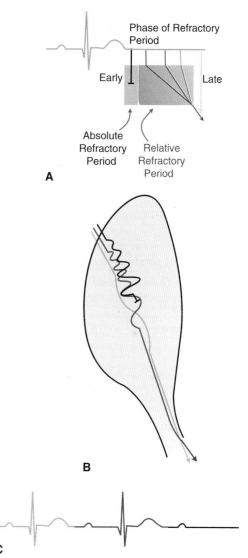

Phase of Refractory Period

Early   Late

Absolute Refractory Period   Relative Refractory Period

A

B

C

FIGURE 4.3 A. Schematic of refractory periods. The earlier in the refractory period that a sinus impulse arrives, the longer the conduction time. **B.** Diagram of Mobitz I block at the AV node. **C.** ECG appearance of Mobitz I block

Second Degree AV Block: Mobitz II

This is an unstable form of conduction that most often occurs in the bundle branches. This progresses to complete heart block.

Mechanism   In Mobitz II block, one bundle branch is continuously blocked while the other is only intermittently blocked. Intermittent block results in QRS complexes that are dropped (Figs. 4.5A and 4.6A).

Location   This is typically an infranodal block. Typically it occurs at the level of the bundle branches. Only rarely does it occur more proximally at the His bundle.

- **Bundle Branch**
- **Bundle of His**

ECG Features

- **Constant PR Length**   The PR interval is fixed and does not shorten or lengthen before a dropped beat.
- **Wide QRS Complexes**   The QRS complexes of conducted beats typically appear similarly to those associated with right or left bundle branch block (Figs. 4.5B and 4.6B).

Causes   Causes of type II block are less likely to be reversible. Common causes include calcification or fibrosis of the conduction system. Infiltrative diseases and ischemia are also notable causes.

Pitfalls   A common mistake is to classify 2 to 1 AV block as Mobitz II because the PR intervals across the ECG appear fixed. It is best to classify this rhythm as "2:1 AV block."
It is important to be able to distinguish between the different types of second degree block. The natural history and management differ.

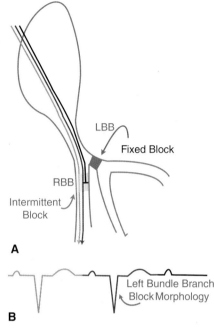

A

FIGURE 4.5 **A**. Mobitz II block with a fixed block in the left bundle. Conducted beats proceed down the right bundle. **B**. They appear as wide QRS complexes with an LBBB morphology on the ECG. A nonconducted beat occurs when conduction fails to pass through the right bundle branch (in addition to the fixed left bundle branch block).

Table 4.1 Comparison of Mobitz 1 and Mobitz II Second Degree AV block

	Mobitz I	Mobitz II
Typical Location	Intranodal (within the AV node)	Infranodal (at the level of the bundle branch)
QRS Morphology	Narrow	Wide, often displays a RBBB or LBBB pattern
PR Interval	Varies (most often progressively lengthens until a beat is dropped)	Constant
Natural History	Transient	Progresses to third degree block
Treatment	Usually not necessary. Atropine may work if symptomatic.	Pacemaker. Atropine will be ineffective.

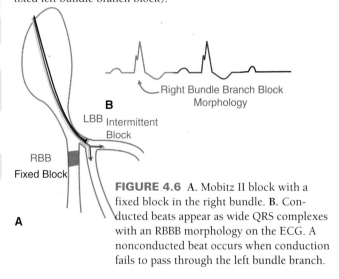

FIGURE 4.6 **A**. Mobitz II block with a fixed block in the right bundle. **B**. Conducted beats appear as wide QRS complexes with an RBBB morphology on the ECG. A nonconducted beat occurs when conduction fails to pass through the left bundle branch.

Advanced Second Degree Block

A block is considered "high grade" or "advanced" if there are two or more P waves for every QRS complex (i.e., the conduction ratio is greater than or equal to 2:1) (Fig. 4.7). The appearance of consecutively dropped QRS complexes is a clear sign of high-grade block. The terms advanced-grade and high-grade block are *not* synonymous with Mobitz II block.

Location

AV Nodal QRS complexes are typically narrow. Advanced second degree block is usually localized to the AV node in patients on AV nodal blocking agents. In the setting of an *inferior* MI, the advanced AV block is likely within the AV node.

Infranodal QRS complexes are typically wide. In the setting of an *anterior* MI, the block is likely infranodal.

Clinical Significance Advanced AV block at the level of the AV node is often transient and has a good prognosis. Infranodal advanced AV block is less stable. Permanent pacemaker may be indicated in symptomatic patients and in asymptomatic patients considered to be high risk.

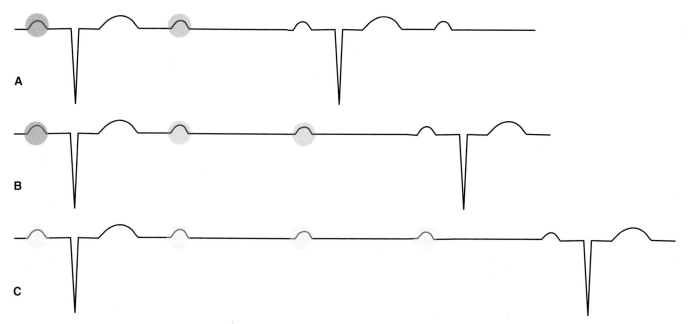

A

B

C

FIGURE 4.7 Different conduction ratios of advanced second degree block. **A.** 2:1 AV Block; **B.** 3:1 AV Block; **C.** 4:1 AV Block

Third Degree AV Block

Third degree AV block is also referred to as complete heart block. Complete heart block is one form of AV dissociation in which the atria and ventricles are controlled by independent pacemakers and contract irrespective of each other. In complete heart block, the atrial rate is faster than the ventricular rate. P waves "march out" through the ECG, unrelated to QRS complexes. The ventricular rhythm is an escape rhythm (from a junctional focus or more distal in the Purkinje system). Escape rhythms are notably regular as they are less influenced by autonomic control.[2]

Causes

Infiltrative Amyloidosis, sarcoidosis, hemochromatosis, hypothyroidism

Drug Toxicity Digitalis, beta-blocker, calcium channel blocker, antiarrhythmics

Ischemia Inferior MI and anterior MI

Infection/Autoimmune Lyme carditis, Chagas disease, diphtheria, acute rheumatic fever, infectious endocarditis, tuberculosis

Fibrosis Lenegre disease, Lev disease

Congenital Anti-Ro and Anti-La antibodies (maternal Sjögren disease or lupus)

Electrolyte Disturbance Severe hyperkalemia

Location

Complete heart block can occur at the AV node or anywhere more distal to it. Block at the level of the AV node is most often congenital. Acquired causes of AV block are usually distal to the His bifurcation and reflect trifascicular conduction disturbance.[1]

AV Node If complete block is at the level of the AV node, a junctional escape rhythm will likely take over (Fig. 4.8).

His Bundle The escape rhythm for infranodal block is ventricular. Prior ECGs demonstrating bundle branch block favors the likelihood of infranodal block.

Bundle Branches

Clinical Significance

Cardiac conduction and contraction become dependent on an escape rhythm. If an escape rhythm fails to take over and to provide sufficient cardiac output, the patient will develop syncope or sudden death.

Pitfalls

A common pitfall is to assume that complete heart block is the cause of all forms of AV dissociation. Complete heart block is one of several causes of AV dissociation. Complete absence of atrial activity is not synonymous with complete heart block. Junctional rhythms are often mistakenly referred to as complete heart block. Another pitfall is failure to recognize atrial fibrillation with a regular ventricular response (also known as "regularized afib") as complete heart block.

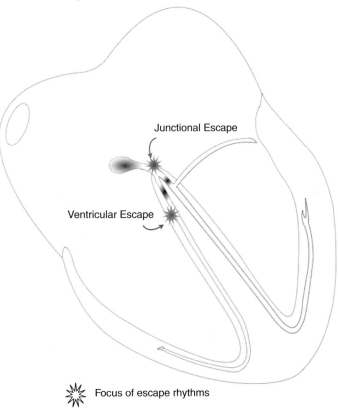

Junctional Escape

Ventricular Escape

✳ Focus of escape rhythms

FIGURE 4.8 Possible locations of third degree AV block (highlighted in gray) include the AV node, bundle of His, and below the His bifurcation. The focus of escape typically occurs just below the site of the block.

Lev and Lenegre

Lev Disease: Calcification and fibrosis of the proximal bundle branches. Seen in the elderly population.

Lenegre Disease: Idiopathic sclerosis and fibrosis of the His-Purkinje system leading to widening of the QRS and development of AV block. Seen in a younger population.

Atrial Fibrillation with Complete Heart Block

This is an important rhythm to recognize. In patients with chronic atrial fibrillation, this is complete heart block secondary to digoxin (or other nodal agent) toxicity until proven otherwise. Most striking about this ECG pattern is the regularity of the ventricular rate. This regularity allows you to infer that the ventricular rhythm is completely dissociated from the irregular supraventricular rhythm of atrial fibrillation.

ECG 4.1

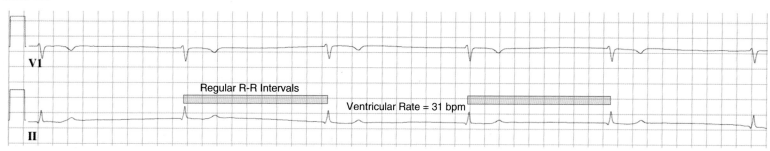

ECG 4.2

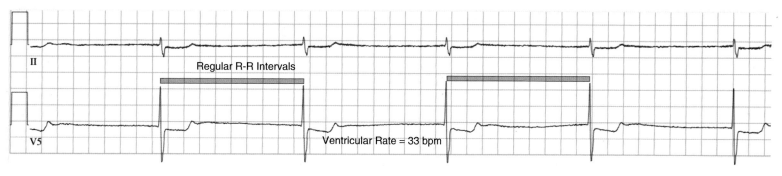

ECG 4.3

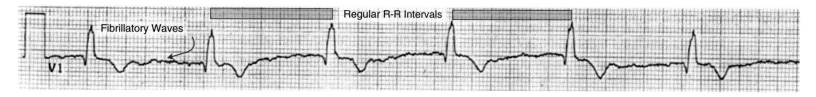

Atrial Fibrillation with Complete Heart Block secondary to Digoxin Toxicity

These ECGs are from three patients who take digitalis for atrial fibrillation. In each ECG, the R-R complexes are constant. This phenomenon can be referred to as "regularized afib." The fibrillatory waves between the QRS complexes can be extremely fine and impossible to appreciate, as in ECGs 4.1 and 4.2.

The patient represented by ECG 4.1 had a digoxin level of 2.8 ng/mL and a potassium level of 6.4 mg/dL. The patient represented by ECG 4.2 was also found to have hyperkalemia associated with digoxin toxicity (potassium 6.5 mg/dL).

AV Dissociation

This is a semantically confusing topic. Complete AV dissociation can be thought of as a broad term to describe any rhythm in which the atria and ventricles conduct independently of each other. Complete heart block is only one form of AV dissociation. Other mechanisms can cause AV dissociation.

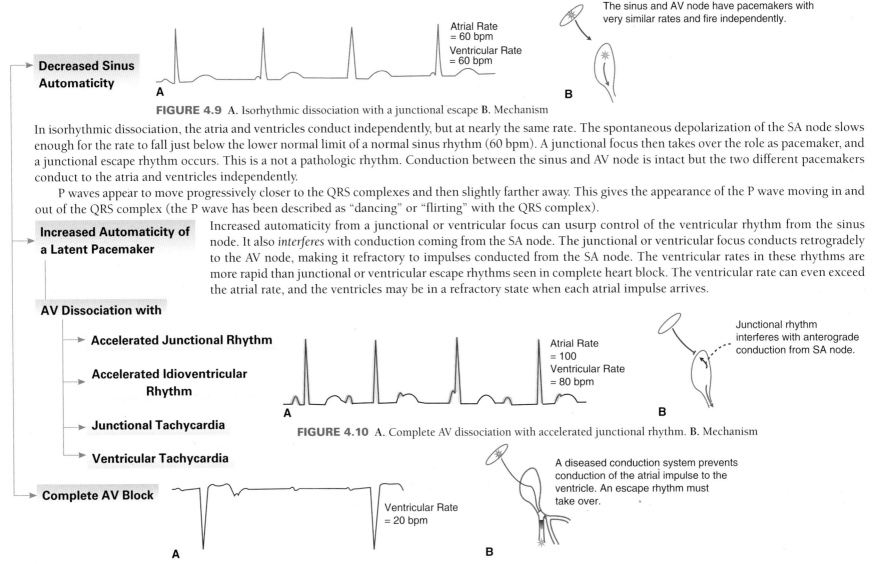

Decreased Sinus Automaticity

Atrial Rate = 60 bpm

Ventricular Rate = 60 bpm

The sinus and AV node have pacemakers with very similar rates and fire independently.

A   B

FIGURE 4.9 A. Isorhythmic dissociation with a junctional escape B. Mechanism

In isorhythmic dissociation, the atria and ventricles conduct independently, but at nearly the same rate. The spontaneous depolarization of the SA node slows enough for the rate to fall just below the lower normal limit of a normal sinus rhythm (60 bpm). A junctional focus then takes over the role as pacemaker, and a junctional escape rhythm occurs. This is a not a pathologic rhythm. Conduction between the sinus and AV node is intact but the two different pacemakers conduct to the atria and ventricles independently.

P waves appear to move progressively closer to the QRS complexes and then slightly farther away. This gives the appearance of the P wave moving in and out of the QRS complex (the P wave has been described as "dancing" or "flirting" with the QRS complex).

Increased Automaticity of a Latent Pacemaker

Increased automaticity from a junctional or ventricular focus can usurp control of the ventricular rhythm from the sinus node. It also *interferes* with conduction coming from the SA node. The junctional or ventricular focus conducts retrogradely to the AV node, making it refractory to impulses conducted from the SA node. The ventricular rates in these rhythms are more rapid than junctional or ventricular escape rhythms seen in complete heart block. The ventricular rate can even exceed the atrial rate, and the ventricles may be in a refractory state when each atrial impulse arrives.

AV Dissociation with

Accelerated Junctional Rhythm

Accelerated Idioventricular Rhythm

Junctional Tachycardia

Ventricular Tachycardia

Atrial Rate = 100

Ventricular Rate = 80 bpm

Junctional rhythm interferes with anterograde conduction from SA node.

A   B

FIGURE 4.10 A. Complete AV dissociation with accelerated junctional rhythm. B. Mechanism

Complete AV Block

Ventricular Rate = 20 bpm

A diseased conduction system prevents conduction of the atrial impulse to the ventricle. An escape rhythm must take over.

A   B

FIGURE 4.11 A. Complete heart block with ventricular escape. B. Mechanism.

To define a rhythm as complete heart block, the ventricular rate has to be slower than the atrial rate. The ventricular rate must be slow enough for the AV node and ventricles to be out of their refractory periods when atrial impulses arrive. If the atrial impulse fails to conduct to the ventricles when the ventricular rate is slow (<50 bpm), then complete heart block is the cause of the AV dissociation. (Fig. 4.11)

ECG 4.4a

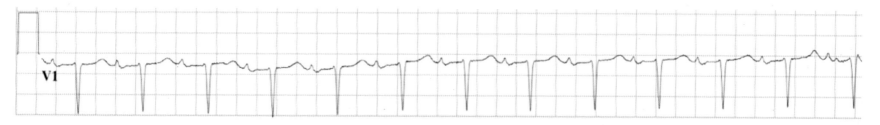

ECG 4.5a

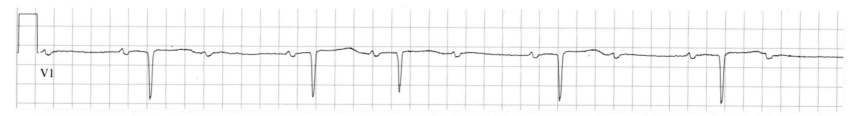

ECG 4.6a A 92-year-old male presents with back-to-back episodes of syncope.

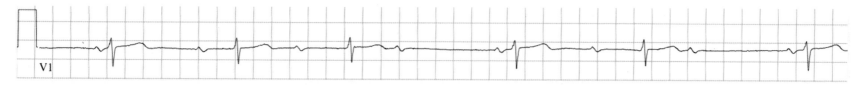

ECG 4.7a A 69-year-old male complains of weakness and fatigue.

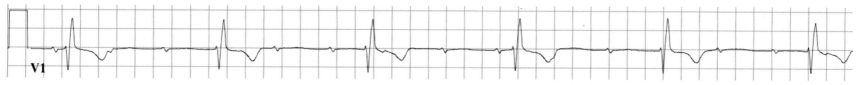

ECG 4.4b

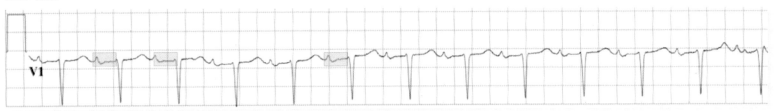

First Degree AV Block

ECG 4.5b

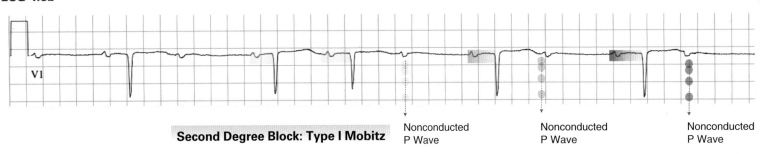

Second Degree Block: Type I Mobitz   Nonconducted P Wave   Nonconducted P Wave   Nonconducted P Wave

ECG 4.6b A 92-year-old male presents with back-to-back episodes of syncope.

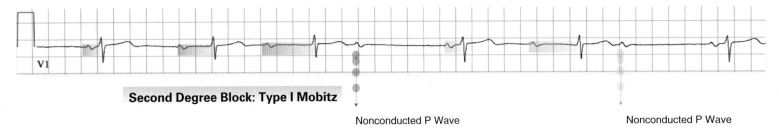

Second Degree Block: Type I Mobitz

Nonconducted P Wave   Nonconducted P Wave

ECG 4.7b A 69-year-old male complains of weakness and fatigue.

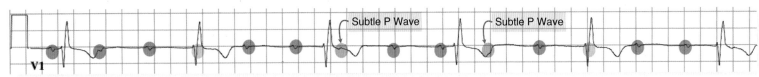

Subtle P Wave   Subtle P Wave

Complete Heart Block

Note how P waves march through at regular intervals. Some P waves are completely masked by QRS complexes and others make discrete deflections in the ST segments or T waves.

ECG 4.8a A 56-year-old asymptomatic male is med-flighted to a tertiary care hospital for "possible junctional rhythm."

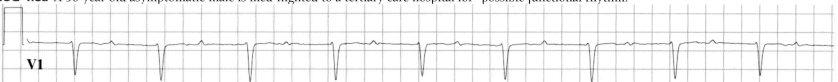

ECG 4.9a An 83-year-old female presents with several days of severe lethargy.

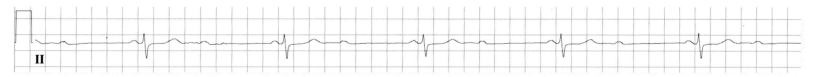

ECG 4.10a

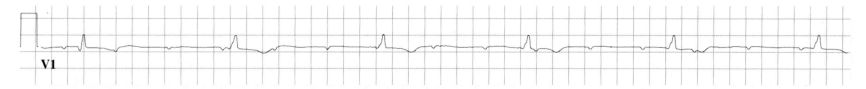

ECG 4.11a An 81-year-old with coronary artery disease and a prosthetic aortic valve presents with two days of dyspnea and fatigue.

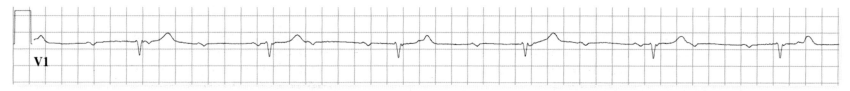

ECG 4.8b A 56-year-old asymptomatic male is med-flighted to tertiary care hospital for "possible junctional rhythm."

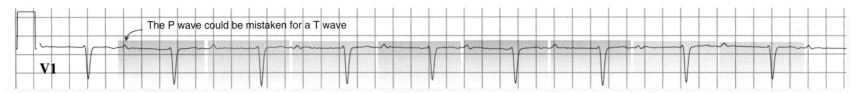

The P wave could be mistaken for a T wave

Extreme First Degree Block

ECG 4.9b An 83-year-old female presents with several days of severe lethargy.

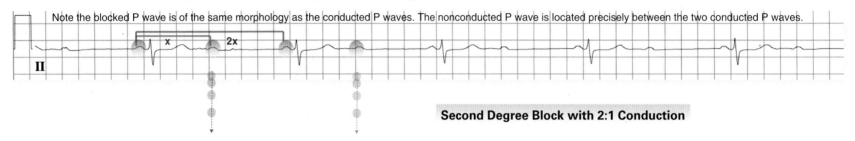

Note the blocked P wave is of the same morphology as the conducted P waves. The nonconducted P wave is located precisely between the two conducted P waves.

Second Degree Block with 2:1 Conduction

ECG 4.10b

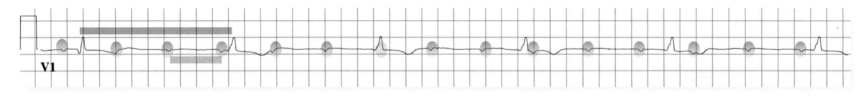

The atrial rate is faster than the ventricular rate. P waves march out at regular intervals. Wide QRS complexes represent a ventricular escape rate of 33 bpm.

Complete Heart Block

ECG 4.11b An 81-year-old with coronary artery disease and a prosthetic aortic valve presents with two days of dyspnea and fatigue.

Look for subtle distortions in QRS complexes and T waves where P waves would be expected to leave a footprint.

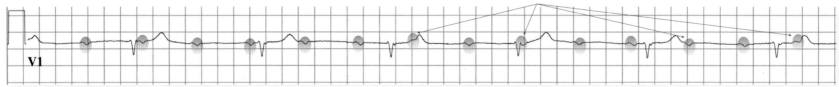

Complete Heart Block

ECG 4.12a A 52-year-old male from El Salvador was incidentally found to be bradycardic during an urgent care visit.

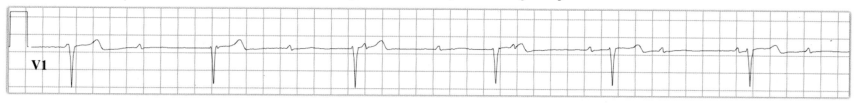

ECG 4.13a

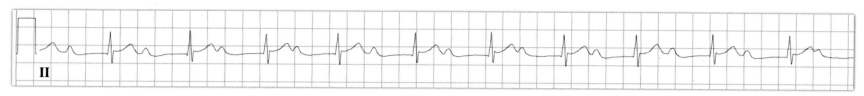

ECG 4.14a A 90-year-old male with a history of hypertension presents with three days of "dizziness."

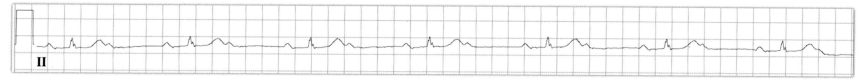

ECG 4.15a A 23-year-old male returns from a camping trip in Maine.

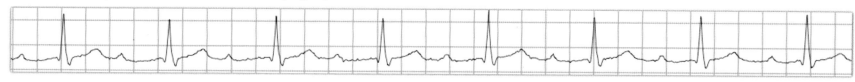

Image courtesy of Eric Antonsen, MD.

ECG 4.12b A 52-year-old male from El Salvador was incidentally found to be bradycardic during an urgent care visit.

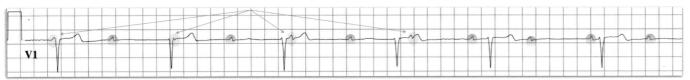

Distortions in QRS complexes and T waves

Complete Heart Block

Note that despite the rate being as slow as 36 bpm, the escape complexes are narrow. This patient was ultimately diagnosed as having congenital heart block at the level of the AV node. He underwent placement of a pacemaker.

ECG 4.13b

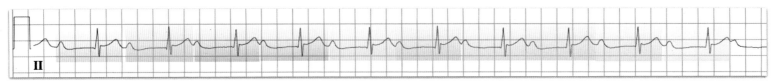

Extreme First Degree Block

ECG 4.14b A 90-year-old male with a history of hypertension presents with three days of "dizziness."

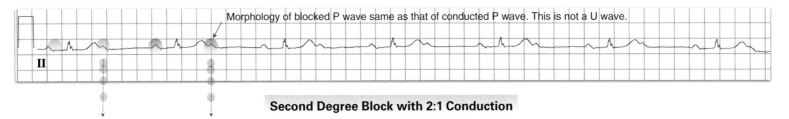

Morphology of blocked P wave same as that of conducted P wave. This is not a U wave.

Second Degree Block with 2:1 Conduction

The ventricular escape rate is 41 bpm in this ECG. The QRS morphology is that of an RBBB. During telemetry monitoring, the patient was found to have QRS complexes that switched to a left bundle branch morphology. Given the patient's demonstration of trifascicular conduction disease, the rhythm above most likely represents a Mobitz II block. He underwent pacemaker placement during this hospitalization.

ECG 4.15b A 23-year-old male returns from a camping trip in Maine.

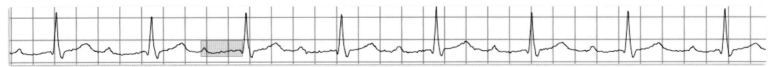

First Degree Block

This patient was diagnosed with Lyme carditis. Approximately 4% to 10% of patients with Lyme disease develop Lyme carditis.[4] Lyme carditis most commonly manifests as AV conduction disturbance. Approximately 50% of patients with conduction disturbance have complete heart block, and this typically resolves within one week. Mobitz I block occurs in 40% of patients with Lyme carditis.[5]

ECG 4.16a A 92-year-old male on atenolol presents with a rash consistent with zoster.

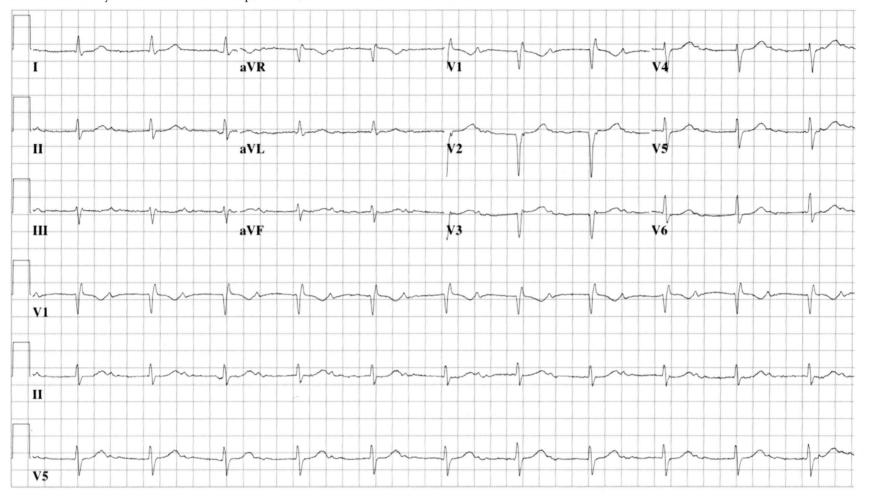

ECG 4.16b A 92-year-old male on atenolol presents with a rash consistent with zoster.

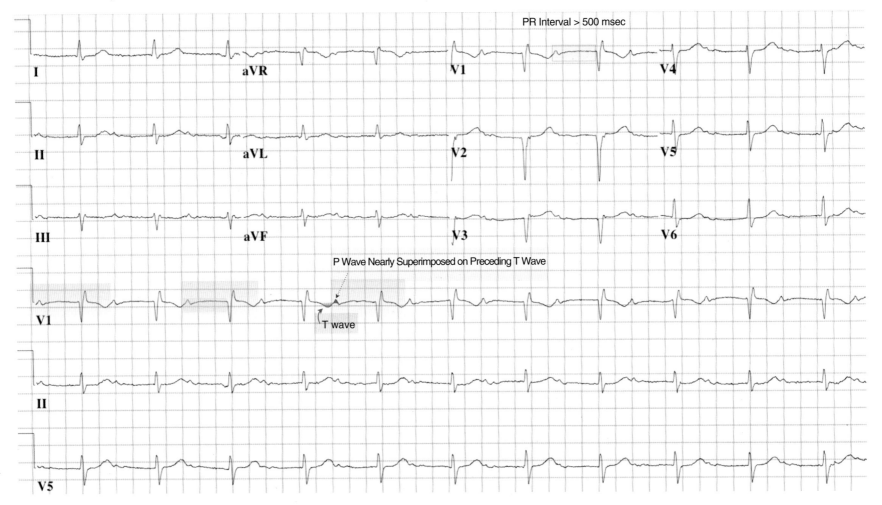

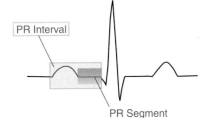

FIGURE 4.12 PR segment and interval

Extreme First Degree AV Block

PR prolongation is not commonly this extreme. One might be tempted to call this AV dissociation or accelerated junctional rhythm, but a closer look shows that the PR relationship here is constant and that P waves immediately follow T waves.

Upper limit of normal PR interval length: 200 msec

PR interval in this patient: approximately 550 msec

ECG 4.17a

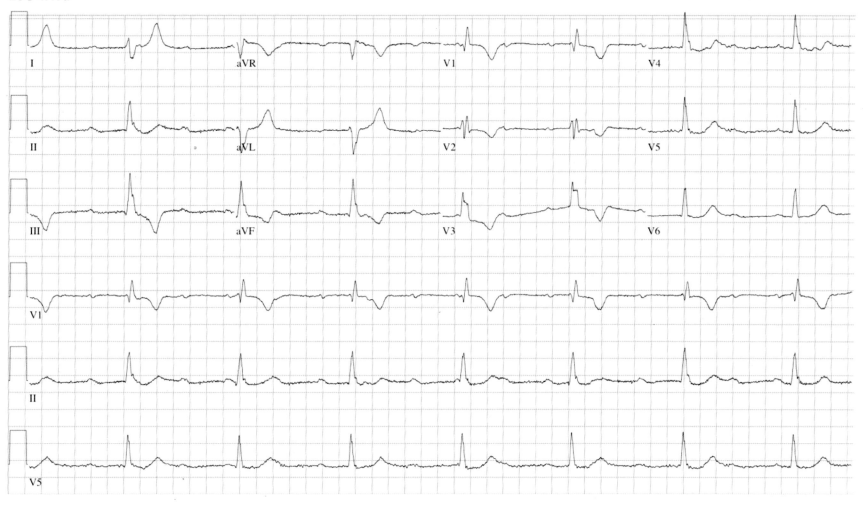

ECG 4.17b

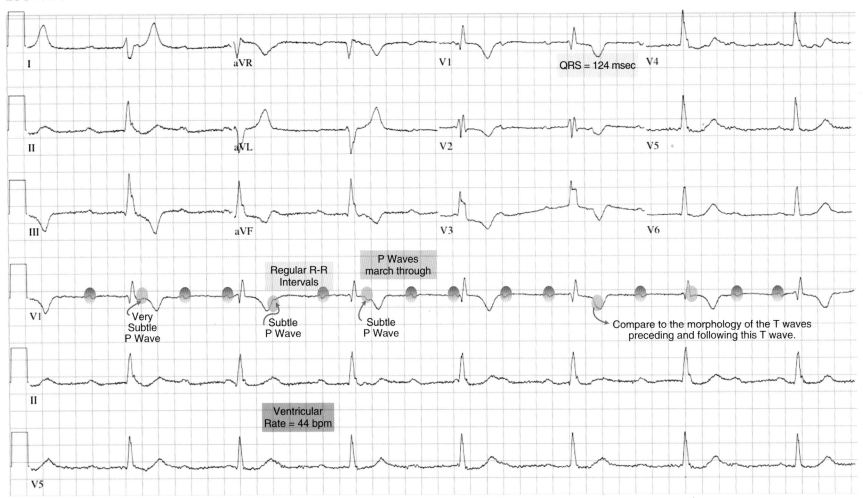

Complete Heart Block

ECG 4.18a

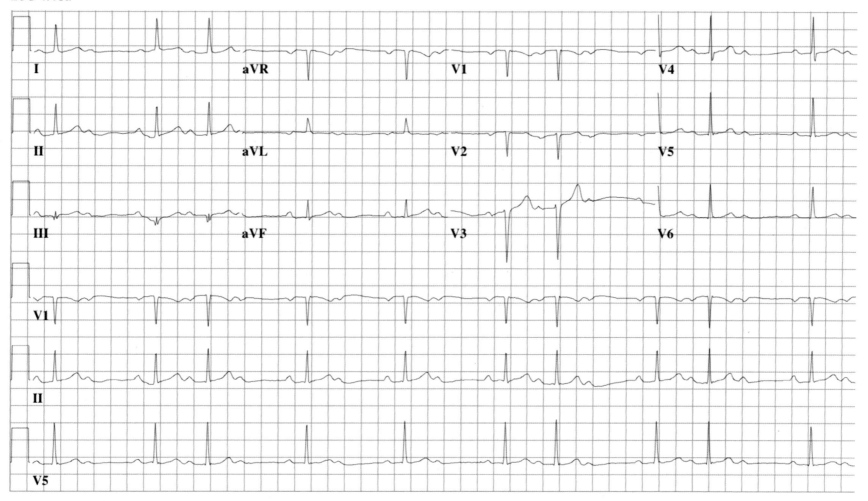

ECG 4.18b

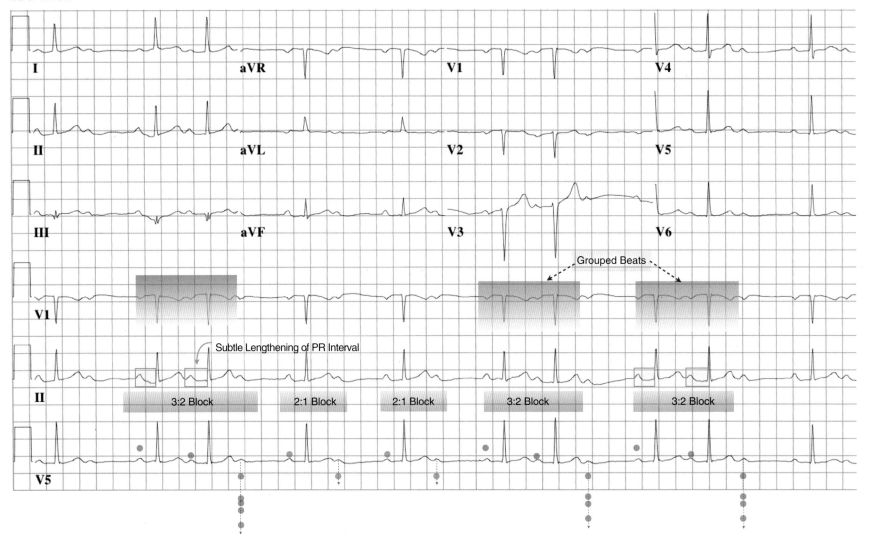

Second Degree AV Block: Mobitz I with Variable Conduction

The ratio of P waves to QRS complexes in second degree AV block may be variable within a single electrocardiogram. The presence of 3:2 block allows you to appreciate the gradual lengthening of PR segments and to infer that the 2:1 block in this ECG is Mobitz I type.

This cycle of progressively increasing in AV node refractoriness tends to group QRS complexes together. Grouped beats (highlighted in red boxes) are separated by dropped QRS complexes.

ECG 4.19a A 69-year-old male with hypertension and Parkinson's disease presents with lower extremity cellulitis.

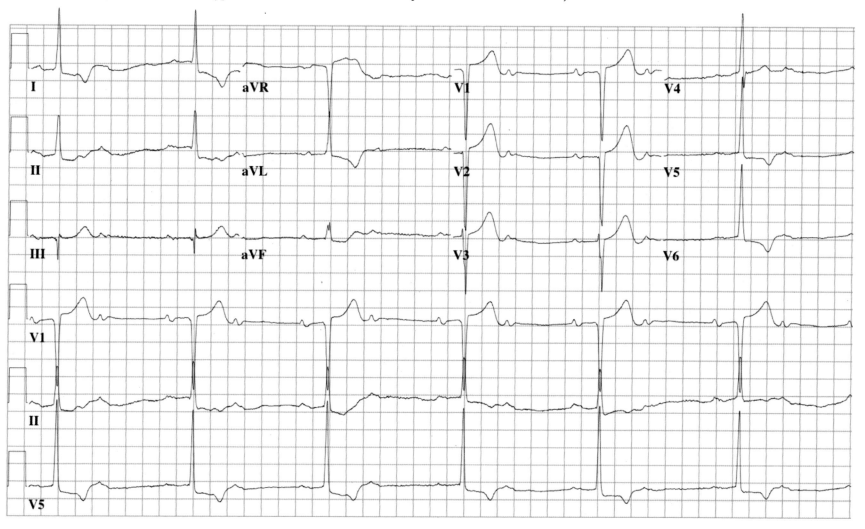

ECG 4.19b A 69-year-old male with hypertension and Parkinson's disease presents with lower extremity cellulitis.

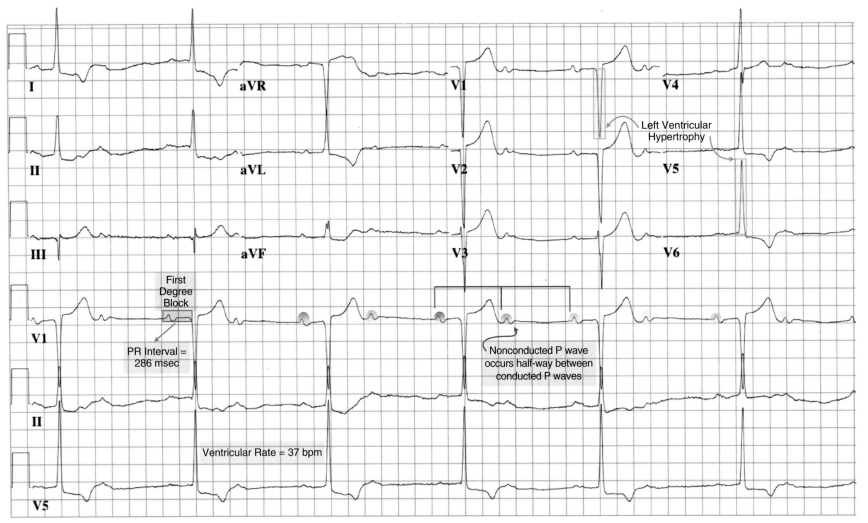

Second Degree AV Block with 2:1 Conduction

2:1 AV block makes Mobitz classification impossible because there are no two consecutive PR intervals to compare. One can't tell if the PR segment is constant or lengthening. The QRS complex here is of a left bundle branch morphology but is only 102 msec wide. The ventricular rate is 37 bpm. Subsequent ECGs from this patient demonstrated type I Mobitz block. He underwent placement of a pacemaker once his cellulitis completely resolved.

This ECG also demonstrates left ventricular hypertrophy and left ventricular strain pattern (downsloping ST depressions and T wave inversions in I, aVL, V5 and V6).

ECG 4.20a A 103-year-old male with a history of myocardial infarction 30 years ago and left bundle branch block was found by his home health aide to be bradycardic and somnolent.

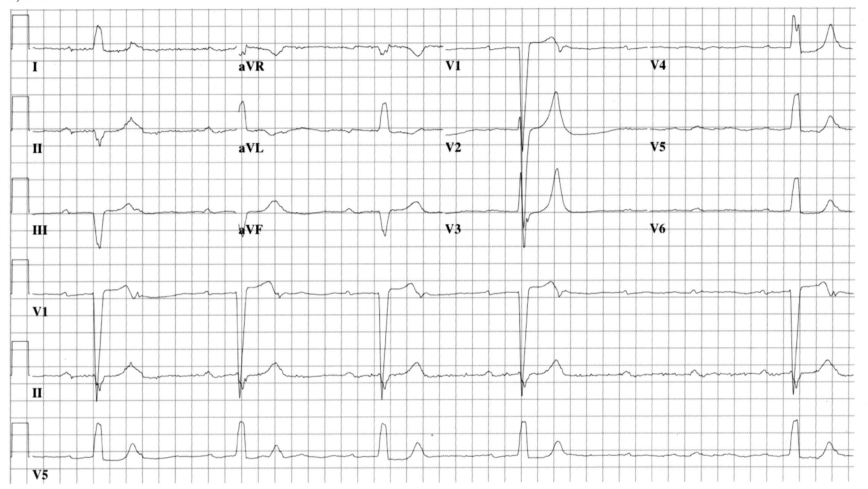

ECG 4.20b A 103-year-old male with a history of myocardial infarction 30 years ago and left bundle branch block was found by his home health aide to be bradycardic and somnolent.

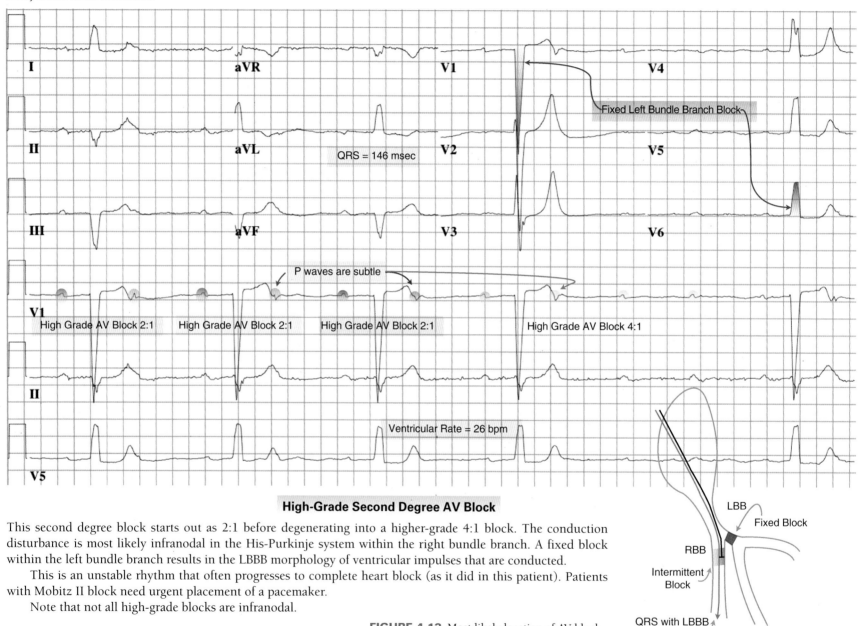

High-Grade Second Degree AV Block

This second degree block starts out as 2:1 before degenerating into a higher-grade 4:1 block. The conduction disturbance is most likely infranodal in the His-Purkinje system within the right bundle branch. A fixed block within the left bundle branch results in the LBBB morphology of ventricular impulses that are conducted.

This is an unstable rhythm that often progresses to complete heart block (as it did in this patient). Patients with Mobitz II block need urgent placement of a pacemaker.

Note that not all high-grade blocks are infranodal.

FIGURE 4.13 Most likely location of AV block.

ECG 4.21a A 79-year-old male with a history of two prior myocardial infarctions presents with fatigue and nausea for the past 5 days.

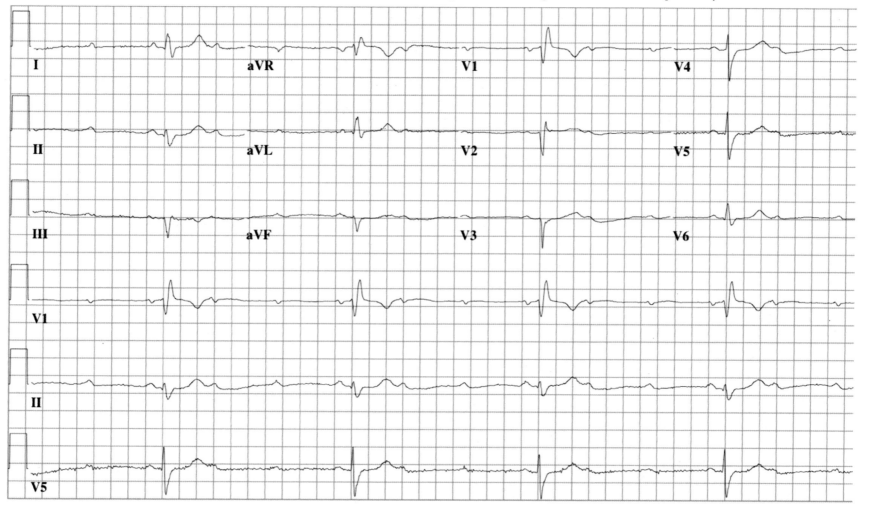

ECG 4.21b A 79-year-old male with a history of two prior myocardial infarctions presents with fatigue and nausea for the past 5 days.

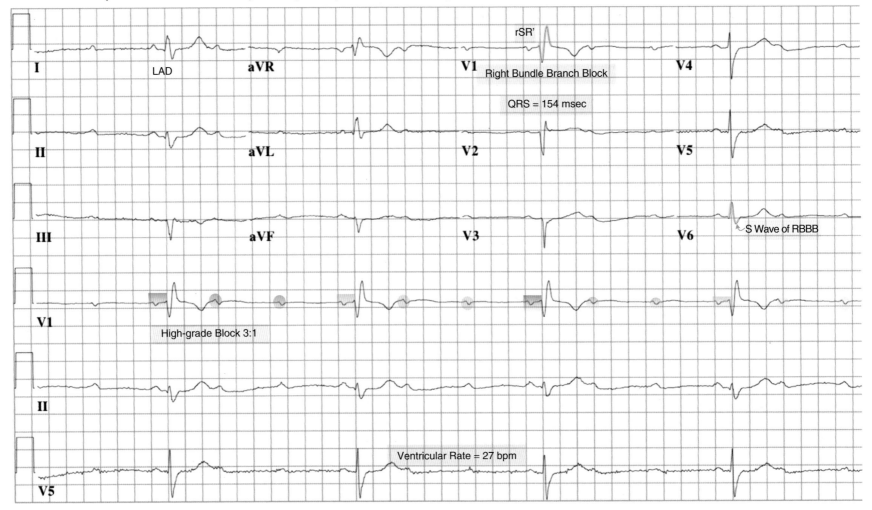

Advanced Second Degree AV Block with 3:1 Conduction

Because there are no consecutively conducted P waves to determine if the PR interval is lengthening, it's difficult to classify this block as Mobitz I or II. This block is likely infranodal, located within the left posterior fascicle. There appear to be fixed blocks in the right bundle branch and in left anterior fascicle (note the left axis deviation, rS waves in the inferior limb leads and qR wave in lead aVL. P waves followed by dropped QRS complexes represent trifascicular block. QRS complexes represent conduction down the left posterior fascicle (Fig. 3.19). This is a high-grade AV block with more than one consecutively dropped QRS complex. This patient underwent placement of a permanent pacemaker.

ECG 4.22a

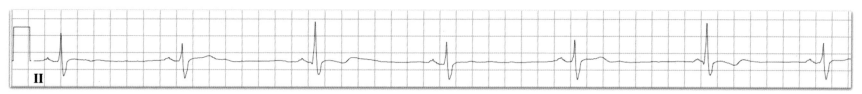

Image courtesy of Chris Kabrhel, MD.

ECG 4.23a An 86-year-old female complains of light-headedness for 2 weeks.

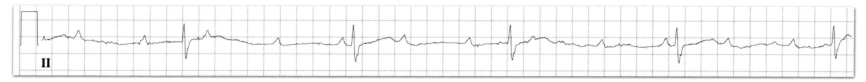

ECG 4.24a

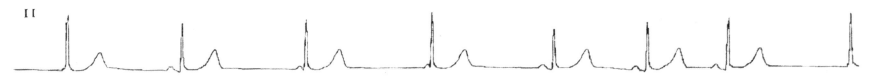

Image courtesy of Thomas Nielan, MD.

ECG 4.25a A 71-year-old female on a beta blocker and calcium channel blocker presents with hypotension, bradycardia, and near-syncope.

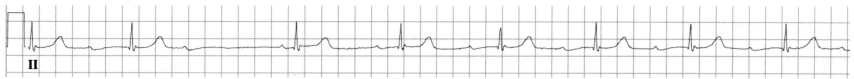

ECG 4.22b

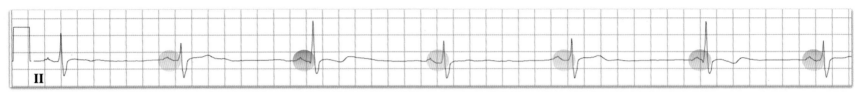

Note the gradual changes in PR interval length.   **Isorhythmic Dissociation**

ECG 4.23b An 86-year-old female complains of light-headedness for 2 weeks.

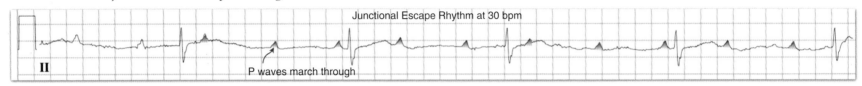

Complete Heart Block

ECG 4.24b

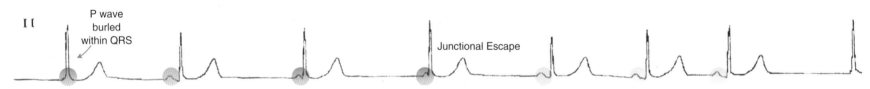

P waves move closer to and then farther from the QRS complex.   **Isorhythmic Dissociation**

ECG 4.25b A 71-year-old female on a beta blocker and calcium channel blocker presents with hypotension, bradycardia, and near-syncope.

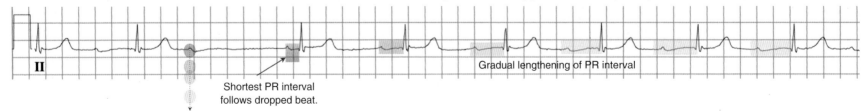

Second Degree Block: Mobitz I

ECG 4.26a A 76-year-old male with diabetes mellitus and coronary artery disease presents after a syncopal episode.

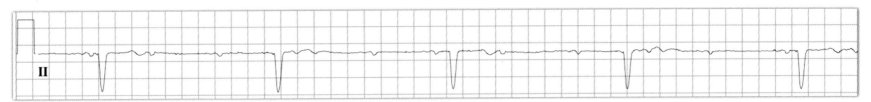

ECG 4.27a

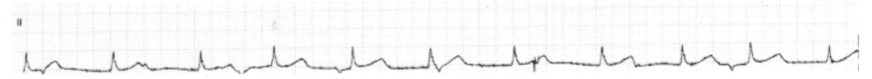

Image courtesy of Josh Kosowsky, MD.

ECG 4.28a A 92-year-old female with chronic atrial fibrillation appears confused and disheveled to her primary care doctor.

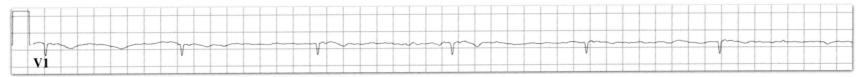

ECG 4.29a

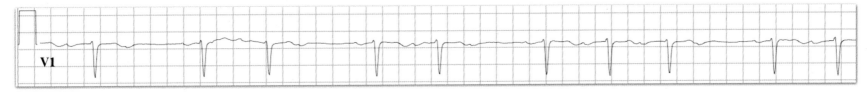

ECG 4.26b A 76-year-old male with diabetes mellitus and coronary artery disease presents after a syncopal episode.

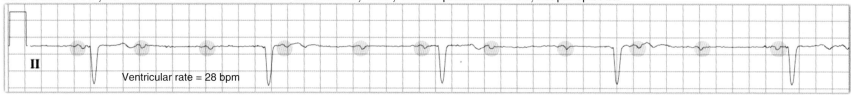

II

Ventricular rate = 28 bpm

Complete Heart Block

ECG 4.27b

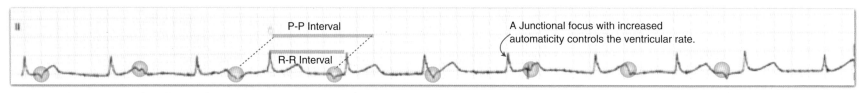

P-P Interval

R-R Interval

A Junctional focus with increased automaticity controls the ventricular rate.

Note that the R-R interval is shorter than the P-P interval.

AV Dissociation: Accelerated Junctional Rhythm

ECG 4.28b A 92-year-old female with chronic atrial fibrillation appears confused and disheveled to her primary care doctor.

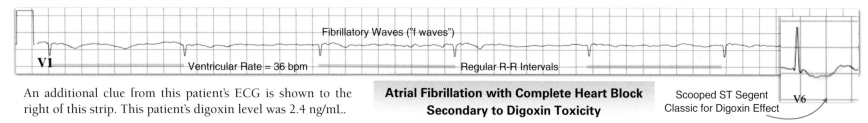

Fibrillatory Waves ("f waves")

V1

Ventricular Rate = 36 bpm

Regular R-R Intervals

V6

An additional clue from this patient's ECG is shown to the right of this strip. This patient's digoxin level was 2.4 ng/mL.

Atrial Fibrillation with Complete Heart Block
Secondary to Digoxin Toxicity

Scooped ST Segent
Classic for Digoxin Effect

ECG 4.29b

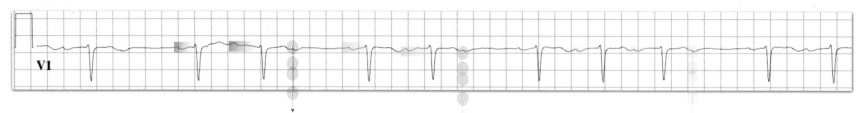

V1

Second Degree AV Block: Mobitz I

References

1. Mirvis DaG A. Electrocardiography. In: Bonow RM, D; Zipes, D; Libby P, eds. *Braunwald's Heart Disease: A Textbook of Cardiovascular Medicine.* 9th ed. Philadelphia, PA: Elsevier; 2011.
2. Wagner GS, ed. *Marriott's Practical Electrocardiography.* 11th ed. Philadelphia, PA: Lippincott Williams & Wilkins; 2008:402–420.
3. Barold SS, Hayes DL. Second-degree atrioventricular block: a reappraisal. Mayo Clin Proc 2001;76:44–57.
4. Schmid GP, Horsley R, Steere AC, et al. Surveillance of Lyme disease in the United States, 1982. *J Infect* Dis 1985;151:1144–1149.
5. McAlister HF, Klementowicz PT, Andrews C, et al. Lyme carditis: an important cause of reversible heart block. *Ann Intern Med* 1989;110: 339–345.

CHAPTER 5

Premature Contractions

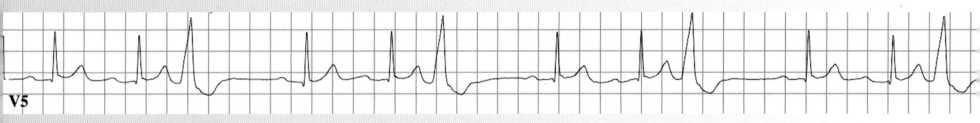

V5

Premature Atrial Contraction

Premature atrial contractions (PACs) arise from an ectopic focus anywhere in the atria, including the coronary sinus and pulmonary veins. PACs simultaneously conduct anterograde to the AV node and in retrograde fashion to the sinus node. Retrograde conduction causes depolarization of the sinus node and the timing of the sinus rhythm to be reset. This results in a noncompensatory pause.

The P wave of a PAC occurs prematurely and has a different morphology than the sinus P wave. A premature atrial complex may occur in isolation in a single ECG. It may also recur in a pattern of bigeminy or trigeminy.

Depending on the state of the AV node from the preceding sinus impulse, these premature atrial complexes have several possible fates.

Blocked   A PAC is blocked when it encounters the AV node still in its refractory period (corresponds to label A in Fig. 5.1). The P wave of a blocked PAC can be very subtle, especially if it is buried in the previous T wave. Because this premature beat resets the sinus node, a pause follows. When the block occurs repeatedly, these pauses can separate QRS complexes into grouped beats.

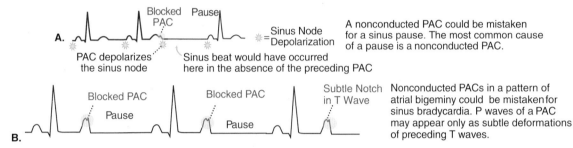

FIGURE 5.2   **A.** ECG appearance of a blocked PAC occurring in isolation and **B.** in a pattern of atrial bigeminy.

Conducted   A premature atrial impulse encounters an AV node that is no longer in its absolute refractory period.

Conducted Normally

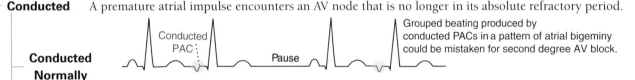

FIGURE 5.3   ECG appearance of a normally conducted PAC (corresponds to label B in Fig. 5.1).

Conducted with PR Prolongation   An ectopic atrial impulse may encounter the AV node in its relative refractory period. Conduction is delayed somewhere within the AV node or bundle of His and PR prolongation results (C in Fig. 5.1). Conduction then proceeds down the bundle branches resulting in a normal-appearing QRS complex.

Conducted with Aberration   An ectopic atrial impulse may encounter the right bundle branch in its absolute refractory period (D in Fig. 5.1). The right bundle branch tends to have a longer refractory period than the left bundle branch. QRS complexes are wide and have an RBBB pattern (Fig. 5.4). PACs with aberrant conduction could be confused with PVCs, especially when the P wave of a PAC is buried within the preceding T wave.

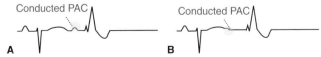

FIGURE 5.4   ECG appearances of a PAC conducted with aberration.

Atrial Tachycardia   When three or more consecutive PACs from the same atrial focus occur at a rate greater than 100 bpm.

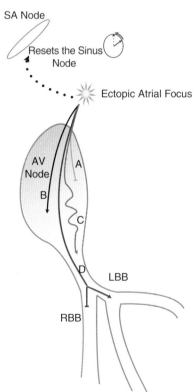

FIGURE 5.1.   Different conduction fates of a premature atrial impulse.

Premature Junctional Contraction

The AV junction includes the AV node and the Bundle of His. Premature junctional complexes (PJCs) are less common than premature atrial and ventricular complexes. Nonsustained PJCs are considered benign.

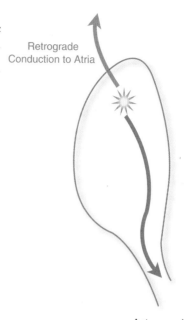

Retrograde Conduction to Atria

ECG Features

Narrow QRS Complex Anterograde conduction from a junctional focus results in simultaneous activation of left and right ventricles. The QRS complex of a PJC is narrow.

Inverted P Wave Premature impulses arising from the AV junction can travel in retrograde fashion to activate the atria. Atrial conduction occurs in an inferior-to-superior direction. P waves of junctional impulses are inverted in the inferior limb leads II, III, and aVF.

Narrow P Wave Because both left and right atria are activated simultaneously from the junctional focus, P waves tend to be narrow.[2]

Depending on the relative conduction speeds of the anterograde ventricular conduction and retrograde atrial conduction, this P wave may occur before the QRS complex, buried within the QRS complex, or after the QRS complex.

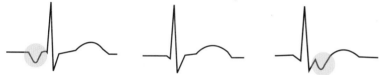

FIGURE 5.6 Different appearances of premature junctional contractions.

Anterograde Conduction to Ventricles

FIGURE 5.5 Anterograde and retrograde conduction coming from a junctional focus.

Retrograde conduction to the atria may or may not reset the sinus node. The next sinus beat may occur on time (fully compensatory pause) as if no premature junctional beat had occurred. If the sinus node is reset, the next sinus beat may occur earlier than expected (noncompensatory pause).

Accelerated Junctional Rhythm

When consecutive junctional impulses occur at a rate greater than the intrinsic rate of the AV junction (40 to 60 bpm), the rhythm is called accelerated junctional rhythm.

Rates greater than 60 bpm are above the upper normal intrinsic rate of the AV junction; the term nonparoxysmal junctional tachycardia is often used interchangeably with accelerated junctional rhythm when the rate of a junctional rhythm exceeds 60 bpm.

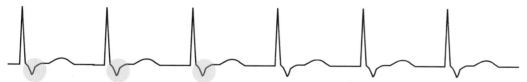

FIGURE 5.7 Accelerated junctional rhythm with retrograde P waves following QRS complexes. Retrograde P waves can also be buried in QRS complexes or appear before the QRS complexes.

AV dissociation can occur in accelerated junctional rhythm. A junctional focus may be able to conduct anterograde to ventricles but fail to conduct retrograde to the atria. When this is the case, atrial conduction is controlled by the sinus node and ventricular conduction by the AV junction.

An important cause of accelerated junctional rhythm is digitalis toxicity.

Premature Ventricular Contraction

A premature ventricular contraction (PVC) is an impulse that arises from the ventricle. The occurrence of PVCs increases with age. The clinical significance and prognostic importance of PVCs remain unclear.

ECG Appearance

Widened QRS   The QRS complex of a PVC is widened because ventricular activation occurs through myocardial spread rather than through the normal conduction system.

Discordance   Abnormal depolarization initiated by a premature ventricular impulse is followed by abnormal repolarization. The ST segment and T wave are therefore opposite the direction of the QRS wave.

Fully Compensatory Pause   A pause will follow each PVC because the ventricle will be refractory to the next incoming supraventricular impulse. The sinus node continues to fire unaffected by the PVC. The sinus impulse that follows a PVC occurs on time. This is called a fully compensatory pause. The distance between the two R waves spanning a PVC is twice the R-R distance between adjacent sinus beats.

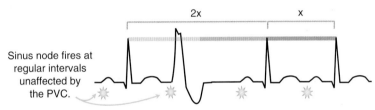

FIGURE 5.8 Fully compensatory pause.

A PVC may conduct retrogradely through the normal AV conduction system to the atria. If this occurs, the retrograde atrial conduction is often concealed by the ST segment and T wave.

Coupling Interval   The interval between a QRS complex and the following PVC is called the coupling interval. The coupling interval is often fixed.

A short coupling interval brings the R wave of the PVC close to the T wave of the preceding beat. A PVC that occurs during the relative refractory period of the previous beat ("R on T phenomenon") can initiate ventricular tachycardia or ventricular fibrillation.

Polymorphic PVCs   Wide QRS complexes with varying morphology may represent PVCs coming from different ventricular foci. These are also referred to as multifocal PVCs. (Fig. 5.10A)

Recurring PVCs   PVCs can occur with regularity throughout an ECG.

Bigeminy

Couplet   Two consecutive PVCs are referred to as a pair or couplet.

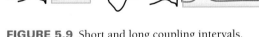

FIGURE 5.9 Short and long coupling intervals.

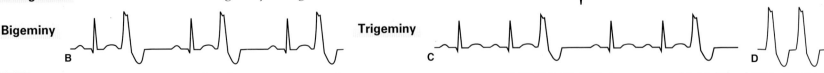

FIGURE 5.10 PVCs in a patterns of A. Multifocal PVCs. PVCS in patterns of B. Bigeminy and C. Trigeminy. D. A PVC couplet.

ECG 5.1a

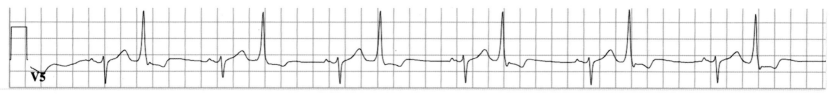

V5

ECG 5.2a

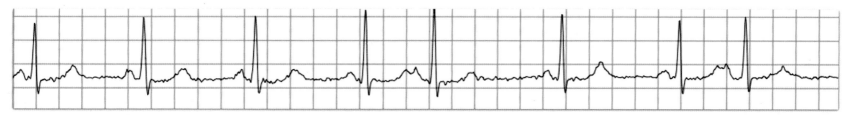

ECG 5.3a

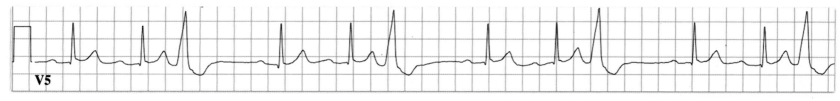

V5

ECG 5.4a

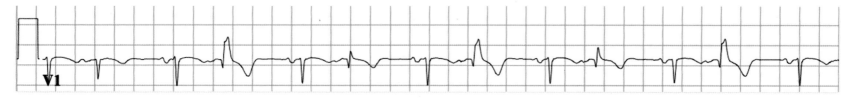

V1

ECG 5.1b

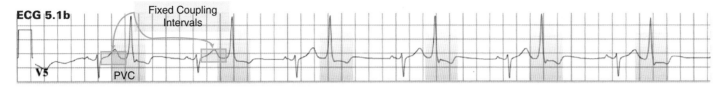

The presence of a fixed coupling interval suggests that reentry is the mechanism underlying these PVCs.

PVCs in a Bigeminy Pattern

ECG 5.2b

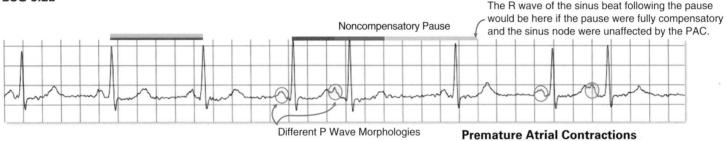

Note that the distance between R waves straddling the conducted PAC is less than twice the distance between two adjacent sinus R waves. This is referred to as a noncompensatory pause. The PAC resets the sinus node to an earlier schedule.

Premature Atrial Contractions

ECG 5.3b

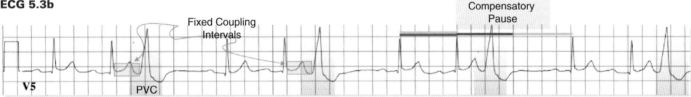

PVCs in a Trigeminy Pattern

ECG 5.4b

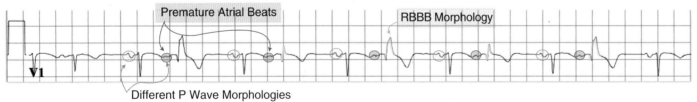

PACs Conducted with Aberration

The wide QRS complexes resulting from premature atrial contractions could easily be mistaken for PVCs by overlooking the P wave preceding each wide QRS complex. Note the alternating QRS morphology of the premature beats. The premature atrial beats are likely arriving at the right bundle branch in different stages of refractoriness; the wider, aberrant QRS complexes result from complexes arriving earlier in the refractory period of the right bundle branch.

Determine the rhythm underlying each series of grouped beating.

ECG 5.5a

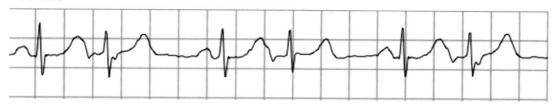

ECG 5.6a

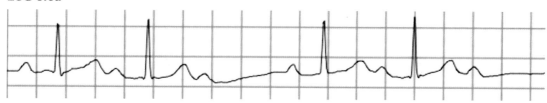

ECG 5.7a

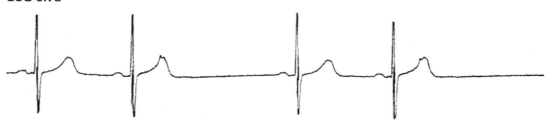

Image courtesy of Thomas Nielan, MD.

Grouped Beats Grouped beating is not only present in AV Block. Premature atrial contractions, whether conducted or blocked, are followed by a pause. When a premature beat comes from an atrial focus, it conducts retrograde to the SA node and interferes with the sinus rhythm. The sinus node discharges ahead of schedule.

ECG 5.5b

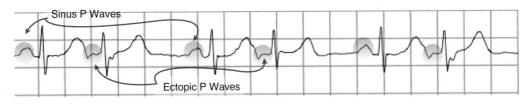

The P waves of the PACs have different contours than those of the sinus P waves.

Here PACs are coupled in a pattern of atrial bigeminy.

Conducted PACs

ECG 5.6b

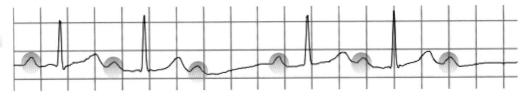

The P wave morphologies are uniform. Lengthening of the PR interval in this example is subtle.

Second Degree: Mobitz I

ECG 5.7b

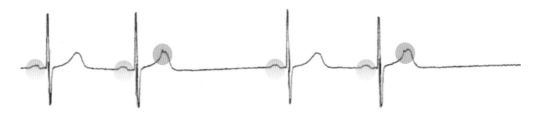

The P waves of atrial premature beats cause notching of the preceding T waves of normal sinus beats.

Nonconducted PACs

PACs that occur very early (shortly after a previous sinus beat) may fail to conduct through an AV node or ventricle that is still refractory from the previous sinus beat. These PACs are still able to conduct retrograde throught the atria to depolarize and reset the sinus node. This results in a pause that sets apart the previous sinus beat from the following normal sinus beat, giving the appearance of grouped beating.

ECG 5.8a

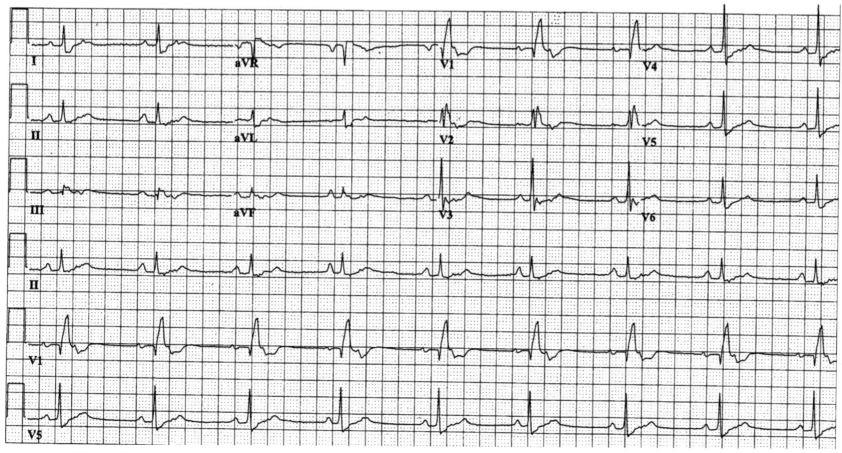

Image courtesy of Thomas Nielan, MD.

ECG 5.8b

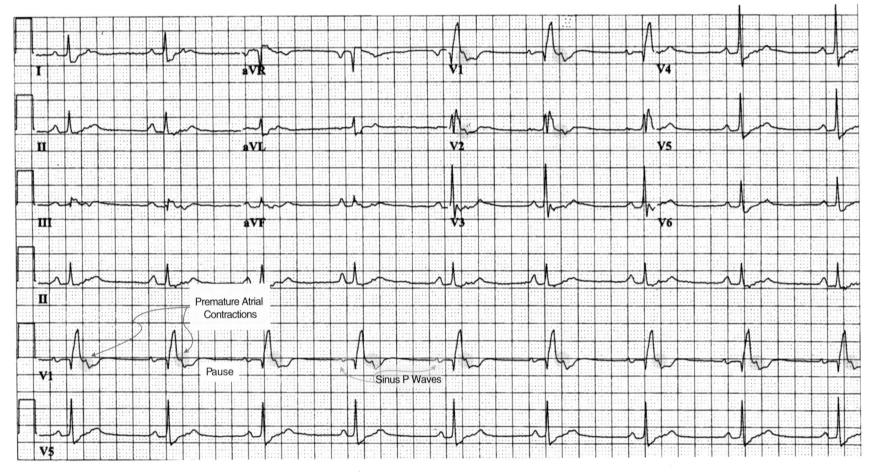

This rhythm could be mistaken for sinus bradycardia by overlooking the P waves in the right precordial leads.

Normal Sinus Rhythm with Nonconducted PACs in a Pattern of Atrial Bigeminy

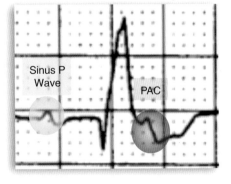

ECG 5.9a

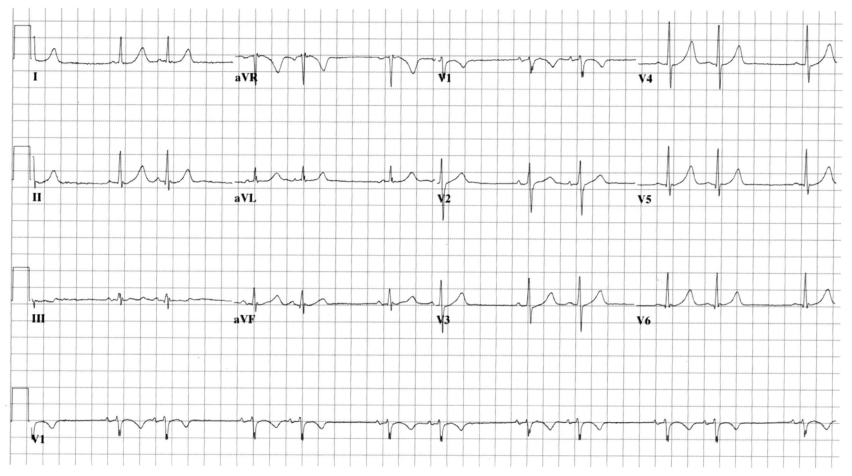

ECG 5.9b

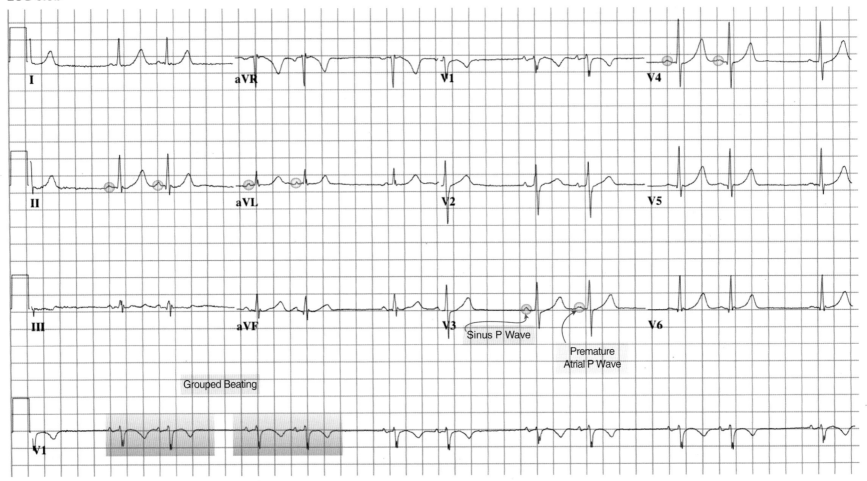

Grouped Beating

Sinus P Wave

Premature
Atrial P Wave

Conducted PACs in a Pattern of Atrial Bigeminy

The P wave morphologies of the sinus and ectopic atrial beats are strikingly similar in lead V1. Subtle differences can be appreciated, however, in other leads. The regular pattern of conducted premature atrial contractions results in grouped beating separated by noncompensatory pauses. Each premature atrial beat causes the sinus node to depolarize and effectively puts the sinus node on an earlier schedule of spontaneous depolarization. The sinus beat following a premature atrial contraction arrives earlier than it would if the sinus node had continued to fire uninterrupted.

ECG 5.10a

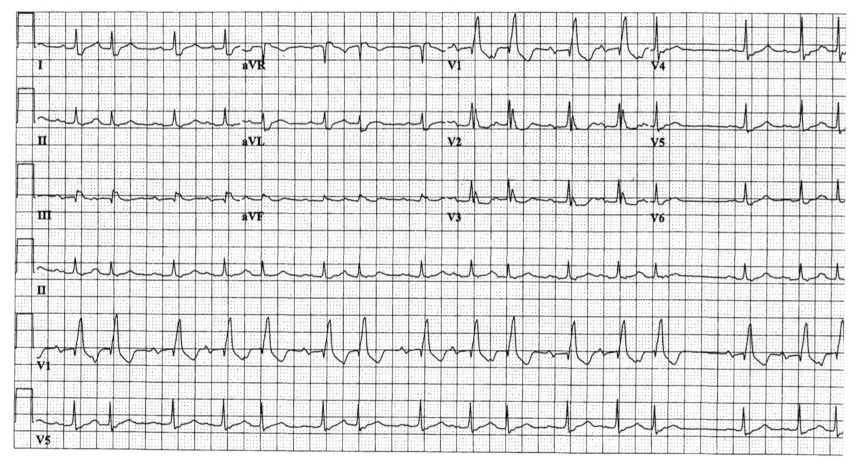

Image courtesy of Thomas Nielan, MD.

ECG 5.10b

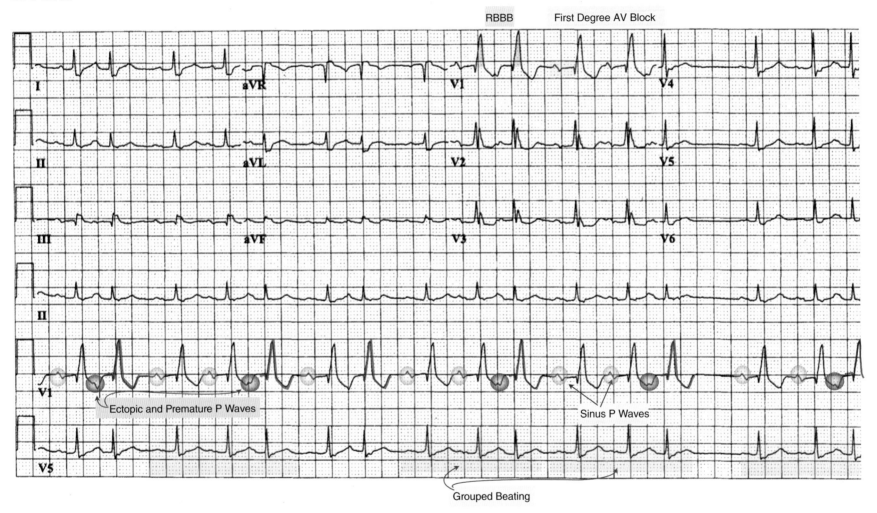

Normal Sinus Rhythm with Frequently Conducted PACs

QRS complexes appear in groups of 2 and 3. The differential for grouped beating includes Mobitz I AV block and PACs. The P waves of the premature atrial beats are subtle as they occur within the preceding T waves. The morphology of the sinus and premature P waves is different. In Mobitz I block, the morphology of the P waves is uniform.

ECG 5.11a

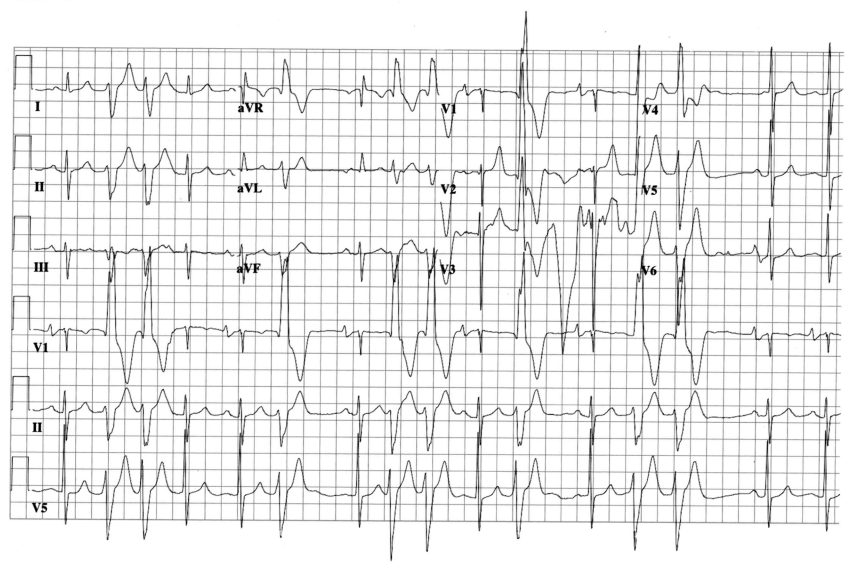

ECG 5.11b

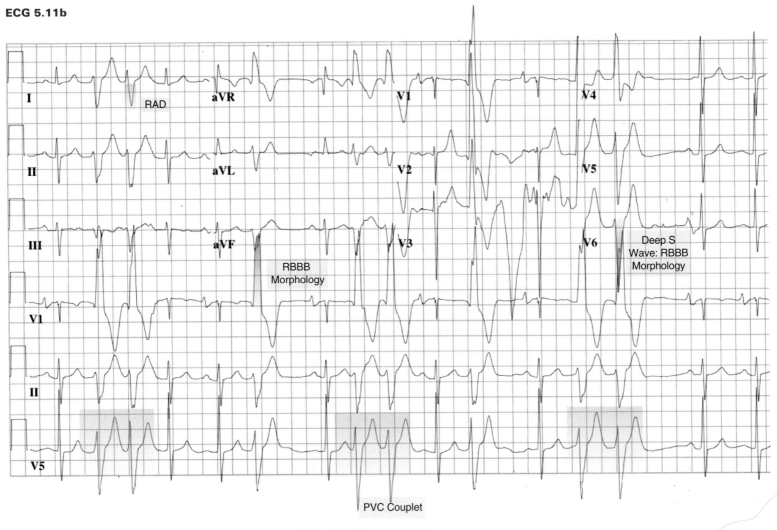

Frequent PVCs and PVC Couplets

The RBBB morphology of the PVCs and right axis deviation indicate that the PVCs in this ECG originate from the left ventricle.

FIGURE 5.11 Pattern of ventricular activation from a left-sided PVC.

ECG 5.12a

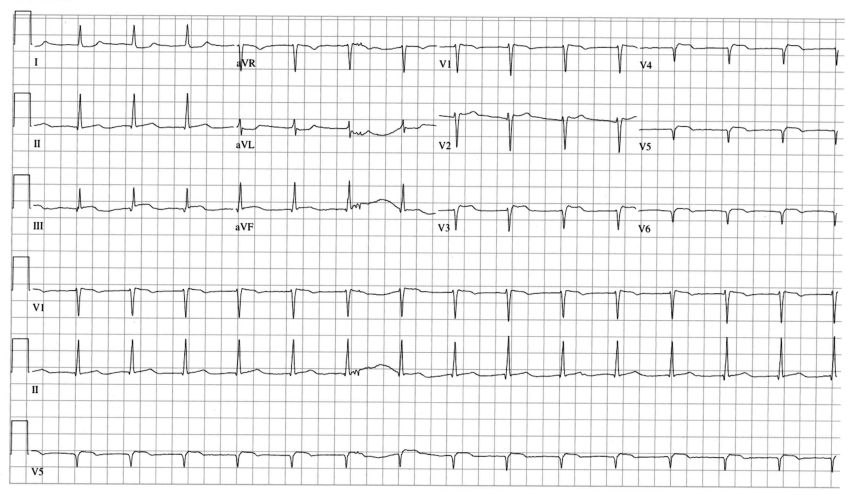

ECG 5.12b

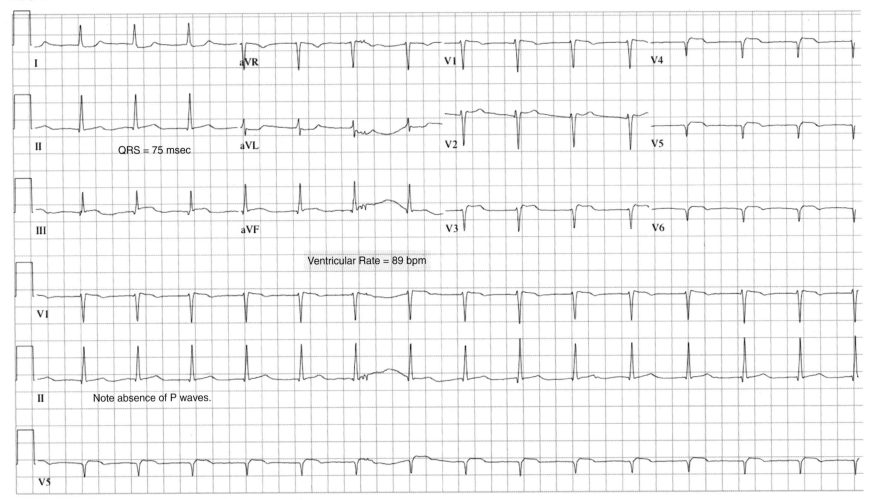

QRS = 75 msec

Ventricular Rate = 89 bpm

Note absence of P waves.

Accelerated Junctional Rhythm

Simultaneous activation of atria and ventricles from a junctional focus can result in P waves that are completely obscured by QRS complexes.

ECG 5.13a

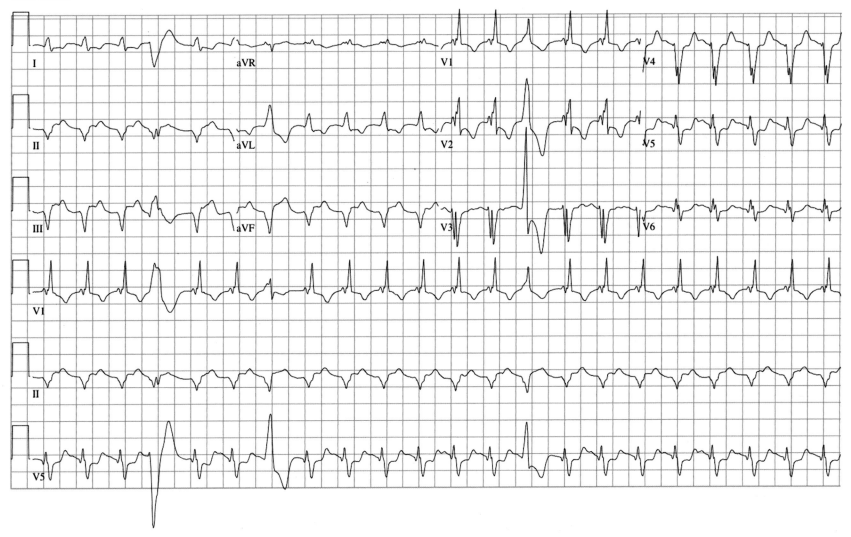

ECG 5.13b

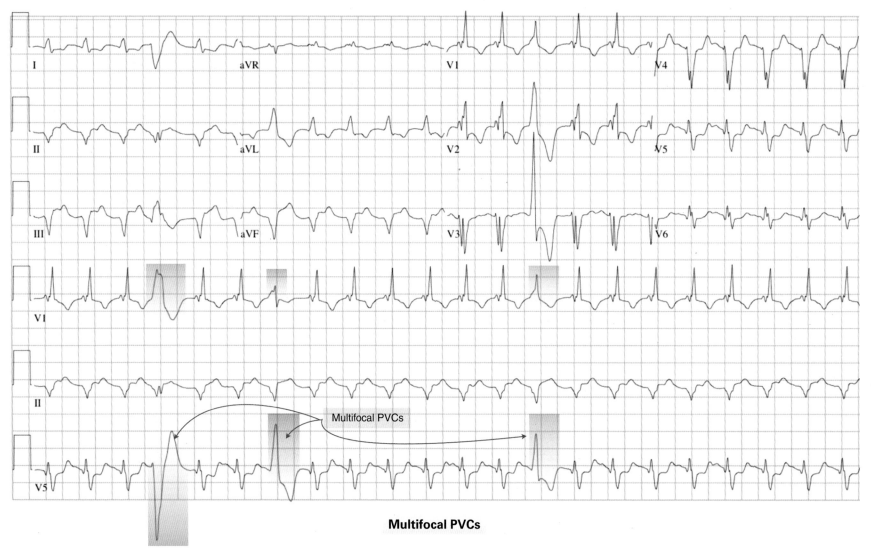

Multifocal PVCs

Multifocal PVCs

References

1. Wagner GaW, T. Premature beats. In: Wagner G, ed. *Marriott's Practical Electrocardiography*. 11th ed. Philadelphia, PA: Lippincott Williams & Wilkins; 2008.
2. Baltazar R. Premature supraventricular complexes. In: *Basic and Bedside Electrocardiography*. Philadelphia, PA: Lippincott Williams & Wilkins; 2009.

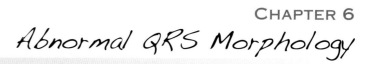

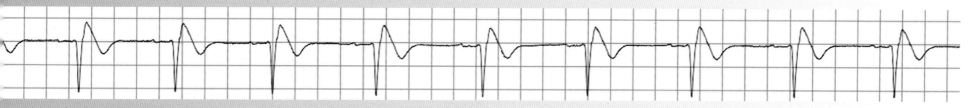

Brugada Pattern and Syndrome

Pathogenesis   Brugada syndrome is an autosomally dominant inherited disease (with incomplete penetrance) known for causing sudden death in patients with structurally normal hearts. More than half of cases, however, are sporadic. The disease has been linked to the *SCN5A* gene that encodes for a subunit of the sodium channel within epicardial cells of the right ventricle.

Clinical Course   Patients present with syncope or sudden cardiac death from polymorphic ventricular tachycardia. Mean age of sudden cardiac death is 41 years. The disease is markedly more predominant in males and, while present worldwide, is endemic in Southeast Asia.[1]

ECG Features   The classic ECG findings are right bundle branch block pattern and ST elevation in V1-V3. These findings in a patient with Brugada syndrome may be absent at any given time. Fever, drugs (sodium channel–blocking medications), electrolyte disturbances, and high vagal tone are known to exaggerate or unmask ST elevation in the right precordial leads.

RBBB Pattern

ST Elevation in V1-V3

There are three different Brugada patterns. Only Type I Brugada pattern is diagnostic of Brugada syndrome. Further testing is required for Types 2 and 3.

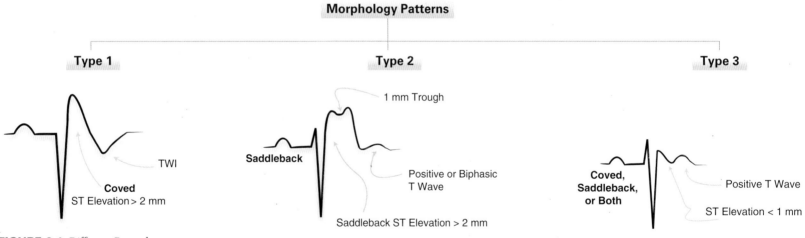

FIGURE 6.1 Different Brugada patterns.

Differential Diagnosis   The differential for ST elevation in right precordial leads should be considered. More common causes of ST elevation such as early repolarization, septal MI, bundle branch block, left ventricular hypertrophy, right ventricular strain, and right ventricular infarction should be ruled out. Toxicity from cocaine and tricyclic antidepressants can mimic the Brugada pattern (through sodium channel–blocking mechanisms). One of the more difficult syndromes to differentiate from Brugada on ECG is arrhythmogenic right ventricular dysplasia. Brugada pattern can also appear for several hours in patients who are cardioverted or defibrillated.

Treatment   The only effective management to date is placement of an implantable cardioverter-defibrillator (ICD).

Arrhythmogenic Right Ventricular Dysplasia (ARVD)

Pathogenesis Arrhythmogenic right ventricular dysplasia is an inherited cardiomyopathy characterized by progressive fatty or fibrofatty infiltration of the right ventricular myocardium. Despite the name given to this disease, involvement of the left ventricle can occur in as many as 60% of patients. Replacement of cardiac myocytes by fibrofatty tissue leads to wall thinning, aneurysm formation of the right ventricle, and conduction abnormalities.[2] Inheritance is most commonly autosomal dominant with variable penetrance although recessive forms have been identified. The most common genetic abnormality identified to date is a mutation in desmosomal proteins that provide mechanical binding between myocytes.

Clinical Course Initially patients with ARVD may have only localized infiltration and involvement of part of the right ventricle. They are asymptomatic but still at risk for sudden cardiac death.[3] As infiltration becomes more diffuse in the right ventricle and starts to involve the left ventricle, patients may develop symptomatic arrhythmias (ventricular tachycardia). In late stages of the disease, patients suffer from biventricular heart failure that becomes difficult to distinguish from that caused by dilated cardiomyopathy.

ECG Features Conduction abnormalities in ARVD are located in the right ventricle. The ECG abnormalities in ARVD can be appreciated in the right precordial leads:

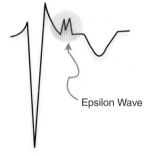

Prolonged QRS Delayed activation of the right ventricle results in prolongation of the QRS. This can take the form of an incomplete or complete right bundle branch block pattern. The QRS in the right precordial leads may be longer than that in the left precordial leads.[4]

Epsilon Wave An epsilon wave is a low-amplitude deflection occurring at the end of the QRS segment or early ST segment. It represents delayed conduction in the right ventricle. This is a subtle finding, but is very specific to ARVD.

T Wave Inversion Inverted T waves in the right precordial leads (V1-V3) is the most common repolarization abnormality seen.[2]

FIGURE 6.2 Incomplete RBBB morphology and epsilon wave.

Arrhythmias

PVCs Frequent PVCs in younger adults may indicate myocardial disease.

Ventricular Tachycardia Nonsustained or sustained VT with left bundle branch morphology results from an ectopic focus in the right ventricle. ARVD should be considered as an underlying cause of an ECG demonstrating right ventricular outflow tract (RVOT) tachycardia.

Ventricular Fibrillation This is the mechanism of sudden cardiac death in athletes and young adults.

Diagnosis The diagnosis of ARVD is based on ECG findings, histopathology from endomyocardial biopsy, family history, and imaging findings. Cardiac MRI, 2D echocardiography, and RV angiography are all used to identify RV dysfunction.

Management Young adults are advised to refrain from vigorous exercise as ventricular arrhythmias are more likely to occur in the setting of an adrenergic surge. Some patients are advised to undergo placement of an ICD.

Wolff-Parkinson-White Pattern

Pathogenesis
In WPW syndrome, atrial conduction is able to reach the ventricles through an accessory pathway that bypasses the normal AV conduction system. Because this pathway bypasses AV nodal tissue where conduction is delayed, a portion of the ventricle becomes prematurely excited.

ECG Features

Wide QRS
The QRS wave can be thought of as a fusion complex. It reflects ventricle that is preexcited by the bypass tract and depolarized by the normal conduction system.

Short PR Interval
Time from atrial to ventricular conduction, represented by the PR interval, is shorter because the accessory pathway bypasses the AV node.

Delta Wave
Represents early depolarization (preexcitation) of the ventricle by the bypass tract. Though ventricular activation is premature, conduction through this tissue is slower, making the slope of the inscribed delta wave less steep than the rest of the QRS complex.

ST/TW Changes
Secondary to the abnormal depolarization pattern of the ventricles. These changes are discordant with the delta wave (e.g., T waves following a positive delta wave are inverted).

Location

The bypass tract can be left-or right-sided. If the tract is left-sided, conduction will travel from left ventricle to right ventricle and result in a positive delta wave or tall R wave in V1. Left-sided free-wall bypass tracts are most common.[5] When the tract is right-sided, conduction spreads from the right to left ventricle, and a negative delta wave with a deep S is present in V1. Patients with Ebstein anomaly commonly have right-sided bypass tracts.

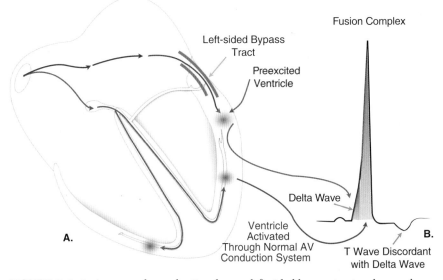

FIGURE 6.4 A. Anterograde conduction down a left-sided bypass tract and normal conduction system. B. Resultant ECG morphology (from the view of a right-sided lead).

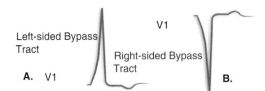

FIGURE 6.3 Appearance of A. left- and B. right-sided bypass tracts in V1.

Direction of Conduction
The bypass tract can be limited to conducting in a single direction or have the ability to conduct in both directions. Bypass tracts that conduct antero-grade from atria to ventricle are recognizable by their ventricular preexcitation patterns on ECG. Bypass tracts capable of only retrograde conduction are considered to be *concealed* pathways with no characteristic ECG findings.

Arrhythmias
A patient who has symptoms of tachycardia related to one of these bypass tracts has WPW *syndrome*.

Atrial Fibrillation
Most feared arrhythmia associated with WPW because it can rarely degenerate into ventricular fibrillation. QRS complex morphology varies dramatically from beat to beat.

AV Reciprocating Tachycardia (AVRT)
Most common arrhythmia associated with WPW. QRS complexes may be wide or narrow depending on the direction of conduction in the bypass tract.

The J Wave (Osborn Wave) and Hypothermia

The J wave is a deflection in the same direction of the R wave in the terminal portion of the QRS complex. J waves are most commonly seen in leads II, III, aVF, V5, and V6; they may be seen more diffusely when hypothermia becomes more severe. In general, the lower the temperature, the larger the amplitude of the J wave.[6,7] J waves start to appear when the temperature drops to 32 degrees celsius.[8] They start to become larger in amplitude as the temperature approaches 30 degrees celsius.[7]

Other Causes   J waves are highly suggestive of hypothermia. They have been described in the following other conditions[6,9]:

Subarachnoid Hemorrhage

Acute Myocardial Infarction

Hypercalcemia

Sepsis

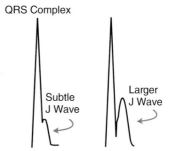

FIGURE 6.5 Appearance of small and large J waves.

ECG Findings in Hypothermia   The conduction system is more sensitive to cold temperatures than the myocardium. With progressive hypothermia, the action potential duration becomes prolonged. PR prolongation results from delay at the AV node. QRS widening and QTc prolongation then develop. P waves may disappear or become difficult to identify when obscured by tremor artifact. The most common rhythm in hypothermic patients is atrial fibrillation with slow ventricular response.[10]

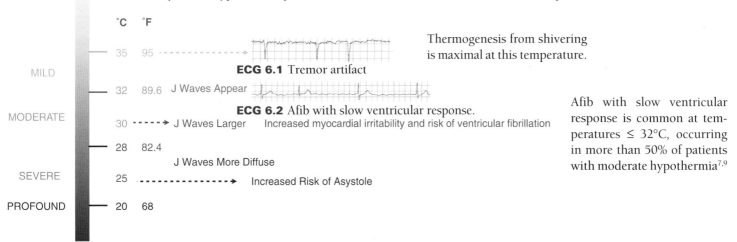

ECG 6.1 Tremor artifact

Thermogenesis from shivering is maximal at this temperature.

ECG 6.2 Afib with slow ventricular response.

Afib with slow ventricular response is common at temperatures ≤ 32°C, occurring in more than 50% of patients with moderate hypothermia[7,9]

FIGURE 6.6 Scale depicting different degrees of hypothermia.

J Wave Mimics   J waves can mimic the ST elevation pattern in acute myocardial infarction.[9] As J waves increase in amplitude, they may also be mistaken for the R' wave of a right bundle branch block.

Hyperkalemia   The ECG findings of hyperkalemia may be masked by hypothermia. Hyperkalemia is more cardiotoxic in hypothermic patients.[11]

The R in aVR and Na⁺ Channel Blockade

Mechanism   Drugs that block myocardial fast sodium channels slow phase 0 depolarization of the action potential. The QRS complex consequently widens. (Fig. 6.7).

The right bundle branch is more sensitive to sodium channel blockade. A characteristic waveform in aVR reflects this exaggerated delay. The terminal R wave is prolonged; unopposed rightward forces can make this R wave especially tall (> 3 mm) and can result in right axis deviation. (Fig. 6.8)

Common Culprit Drugs   Cocaine
Tricyclic antidepressants (TCAs)
Diphenhydramine
Type IA antiarrhythmics (procainamide, quinidine, disopyramide)
Type IC antiarrhythmics (flecainide, propafenone)

ECG Features

Wide QRS   Severe widening can make it difficult to tell if the rhythm is ventricular or supra-ventricular. In TCA overdose, QRS widening has been shown be associated with higher incidence of seizures and ventricular dysrhythmias.[12,13]

R in aVR   The right bundle branch has a longer refractory period and is more sensitive to the effects of intraventricular conduction delay. An R wave in aVR greater than 3 mm is a specific sign for cardiotoxicity by Na⁺ channel–blocking drugs. Sometimes there is a right bundle branch block pattern in aVR.

Mimics   Overdose of Na⁺ channel blockers can produce a Brugada pattern on ECG. Sodium channel blockers can also unmask the Brugada pattern in patients with Brugada Syndrome. Administration of sodium channel blockers is sometimes performed to help confirm the diagnosis of Brugada Syndrome.

Arrhythmias

Sinus Tachycardia   Many of these drugs are associated with tachycardia through other pharmacologic effects. The anticholinergic properties of TCAs and diphenhydramine and the sympathomimetic effects of cocaine cause tachycardia. Toxicity from Na⁺ channel–blocking drugs should be included in the differential of regular wide-complex tachycardias.

Ventricular Tachycardia   Prolongation of intraventricular conduction can result in reentrant circuits including VT.

Bradydysrhythmias   Rare. Sodium channel blockers can decreased automaticity of pacemaker cells resulting in sinus bradycardia and escape rhythms.

Treatment   Sodium bicarbonate. Increasing the extracellular sodium concentration raises the sodium gradient across sodium channels and increases the speed of the action potential. Binding of tricyclic antidepressants and cocaine to the Na⁺ channel is pH-dependent. Raising the pH removes them from the binding site on the sodium channel.[14]

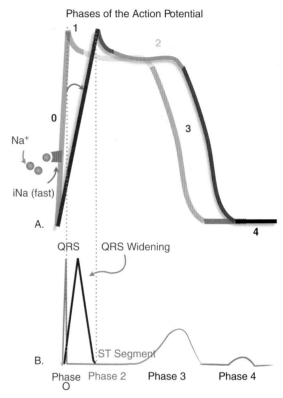

FIGURE 6.7 The action potential affected by sodium channel blockade. The outline of the action potential also represents the cell membrane and depicts blockade of the sodium channels responsible for fast phase 0 depolarization.

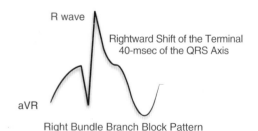

FIGURE 6.8 The R in aVR pattern.

ECG 6.3a A 23-year-old asymptomatic woman.

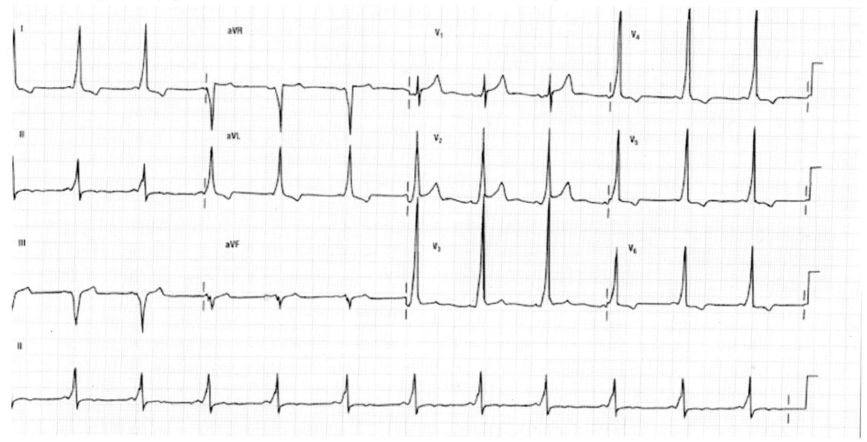

Image courtesy of Josh Kosowsky, MD.

ECG 6.3b A 23-year-old asymptomatic woman.

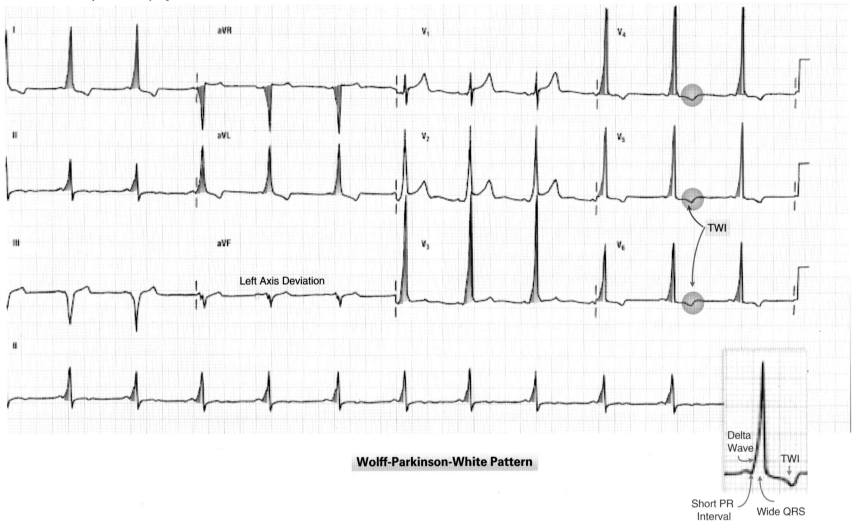

Left Axis Deviation

TWI

Wolff-Parkinson-White Pattern

Delta Wave

TWI

Short PR Interval

Wide QRS

ECG 6.4a A 37-year-old male with a history of palpitations for several years.

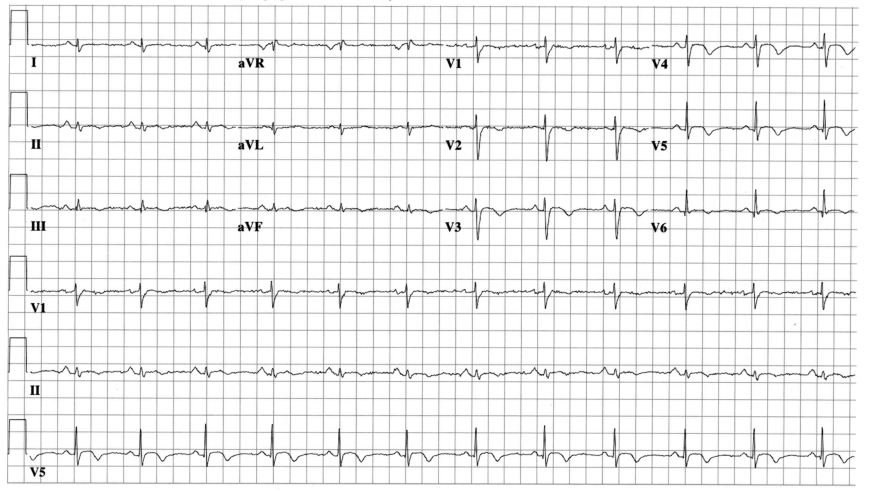

ECG 6.4b A 37-year-old male with a history of palpitations for several years.

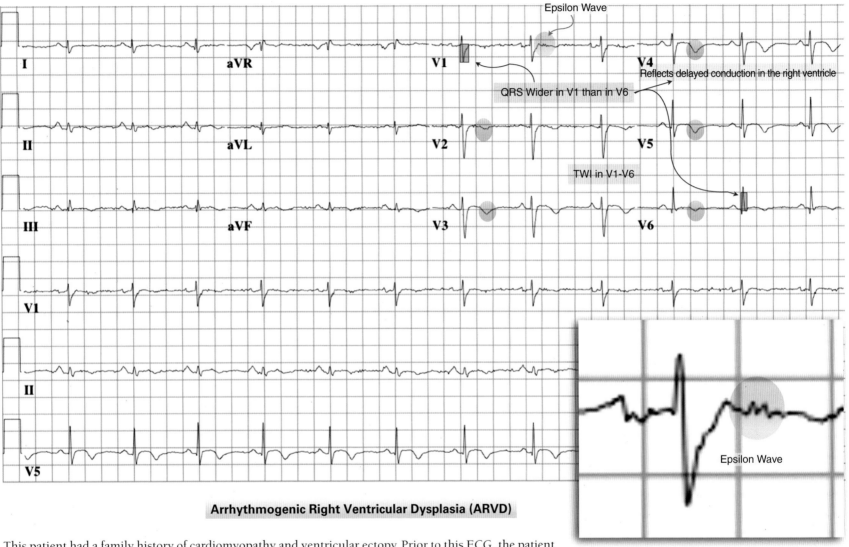

Epsilon Wave

QRS Wider in V1 than in V6

Reflects delayed conduction in the right ventricle

TWI in V1-V6

Epsilon Wave

Arrhythmogenic Right Ventricular Dysplasia (ARVD)

This patient had a family history of cardiomyopathy and ventricular ectopy. Prior to this ECG, the patient was found to be in VT with LBBB morphology. Cardiac MRI revealed fatty changes in the free wall of the RV, and global hypokinesis of the RV with regional variation. Biopsy of his RV revealed myocytic hypertrophy, myocytolysis, and interstitial edema and fibrosis to confirm the diagnosis of ARVD.

ECG 6.5a

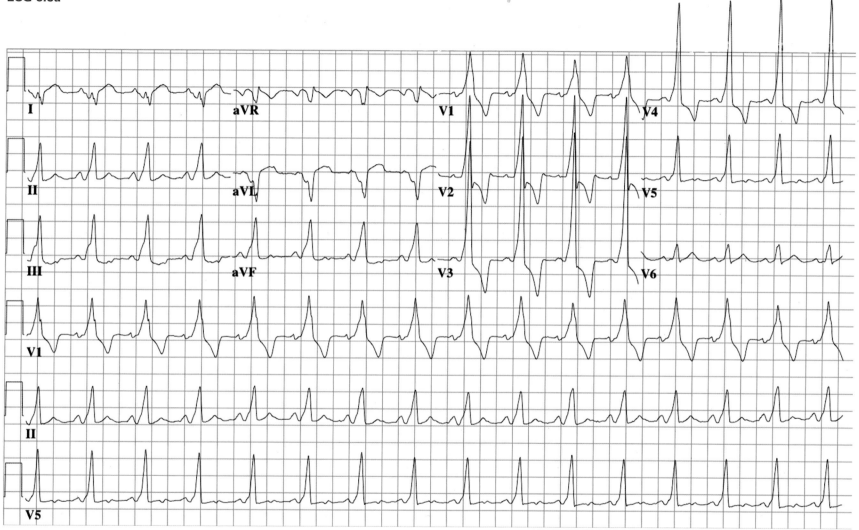

ECG 6.5b

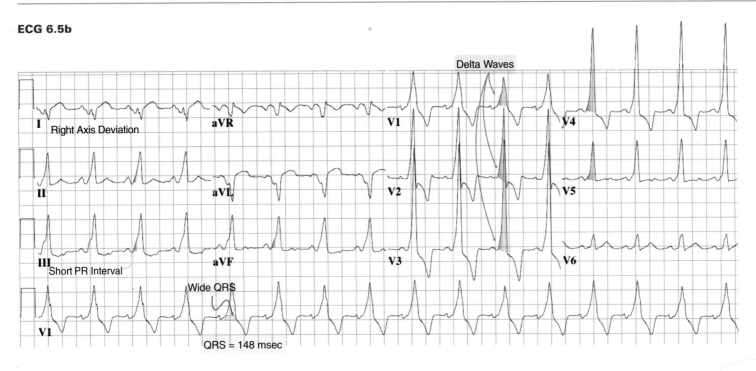

Wolff-Parkinson-White Pattern

This patient has a left-sided bypass tract. A preexcited left ventricle will spread conduction toward the right ventricle. This accounts for the right axis deviation observed in this ECG.

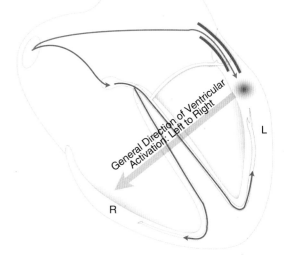

FIGURE 6.9 Pattern of ventricular activation from a left-sided bypass tract.

ECG 6.6a

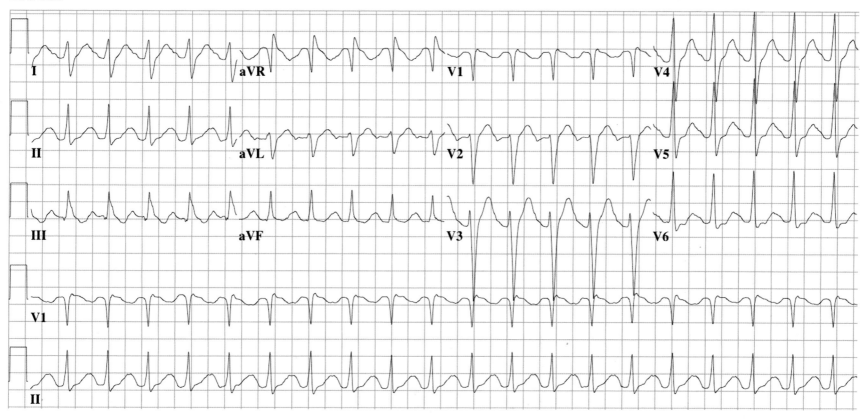

Image courtesy of Chris Kabrhel, MD.

ECG 6.6b

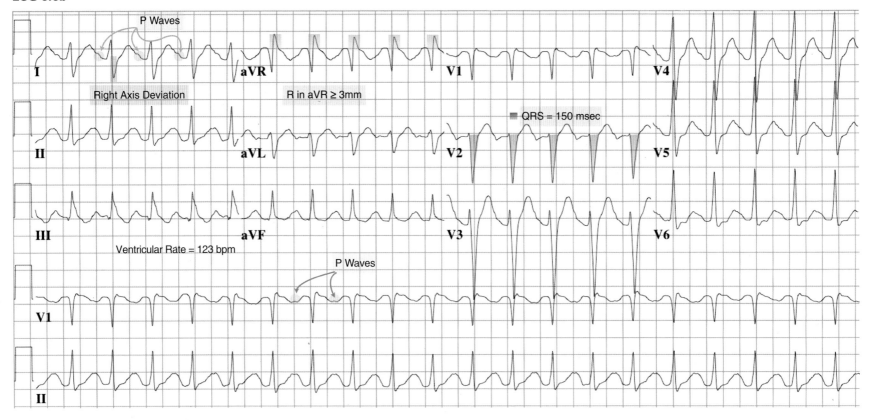

Tricyclic Antidepressant Overdose

The rhythm is sinus tachycardia (P waves are subtle deflections seen best in lead I). The QRS widening, right axis deviation, and R in aVR all normalized after administration of sodium bicarbonate.

ECG 6.3c Same patient… after treatment

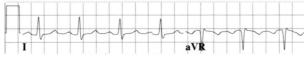

QRS narrowed. R in aVR gone.
Normal axis.

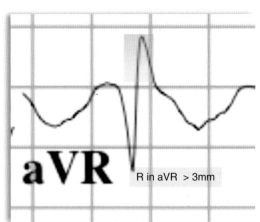

ECG 6.7a

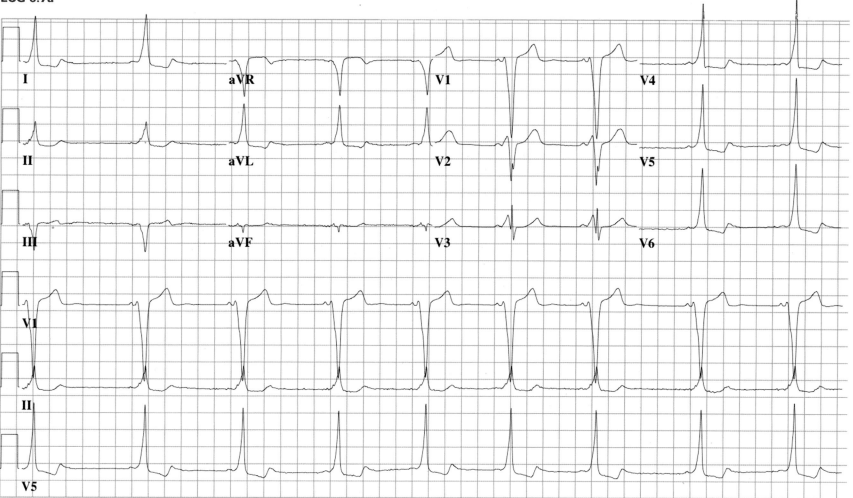

ECG 6.7b

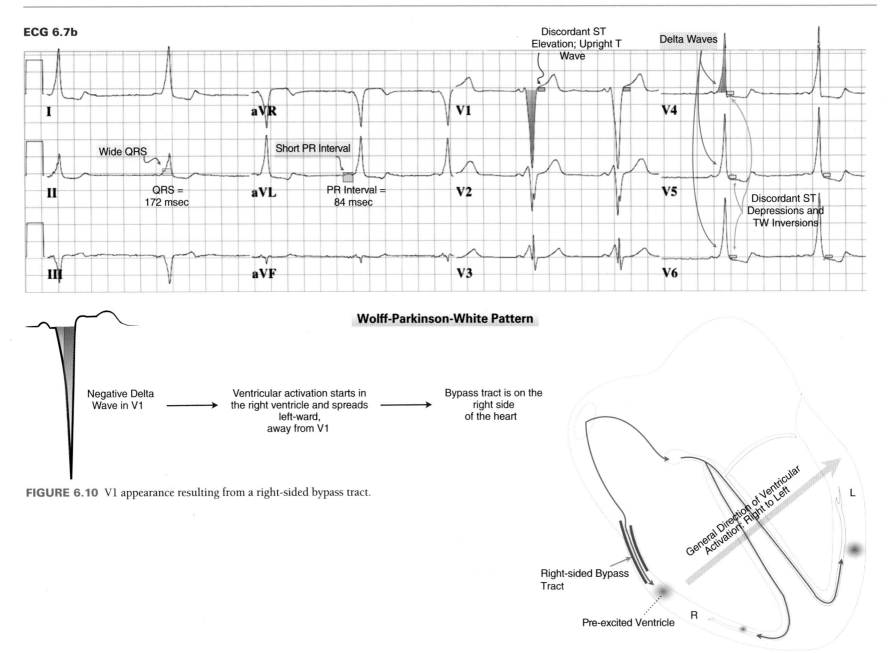

FIGURE 6.10 V1 appearance resulting from a right-sided bypass tract.

FIGURE 6.11 Pattern of ventricular activation from a right-sided bypass tract.

ECG 6.8a An asymptomatic 19-year-old female.

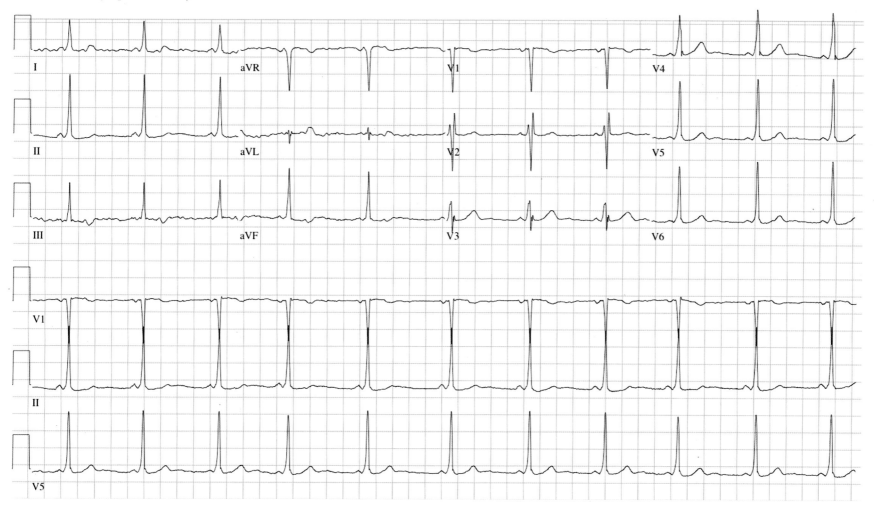

ECG 6.8b An asymptomatic 19-year-old female.

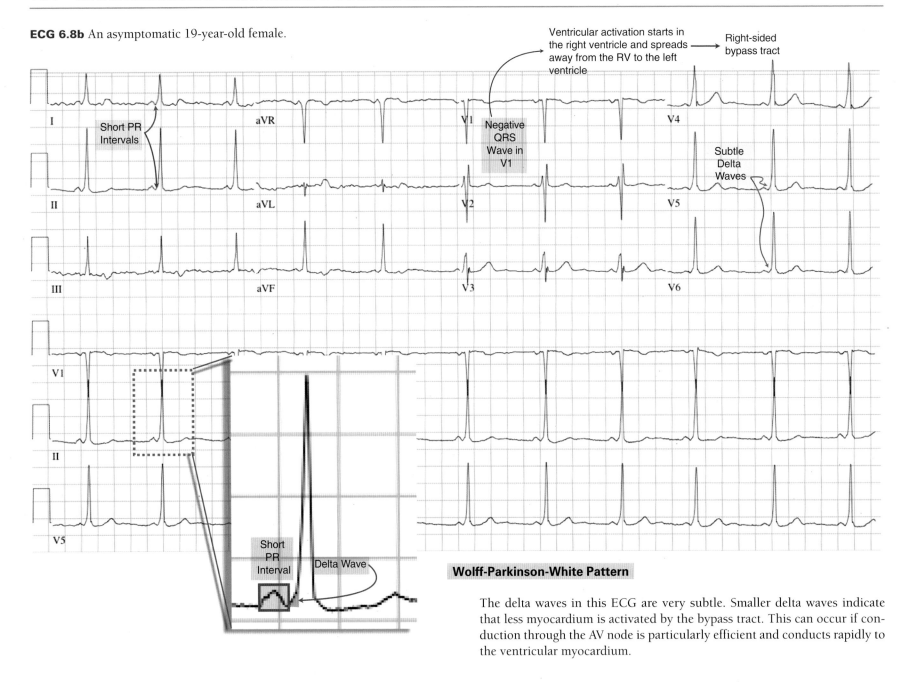

Ventricular activation starts in the right ventricle and spreads away from the RV to the left ventricle

Right-sided bypass tract

Short PR Intervals

Negative QRS Wave in V1

Subtle Delta Waves

Short PR Interval

Delta Wave

Wolff-Parkinson-White Pattern

The delta waves in this ECG are very subtle. Smaller delta waves indicate that less myocardium is activated by the bypass tract. This can occur if conduction through the AV node is particularly efficient and conducts rapidly to the ventricular myocardium.

ECG 6.9a

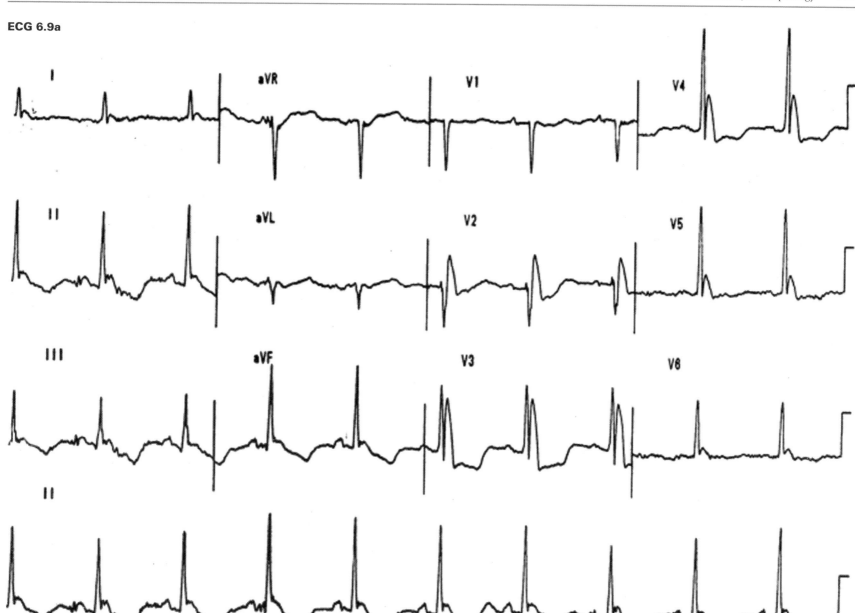

ECG 6.9b

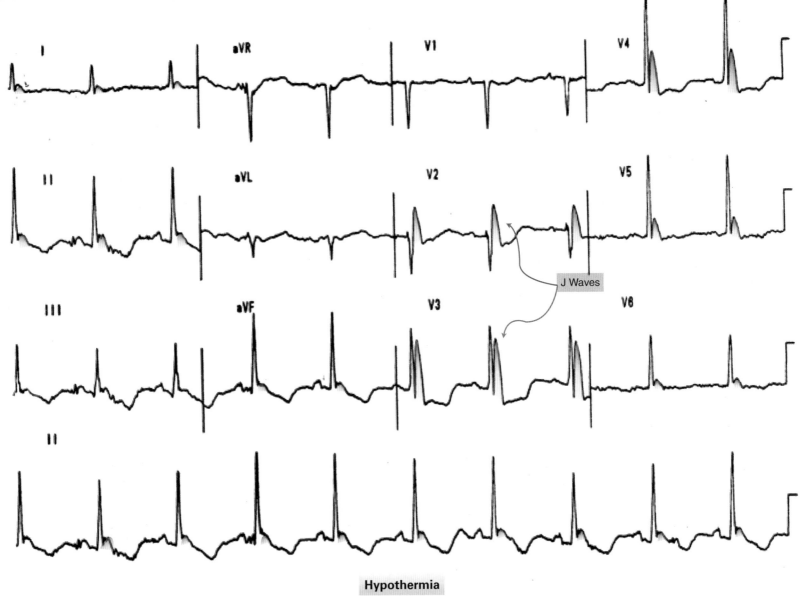

Hypothermia

These are large-amplitude J waves. The amplitude of J waves correlates with the severity of hypothermia. This patient's temperature was 30°C (86°F). J waves become predictably larger at this temperature.

ECG 6.10a A 35-year-old male presents after his AICD fires.

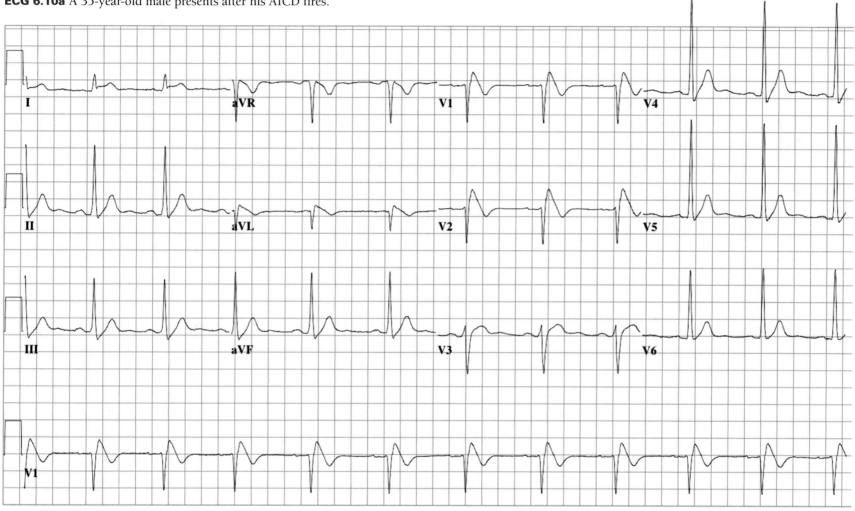

Image courtesy of Liza Gonen, MD.

ECG 6.10b A 35-year-old male presents after his AICD fires.

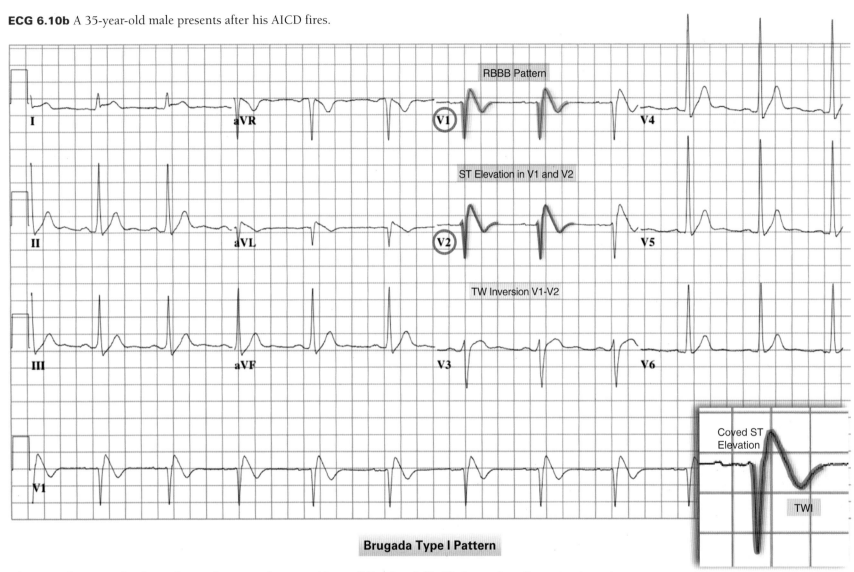

The Brugada pattern has been observed to occur for several hours following defibrillation and cardioversion in patients without this syndrome. Even a type I pattern is nondiagnostic in this setting[15]. This patient underwent placement of an AICD several years prior to this ECG after he was diagnosed with Brugada syndrome.

ECG 6.11a

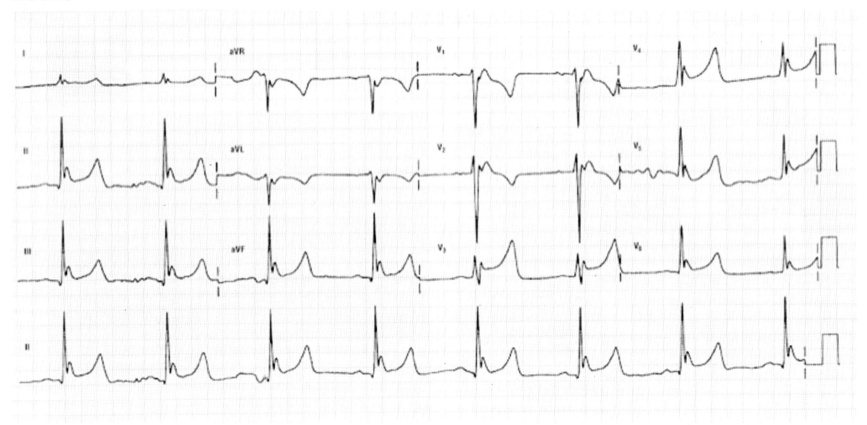

Image courtesy of Josh Kosowsky, MD.

ECG 6.11b

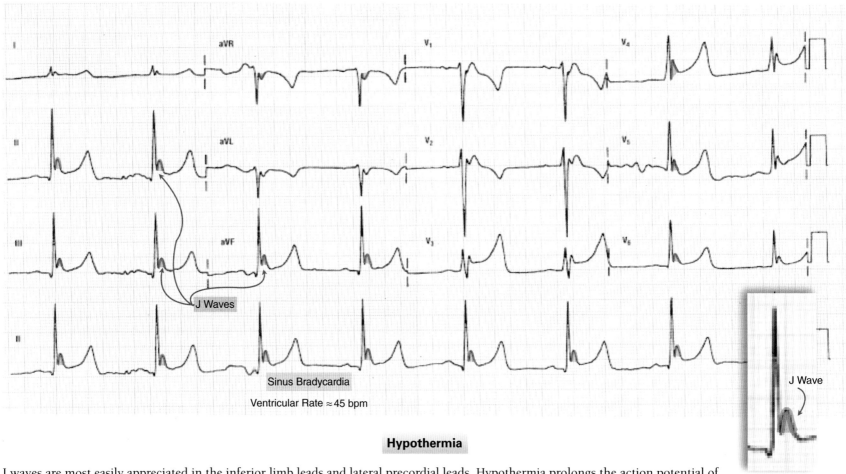

J Waves

Sinus Bradycardia

Ventricular Rate ≈ 45 bpm

J Wave

Hypothermia

J waves are most easily appreciated in the inferior limb leads and lateral precordial leads. Hypothermia prolongs the action potential of pacemaker cells. Bradycardia in hypothermia can be profound.

ECG 6.12a Syncope in a 24-year-old male.

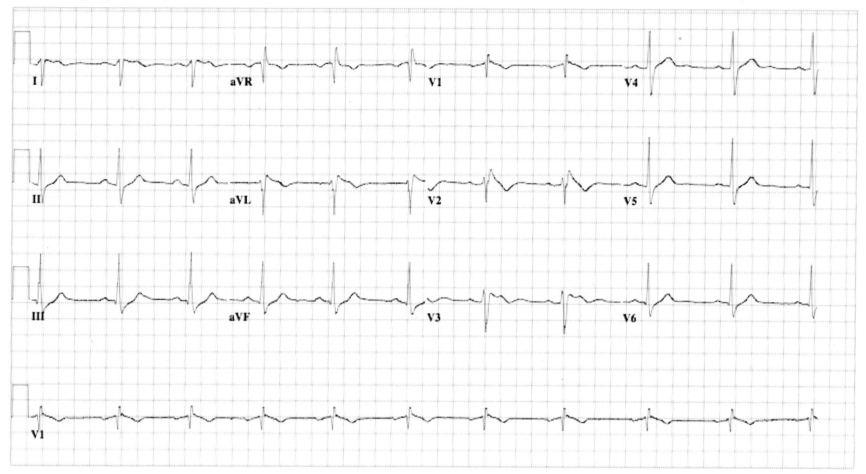

Image courtesy of Josh Kosowsky, MD.

ECG 6.12b Syncope in a 24-year-old male.

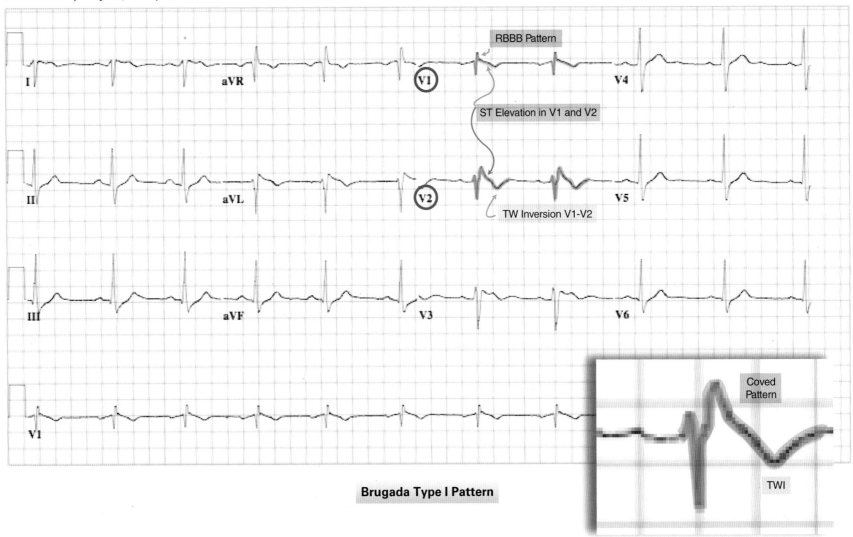

RBBB Pattern

ST Elevation in V1 and V2

TW Inversion V1-V2

Coved Pattern

TWI

Brugada Type I Pattern

ECG 6.13a A 24-year-old presents with seizure.

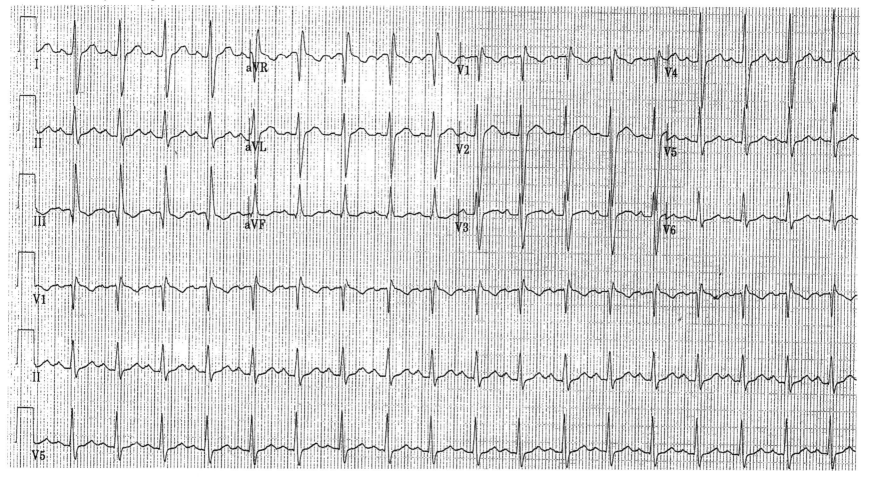

Image courtesy of Chris Kabrhel, MD.

ECG 6.13b A 24-year-old presents with seizure.

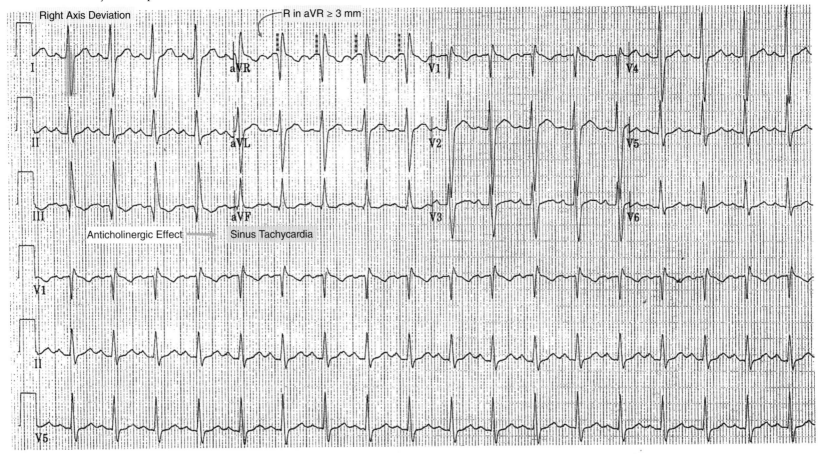

Tricyclic Antidepressant Overdose

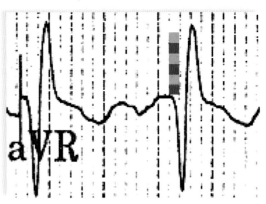

This patient was found to have elevated levels of nortriptyline. He was treated with a sodium bicarbonate drip.

ECG 6.14a

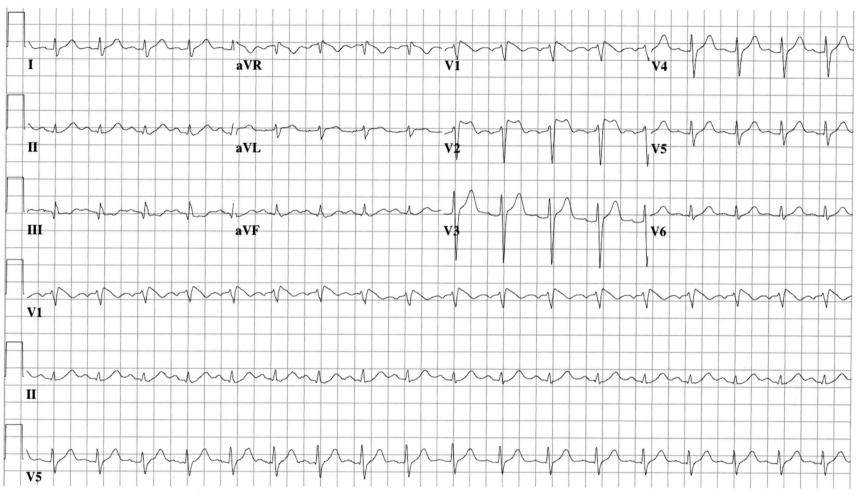

ECG 6.14b

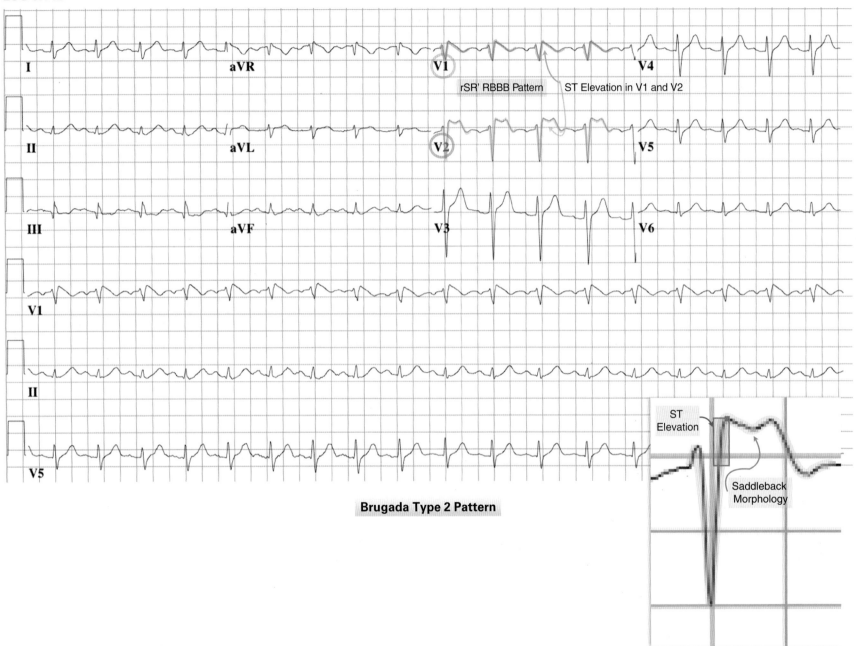

rSR' RBBB Pattern   ST Elevation in V1 and V2

Brugada Type 2 Pattern

ST Elevation

Saddleback Morphology

ECG 6.15a A 28-year-old male presents with tachycardia and diaphoresis.

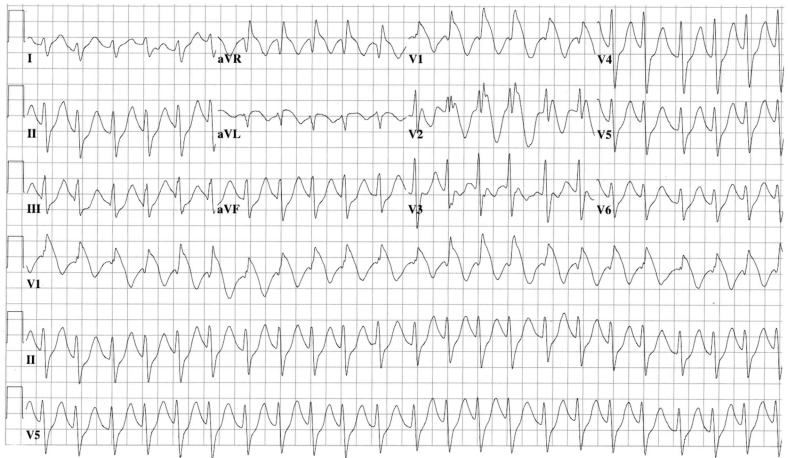

ECG 6.15b A 28-year-old male presents with tachycardia and diaphoresis.

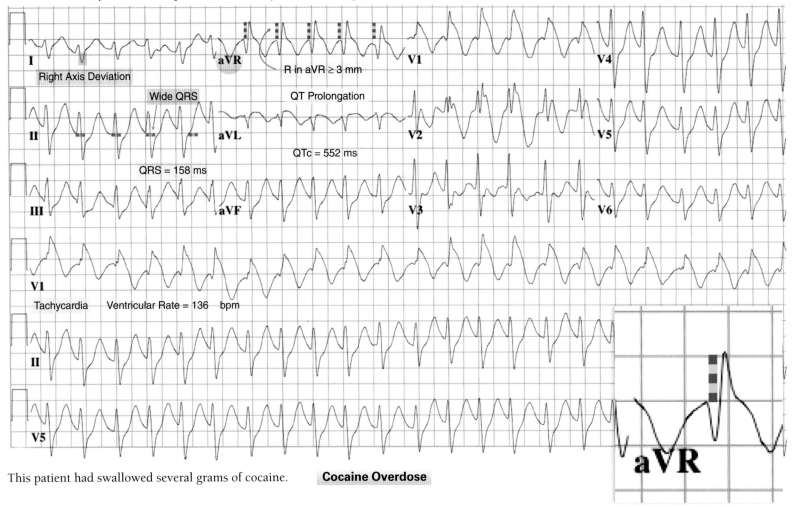

This patient had swallowed several grams of cocaine.   **Cocaine Overdose**

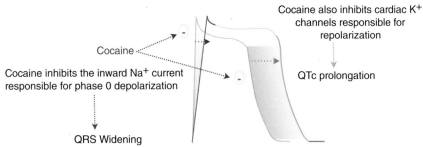

FIGURE 6.12 Cocaine affects the action potential in several ways.

Cocaine also inhibits cardiac K⁺ channels responsible for repolarization

Cocaine

Cocaine inhibits the inward Na⁺ current responsible for phase 0 depolarization

QTc prolongation

QRS Widening

Cocaine Toxicity is much like TCA Toxicity.

Typical ECG features include:

1 QRS widening
2. QTc prolongation
3. R in aVR ≥ 3mm
4. Tachycardia

ECG 6.16a A young patient presents with seizure.

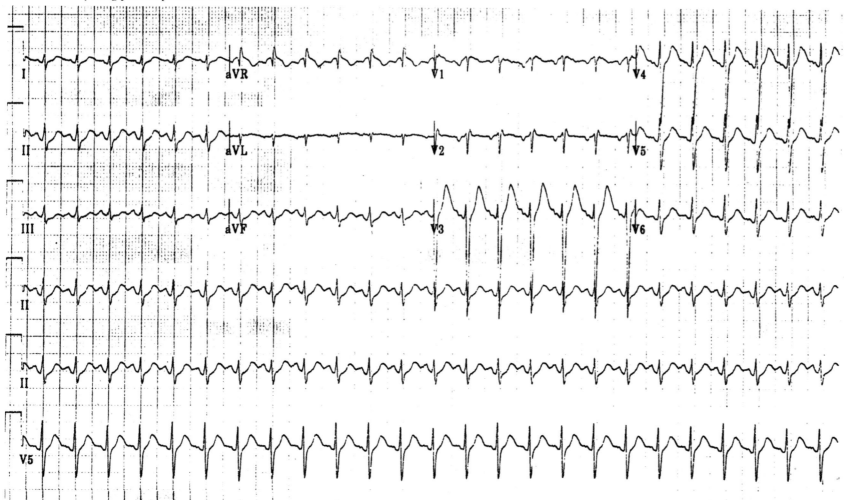

Image courtesy of Keith Marill, MD.

ECG 6.16b A young patient presents with seizure.

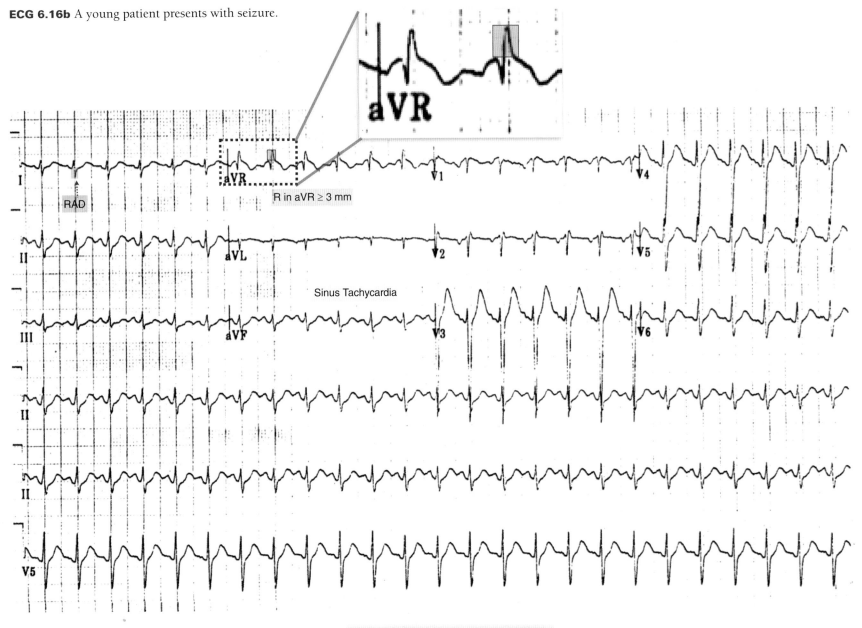

R in aVR ≥ 3 mm

RAD

Sinus Tachycardia

Tricyclic Antidepressant Overdose

This patient ingested 12 75-mg tablets of clomipramine. Note that QRS widening is absent in the ECG.

ECG 6.17a A 37-year-old male presents with recurrent syncopal episodes.

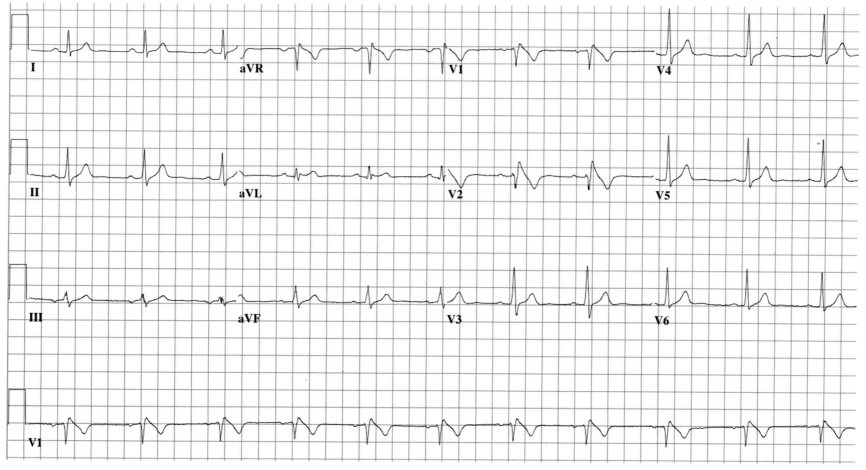

Image courtesy of Justin Hering, MD.

ECG 6.17b A 37-year-old male presents with recurrent syncopal episodes.

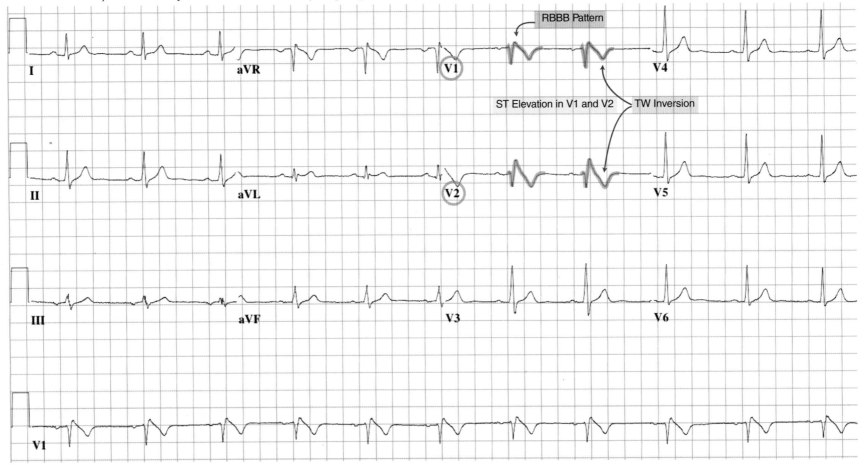

Brugada Type I Pattern

The father of this patient also had a history of multiple syncopal episodes. This patient underwent placement of an ICD soon after this ECG was obtained.

ECG 6.18a A 71-year-old bed-bound woman with multiple sclerosis presents with hypotension.

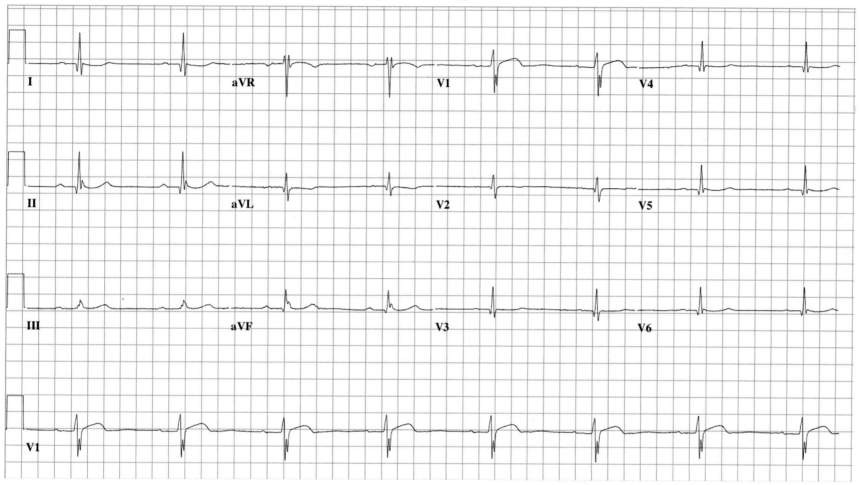

ECG 6.18b A 71-year-old bed-bound woman with multiple sclerosis presents with hypotension.

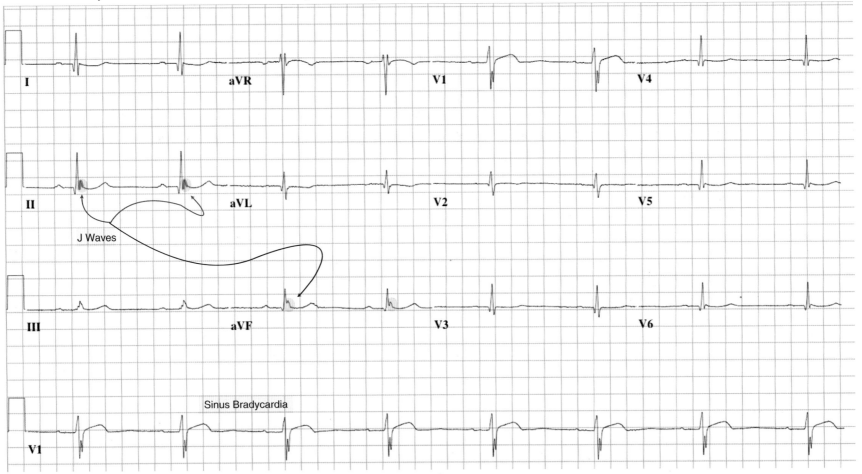

Sepsis and Mild Hypothermia

This patient was found to be in septic shock. The presence of J waves led the treating physician to ask for a rectal temperature (this vital sign was absent on the triage sheet). Rectal temperature was 91°F. Both sepsis and hypothermia can cause J waves. Hypothermia portends a poor prognosis in septic patients.[16]

ECG 6.19a A 63-year-old female with recurrent episodes of light-headedness.

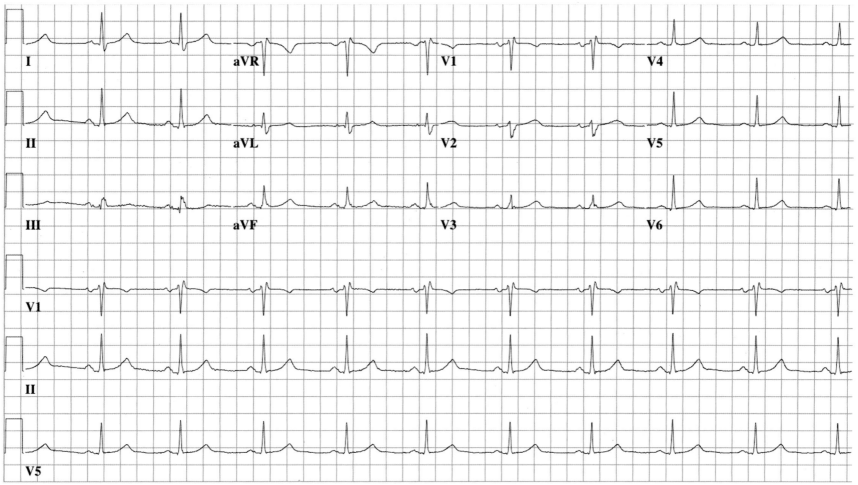

Image courtesy of Patricia Henwood, MD.

ECG 6.19b A 63-year-old female with recurrent episodes of light-headedness.

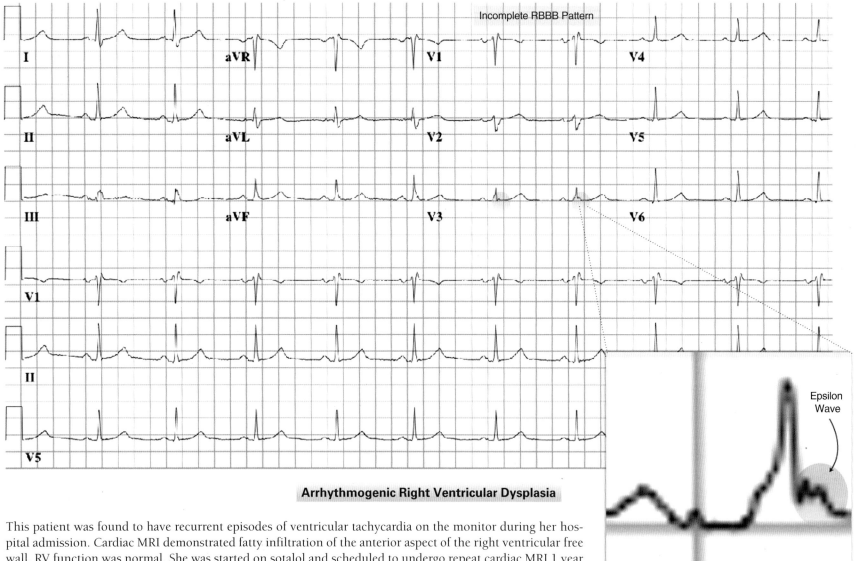

Incomplete RBBB Pattern

Epsilon Wave

Arrhythmogenic Right Ventricular Dysplasia

This patient was found to have recurrent episodes of ventricular tachycardia on the monitor during her hospital admission. Cardiac MRI demonstrated fatty infiltration of the anterior aspect of the right ventricular free wall. RV function was normal. She was started on sotalol and scheduled to undergo repeat cardiac MRI 1 year from presentation.

ECG 6.20a A 47-year-old female with a history of supraventricular tachycardia and depression presents after suicide attempt by drug overdose.

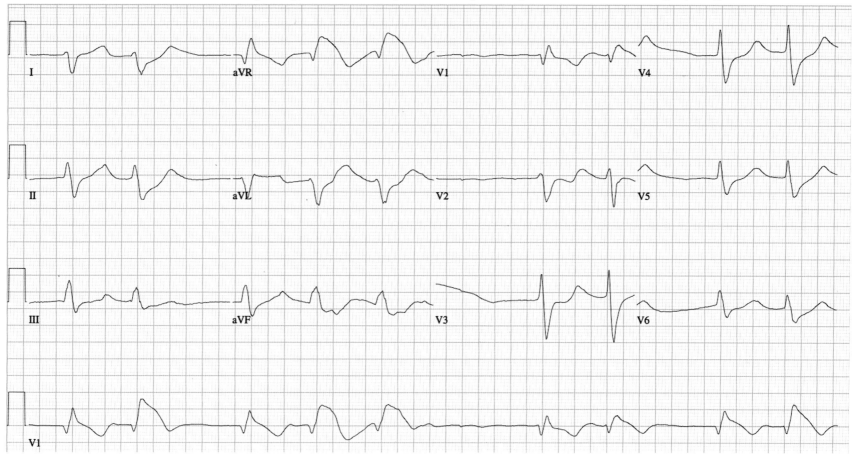

Image courtesy of Liza Gonen, MD.

ECG 6.20b A 47-year-old female with a history of supraventricular tachycardia and depression presents after suicide attempt by drug overdose.

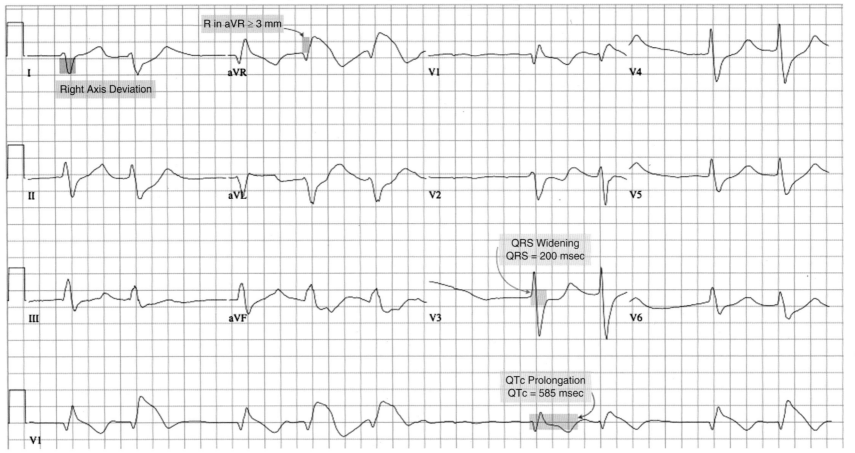

Flecainide Toxicity

This patient ingested more than 4 grams of flecainide. She had recurrent episodes of ventricular tachycardia requiring defibrillation. In the emergency department she was treated with sodium bicarbonate and intravenous fat emulsion (Intralipid ®) therapy. She was discharged from the hospital several days later.

Flecainide is a lipid soluble type 1C antidysrhythmic medication that works by blocking sodium channels during phase 0 depolarization of the action potential. This results in QRS widening and the tall R wave in lead aVR. In toxic doses, it can block slow calcium channels and cause slowed conduction. Flecainide toxicity can cause both bradyarrhythmias and ventricular tachyarrhythmias

References

1. Antzelevitch C, Brugada P, Borggrefe M, et al. Brugada syndrome: report of the second consensus conference: endorsed by the Heart Rhythm Society and the European Heart Rhythm Association. *Circulation* 2005;111:659–670.
2. Basso C, Corrado D, Marcus FI, et al. Arrhythmogenic right ventricular cardiomyopathy. *Lancet* 2009;373:1289–1300.
3. Thiene G, Nava A, Corrado D, et al. ventricular cardiomyopathy and sudden death in young people. *N Engl J Med* 1988;318:129–133.
4. Jain R, Dalal D, Daly A, et al. Electrocardiographic features of arrhythmogenic right ventricular dysplasia. *Circulation* 2009;120:477–487.
5. Olgin JaZD. In: Bonow R MD, Zipes D, Libby P, eds. *Braunwald's Heart Disease: A Textbook of Cardiovascular Medicine*. 9th ed. Philadelphia: PA Elsevier; 2011:771–824.
6. Patel A, Getsos JP, Moussa G, et al. The Osborn wave of hypothermia in normothermic patients. *Clin Cardiol* 1994;17:273–276.
7. Okada M, Nishimura F, Yoshino H, et al. The J wave in accidental hypothermia. *J Electrocardiol* 1983;16:23–28.
8. Danzl D. Accidental Hypothermia. In: Auerbach P, ed. *Wilderness Medicine*. 5th ed. Mosby; 2007.
9. Mattu A, Brady WJ, Perron AD. Electrocardiographic manifestations of hypothermia. *Am J Emerg Med* 2002;20:314–326.
10. Hedayati TaS, S. The ECG in selected noncardiac conditions. In: Mattu ATJB, R, ed. *Electrocardiography in Emergency Medicine*. Dallas: American College of Emergency Physicians; 2007:203–204.
11. Danzl D. Accidental hypothermia. In: Marx JA, ed. *Rosen's Emergency Medicine: Concepts and Clinical Practice*. 6th ed. St. Louis, MA: Mosby; 2006:2236–2253.
12. Boehnert MT, Lovejoy FH Jr. Value of the QRS duration versus the serum drug level in predicting seizures and ventricular arrhythmias after an acute overdose of tricyclic antidepressants. *N Engl J Med* 1985;313:474–479.
13. Shannon MW. Duration of QRS disturbances after severe tricyclic antidepressant intoxication. *J Toxicol Clin Toxicol* 1992;30:377–386.
14. Liebelt EL. Cyclic antidepressants. In: Goldfrank LR, ed. *Goldrank's Toxicologic Emergencies*. 8th ed. New York, NY: McGraw-Hill; 2007:1083–1097.
15. Wilde AA, Antzelevitch C, Borggrefe M, et al. Proposed diagnostic criteria for the Brugada syndrome: consensus report. *Circulation* 2002;106:2514–259.
16. Clemmer TP, Fisher CJ Jr., Bone RC, et al. Hypothermia in the sepsis syndrome and clinical outcome. The Methylprednisolone Severe Sepsis Study Group. *Crit Care Med* 1992;20:1395–1401.

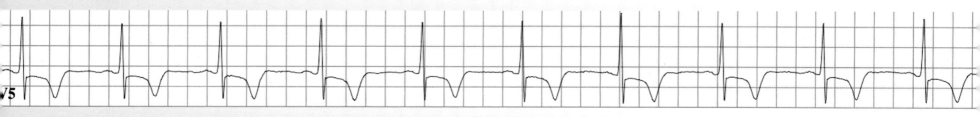

V5

The Normal T Wave

The T wave represents rapid repolarization (phase 3 of the action potential). The normal T wave is asymmetric with a gradual slope followed by a steeper slope. Normal T waves are upright in almost all leads. T waves can be inverted or biphasic in leads III, V1, and V2. The T wave is most often concordant with the QRS wave because the T wave axis is normally within 45 degrees of the QRS axis in adults.

Ischemic T Wave Changes

Hyperacute T Waves

In hyperacute ischemia, the duration of the action potential is shortened, resulting in early repolarization and amplification of the normal T wave. Hyperacute T waves have a broader base than the "peaked T waves" of hyperkalemia. Hyperacute T waves are one of the earliest ECG abnormalities to occur in myocardial infarction. T waves are generally considered hyperacute if they are greater than 10 mm in amplitude in precordial leads or greater than 5 mm in amplitude in limb leads.

Table 7.1

	Hyperacute T Wave	Peaked T Wave
Setting	Acute myocardial infarction	Hyperkalemia
ECG Appearance		
ECG Features	Wide-based	Narrow-based
Location	Localized to several leads	Generally diffuse

T Wave Inversions

- Non–ST-Elevation MI
- Unstable Angina
- Prior MI

T wave inversions can indicate non–ST-elevation MI and unstable angina. They may also be chronic footprints of a past myocardial infarction. The terminal aspect of the ischemic T wave is the first to become inverted, followed by the middle and initial portions after acute infarction. When only the terminal portion of the T wave is inverted, the T wave appears biphasic. Ischemic TW inversions are typically symmetric and narrow (Fig. 7.1 and Table 7.1).

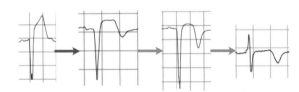

FIGURE 7.1 Progression of T wave changes after acute myocardial infarction.

Pseudonormalization T waves that were previously inverted may become less inverted, flat, or upright during acute ischemia. This is thought to be secondary to acute shortening of the action potential duration.[1]

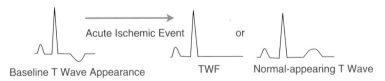

FIGURE 7.2 T wave changes suggestive of pseudonormalization.

Wellens Syndrome

Wellens syndrome refers to a characteristic pattern of ECG changes associated with critical stenosis of the left anterior descending artery. These changes are located in the electrocardiographic distribution of the LAD (leads V2–V4) and consist of deep symmetric T wave inversions (TWI) or less commonly, biphasic T waves.

Criteria for Wellens Syndrome[2]

- **Prior History of Angina**
- **Characteristic T Waves**   Biphasic or deeply inverted T waves in V2 and V3.

| **Normal Precordial R-Wave Progression** | **Minimal or No Elevation in Cardiac Markers** | **Minimal or No ST Elevation** | **Absence of Pathologic Q Waves in Precordium** |

ECG Features

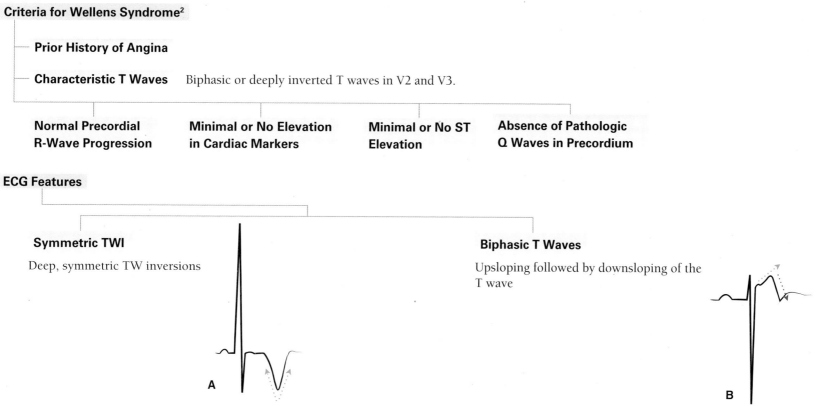

Symmetric TWI

Deep, symmetric TW inversions

Biphasic T Waves

Upsloping followed by downsloping of the T wave

A

B

FIGURE 7.3 Different T wave morphologies in Wellens syndrome.

Timing of ECG Findings	Wellens T waves more commonly occur when patients are free of chest pain. In the setting of chest pain, these T waves may normalize or the ST segments may become elevated. Biphasic T waves and terminal T wave inversions also occur in a majority of patients who have had successful reperfusion of myocardium supplied by a previously occluded left anterior descending artery.[3]
Management	An exercise stress test is contraindicated. These patients may die of cardiac arrest on the treadmill. They should bypass a stress test and undergo urgent cardiac catheterization.
Prognosis	In a study performed by Wellens, 75% of patients with a Wellens pattern who failed to undergo angiography went on to develop extensive anterior wall myocardial infarctions in a mean of 8.5 days.[2]

LV Strain Pattern

ST depression and T wave inversion are commonly seen in patients with left ventricular hypertrophy. This reflects repolarization abnormalities in the thickened left ventricle myocardium. ST depression is minimal and downsloping, running into the gradual descent of the inverted T wave.

ECG Changes

These changes occur in the left precordial (V5 and V6) and limb (I and aVL) leads. ST depression and T wave inversion present in other leads should raise suspicion for myocardial ischemia. A potential pitfall would be to attribute TWIs present in inferior limb leads or diffusely in the precordium to left ventricular strain.[4]

T Wave Morphology   T waves are asymmetric. Gradual downslope and more abrupt upslope.

ST Depression   In leads with tall R waves, the ST segment is depressed and blends with the inverted T wave.

Mechanism

Depolarization from endocardium to epicardium is prolonged in the hypertrophied left ventricle. Depolarization is prolonged enough for the endocardium to become repolarized before the entire myocardium is completely depolarized. Repolarization proceeds from endocardium to epicardium. This results in ST depression and T wave inversion.

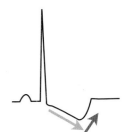

FIGURE 7.4 Appearance of LV strain pattern in leads with tall R waves.

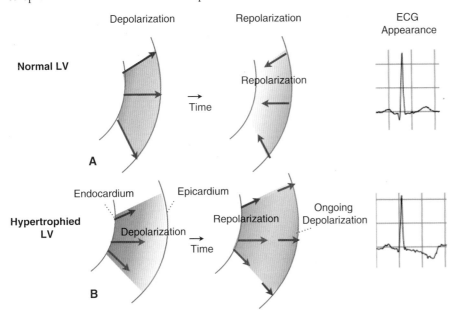

FIGURE 7.5 Depolarization and repolarization patterns in normal versus hypertrophic ventricle. In normal ventricle **A.** depolarization and repolarization vectors are in opposite directions. Despite the opposite directions of these vectors, the QRS and T waves are in the same direction because they represent opposite electrical events (ions flowing in opposite directions). In the hypertrophic left ventricle **B.** these electrically opposite events proceed in the same vector directions. The T wave is therefore opposite in direction to the QRS wave in the hypertrophied heart.

Digitalis Effect

Inverted or flattened T waves following scooped and depressed ST segments are electrocardiographic signs of a patient taking digitalis. They reflect earlier-than-normal repolarization of myocardial cells. These changes occur in patients with normal therapeutic levels of digoxin and *do not* indicate digoxin toxicity.

Morphology

— **Mild ST Depression**   ST depression can mimic myocardial ischemia. ST depression has a scooped appearance (Fig. 7.6).

— **Flat or Inverted T waves**

— **Shortened QTc Interval**   Reflects faster repolarization.

— **Increased U Wave Amplitude**

Location   These changes are most prominent in the lateral precordial leads.

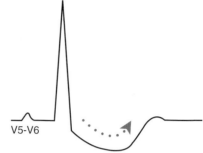

FIGURE 7.6 Appearance of scooped ST segment and inverted T wave associated with digitalis effect.

Persistent Juvenile T Wave Pattern

T wave inversions may be a normal finding in children and can persist into adulthood, more commonly in women than in men. T wave inversions in this pattern can be associated with J-point ST elevations.

Location   These changes occur in leads V1-V3.

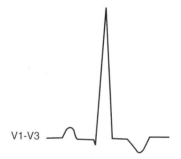

FIGURE 7.7 Appearance of T wave inversions associated with juvenile T wave pattern.

Hyperkalemia

The earliest electrocardiographic sign of hyperkalemia is the presence of peaked T waves. These T waves are typically narrow-based and symmetric. They reflect faster repolarization caused by this electrolyte abnormality. See chapter 8 for more information about the ECG changes associated with hyperkalemia.

Location   These changes are usually diffuse and are most prominent in the precordial leads. (Fig. 7.8)

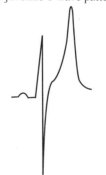

FIGURE 7.8 Appearance of peaked T wave of hyperkalemia.

Cerebral T Waves

ECG abnormalities commonly occur in patients with acute intracranial pathology, especially in patients with acute subarachnoid hemorrhage (SAH). They can also occur in patients with ischemic stroke, intracranial tumors, and transient ischemic attacks. There are several theories regarding the pathophysiology underlying these ECG changes including elevated intracranial pressure, increased sympathetic stimulation, and a surge in catecholamines local to the myocardium.

T Wave Morphology

Some of the largest T waves recorded in electrocardiography are secondary to intracranial causes. These T waves can be upright or inverted. They are referred to as "cerebral T waves," "neurogenic T waves," and "giant T waves." These T waves are very wide and deep. They are often associated with prolongation of the QTc interval.

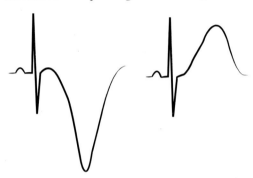

FIGURE 7.9 Appearance of cerebral T waves.

Other ECG Changes Associated with CNS Lesions

T wave changes most commonly reflect repolarization abnormalities. In a study of 406 patients with SAH, T wave abnormalities were noted in 32% of patients, U waves greater than 1 mm in amplitude in 47%, prolonged QTc in 23%, and high-amplitude R waves in 19%.[5]

Changes that Mimic Myocardial Ischemia

Changes in ST segments and T waves can lead to a misdiagnosis of myocardial infarction. Anticoagulation in these patients can have fatal consequences. These changes can persist for weeks, but eventually resolve.

ST Depression   ST depression is far more common than ST elevation.

ST Elevation

Pathologic Q Waves

T Wave Flattening

Prolonged QTc and Arrhythmias

QTc prolongation can occur and increase the risk of torsade de pointes, ventricular tachycardia, and ventricular fibrillation. Arrhythmias typically occur within 48 hours of intracranial hemorrhage. Patients with SAH may die from malignant arrhythmias.[6]

Prominent U Waves   These can be seen as a notch in the terminal aspect of large T waves.

Prolonged QTc   These patients are at risk for torsade de pointes.

Torsade de Pointes

Ventricular Tachycardia

ECG 7.1a

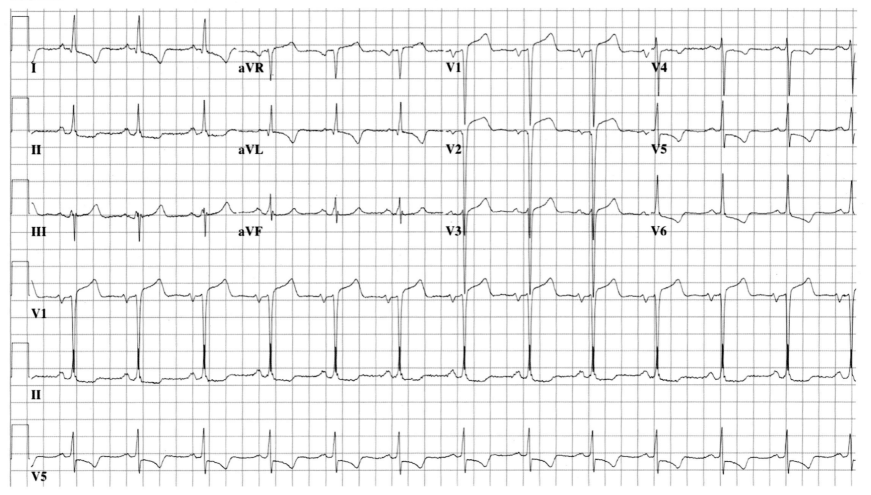

ECG 7.1b

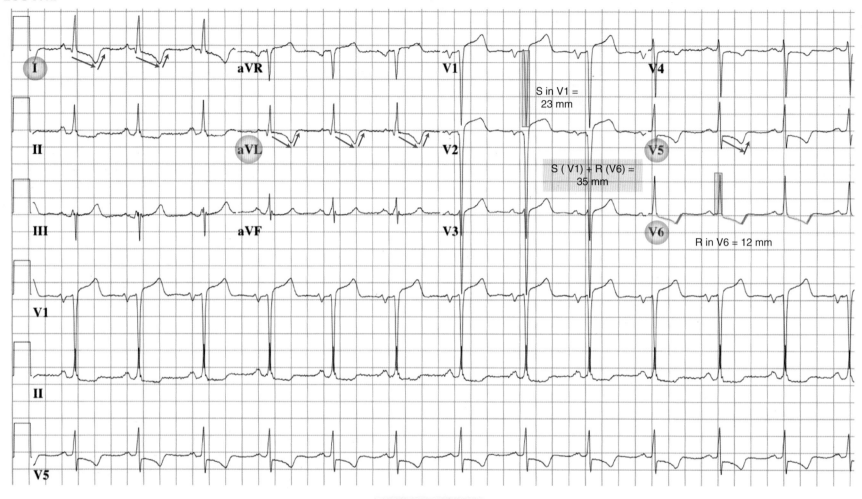

S in V1 = 23 mm

S (V1) + R (V6) = 35 mm

R in V6 = 12 mm

LV Strain Pattern

I, aVL, V5, V6

ECG 7.2a

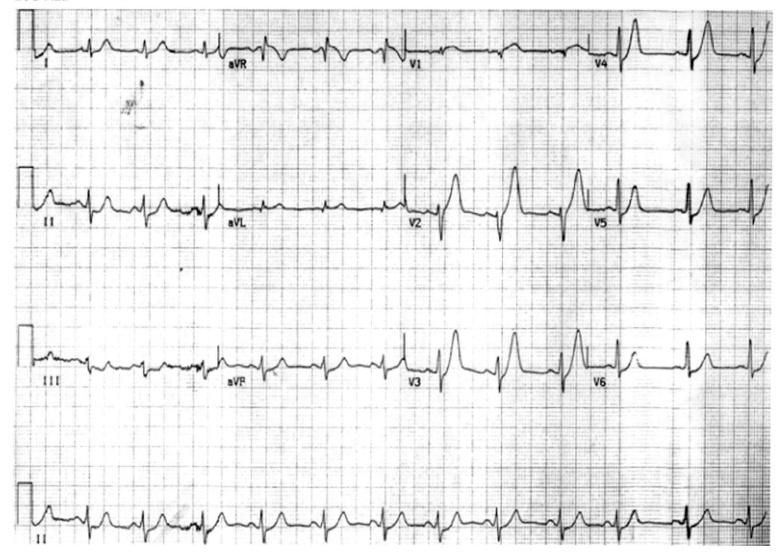

ECG 7.2b

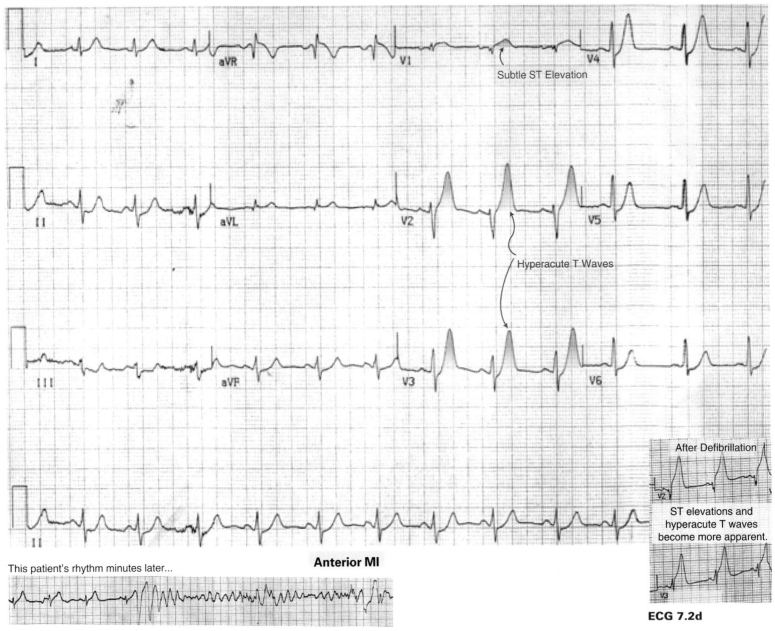

Subtle ST Elevation

Hyperacute T Waves

After Defibrillation

ST elevations and hyperacute T waves become more apparent.

ECG 7.2d

Anterior MI

This patient's rhythm minutes later...

ECG 7.2c

ECG 7.3a A 57-year-old woman presents with frequent episodes of exertional chest pain in the past week.

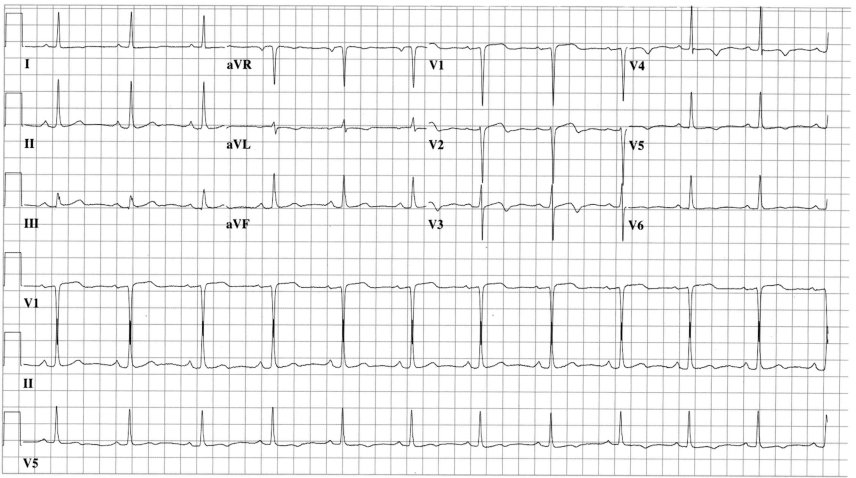

ECG 7.3b A 57-year-old woman presents with frequent episodes of exertional chest pain in the past week

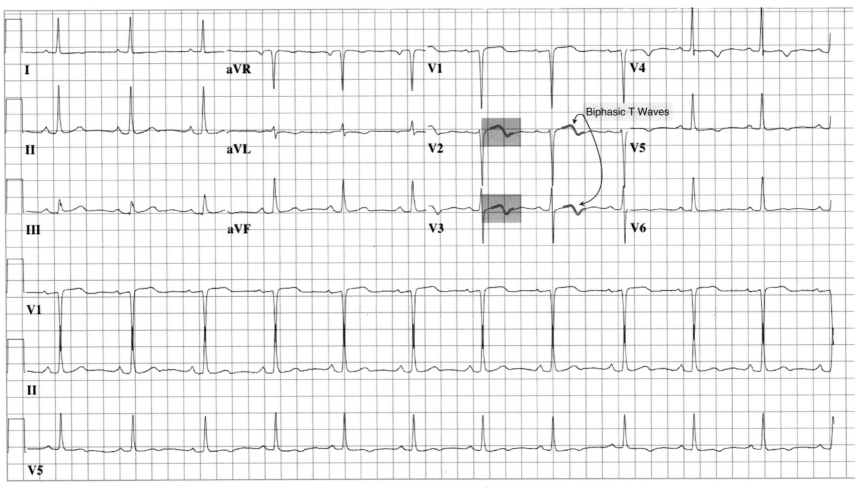

Cardiac catheterization of this patient demonstrated 95% occlusion of the proximal LAD.

Wellens Syndrome

ECG 7.4a A 33-year-old man is intoxicated with alcohol.

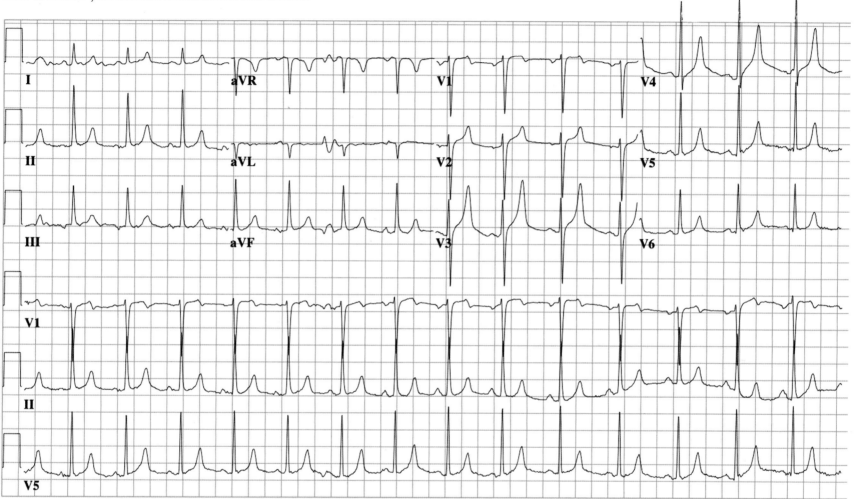

ECG 7.4b A 33-year-old man is intoxicated with alcohol.

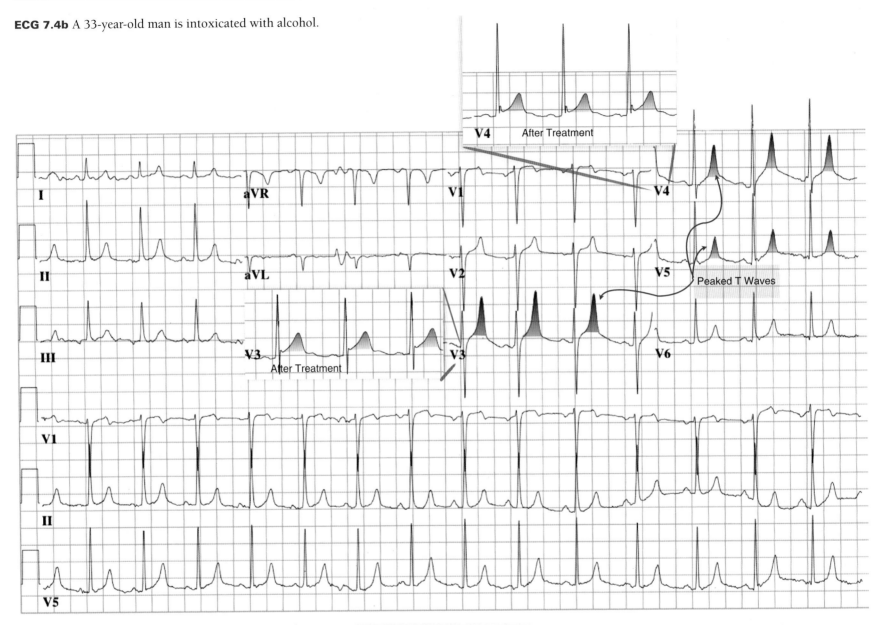

Hyperkalemia; K = 7.8 mg/dL

The T waves of hyperkalemia are narrow-based. In this patient, they become less peaked and more wide-based after treatment.

ECG 7.5a A 57-year-old male has had several episodes of chest pain in the past week.

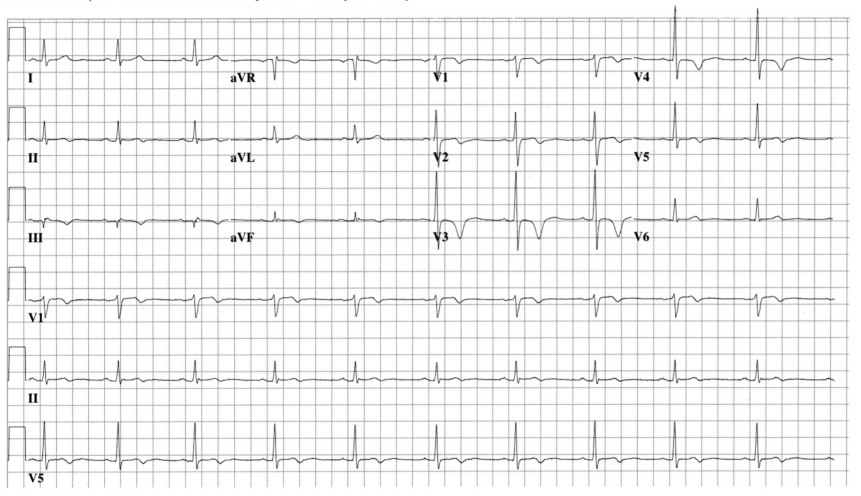

ECG 7.5b A 57-year-old male has had several episodes of chest pain in the past week.

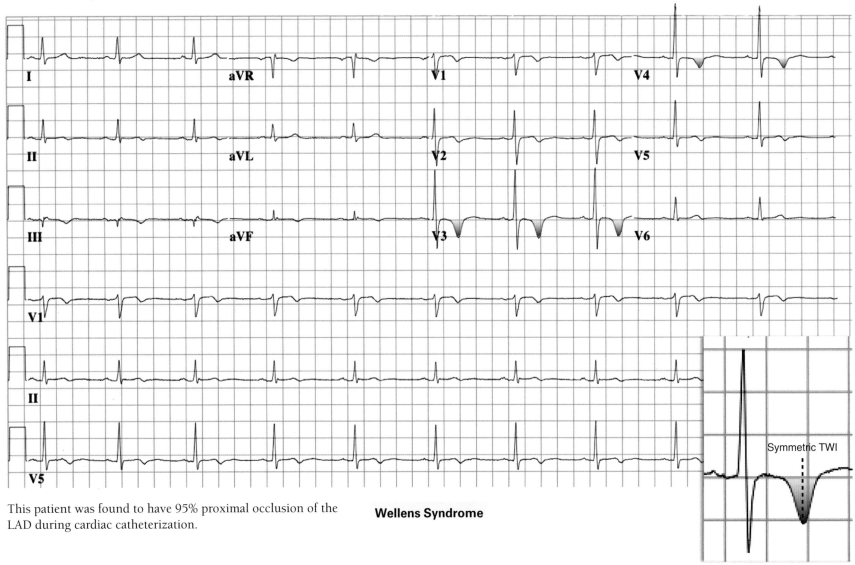

This patient was found to have 95% proximal occlusion of the LAD during cardiac catheterization.

Wellens Syndrome

Symmetric TWI

ECG 7.6a A 46-year-old woman presents with headache, neck stiffness, and confusion after smoking crack cocaine.

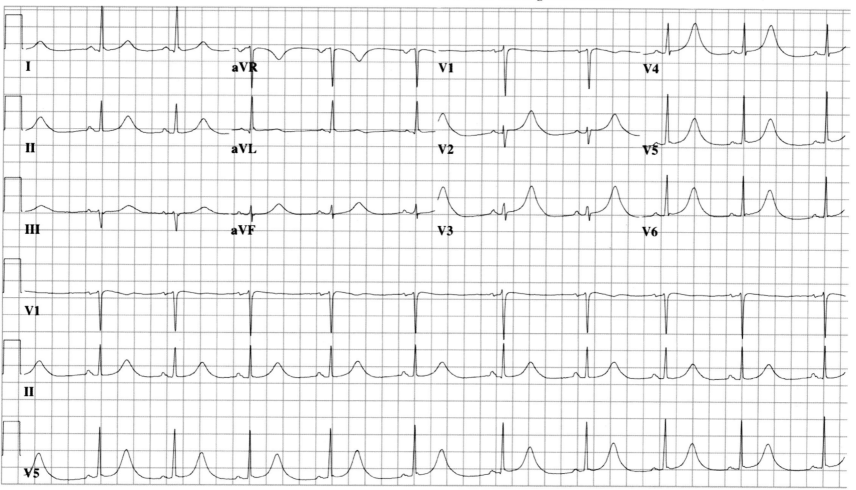

ECG 7.6b A 46-year-old woman presents with headache, neck stiffness and confusion after smoking crack cocaine.

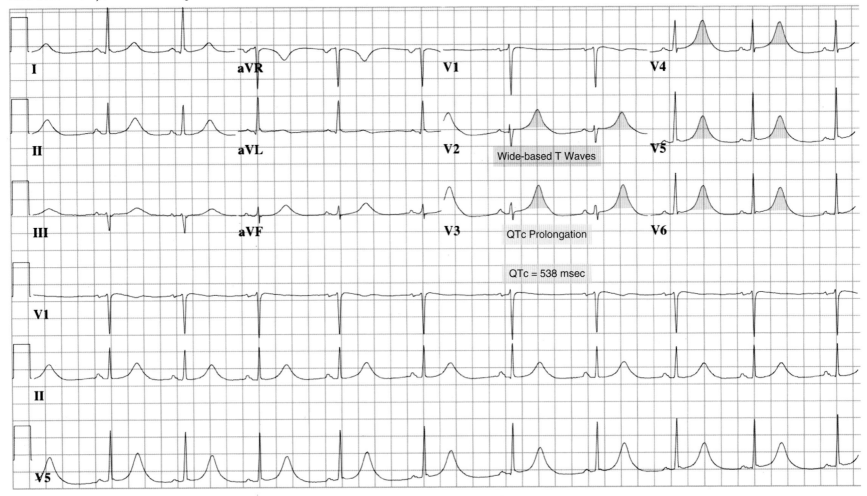

Cerebral T Waves

She was found to have a large subarachnoid hemorrhage from a ruptured right middle cerebral artery aneurysm.

ECG 7.7a A 71-year-old woman with chronic atrial fibrillation.

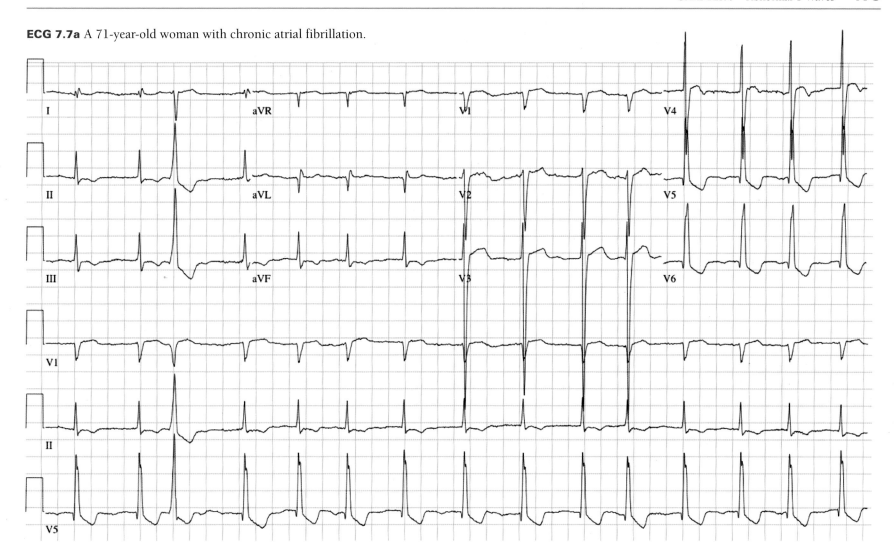

ECG 7.7b A 71-year-old woman with chronic atrial fibrillation.

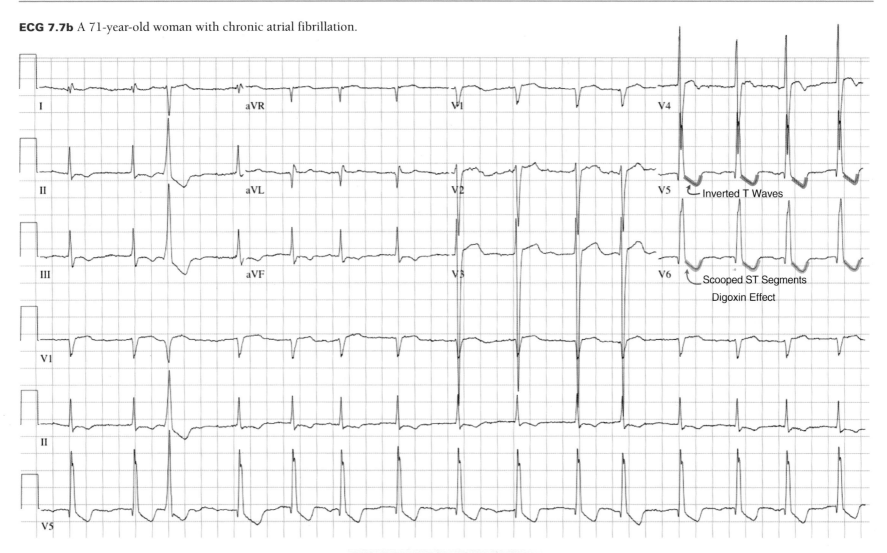

Atrial Fibrillation, Digoxin Effect

The classic appearance of digoxin effect can be appreciated in leads V5 and V6.

ECG 7.8a A 59-year-old male complains of crushing chest pain radiating down both arms.

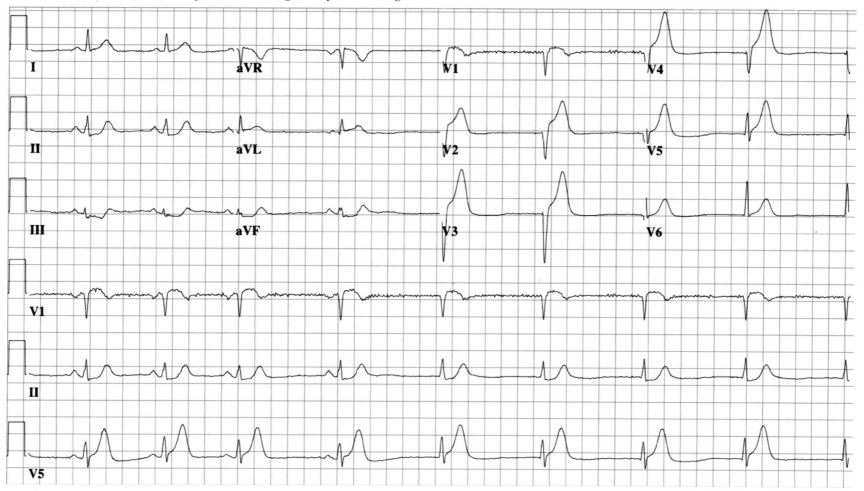

ECG 7.8b 59-year-old male complains of crushing chest pain radiating down both arms.

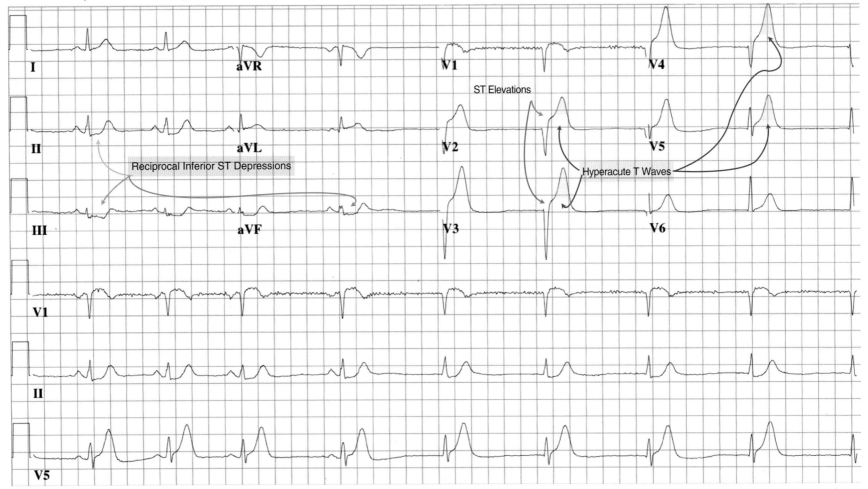

Hyperacute T Waves Secondary to Acute MI

This patient was found to have 100% thrombotic occlusion of his mid-LAD stent. Hyperacute T waves, highlighted in blue, are most prominent in the anterior leads.

ECG 7.9a A 48-year-old man intoxicated with alcohol is found down on a deck.

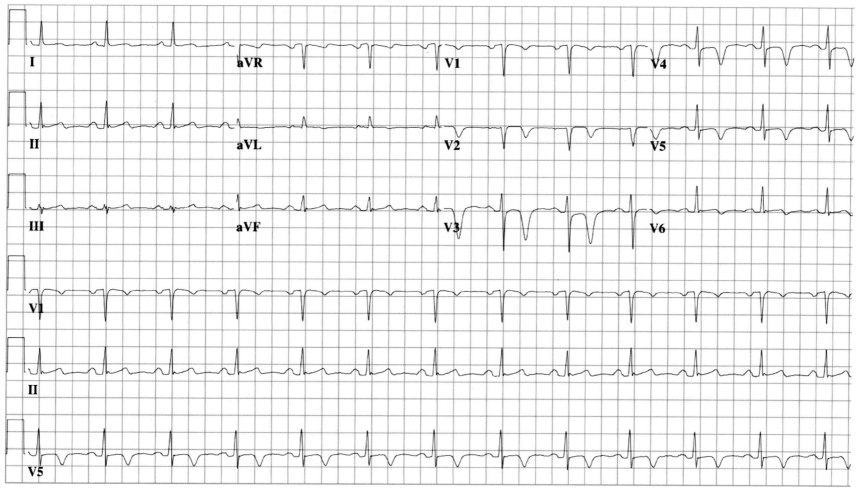

ECG 7.9b A 48-year-old man intoxicated with alcohol is found down on a deck.

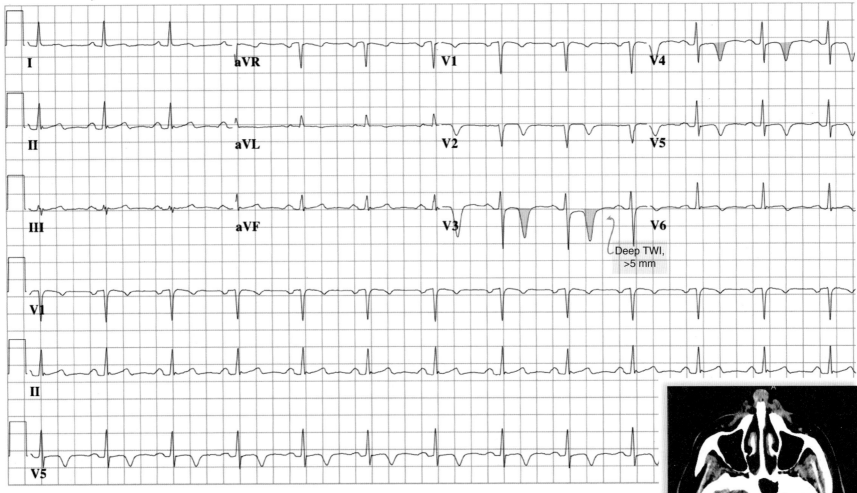

CT Image and ECG courtesy of Susan Wilcox, MD.

Cerebral T Waves

This patient was found on head CT to have traumatic subarachnoid hemorrhage, bilateral hemorrhagic contusions, a right acute subdural hemorrhage, and temporal and parietal bone fractures. His computed tomography scan is shown in Fig. 7.10.

subarachnoid blood

FIGURE 7.10 A noncontrast computerized tomography (CT) scan of the head demonstrates SAH.

ECG 7.10a

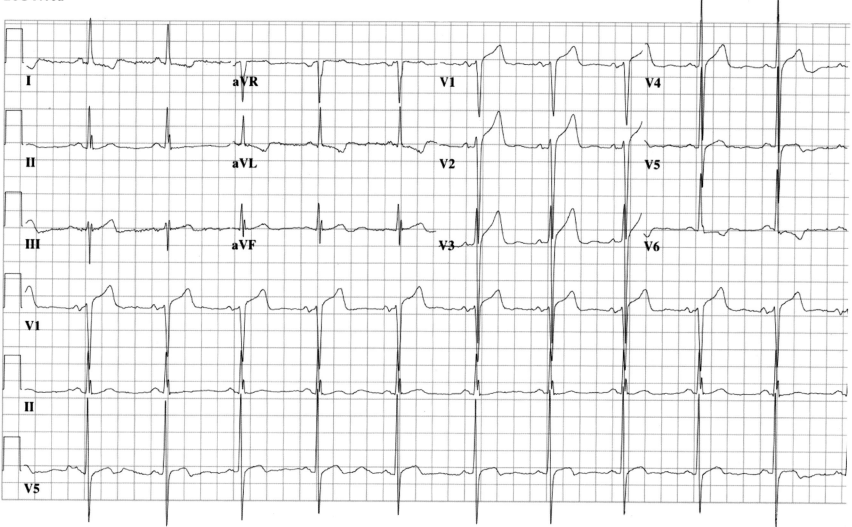

ECG 7.10b

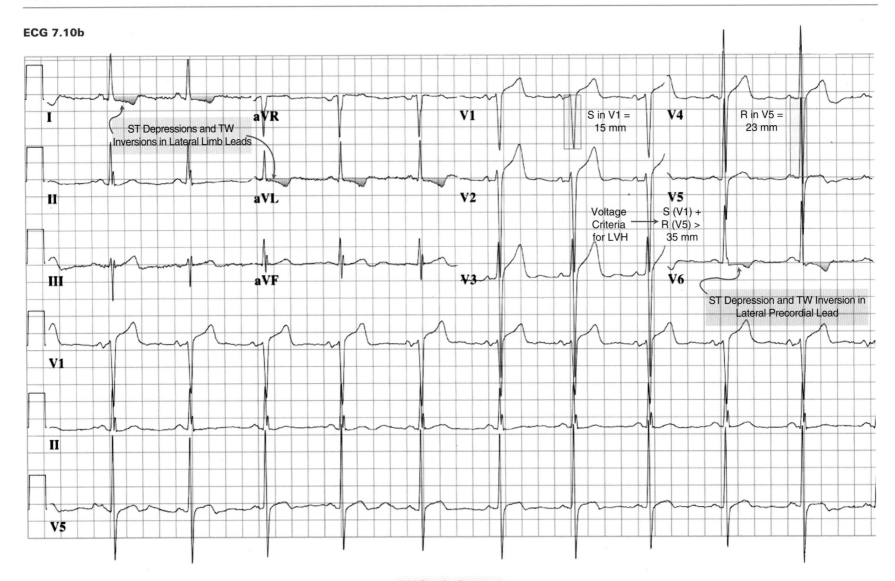

I

ST Depressions and TW
Inversions in Lateral Limb Leads

aVR

V1

S in V1 =
15 mm

V4

R in V5 =
23 mm

II

aVL

V2

V5

Voltage
Criteria
for LVH

S (V1) +
R (V5) >
35 mm

III

aVF

V3

V6

ST Depression and TW Inversion in
Lateral Precordial Lead

V1

II

V5

LV Strain Pattern

ECG 7.11a A 68-year-old male, 24 hours after successful stent placement in an acutely occluded proximal left anterior descending artery.

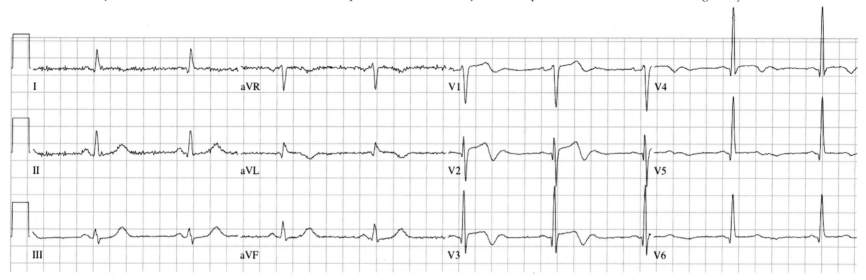

ECG 7.12a 1.5 months later…

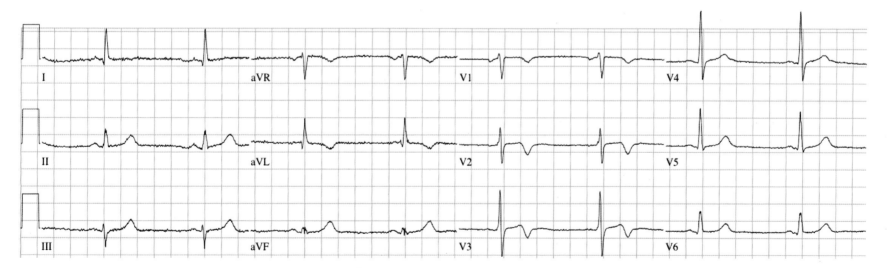

ECG 7.11b A 68-year-old male, 24 hours after successful stent placement in an acutely occluded proximal left anterior descending artery.

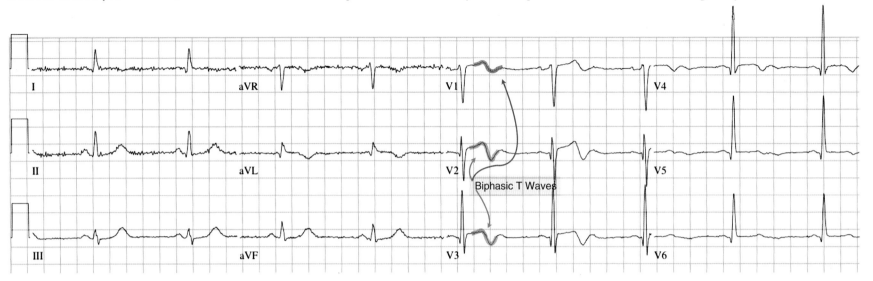

ECG 7.12b 1.5 months later…

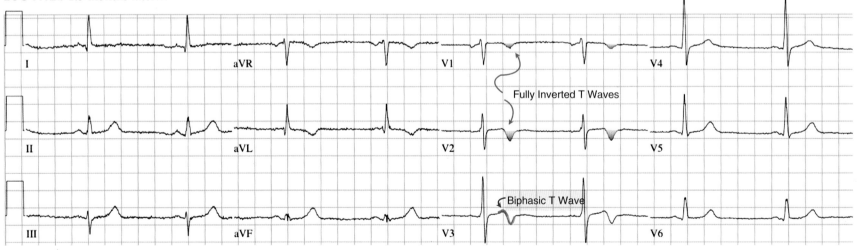

Postinfarction T Waves

Hours after the onset of an acute MI, the terminal portion of T waves will become inverted, and the T wave appears biphasic. Days after infarction, after the middle and initial portions of the T wave become inverted, the post-ischemic T wave appears fully inverted. The inverted T wave may return to its normal upright position or persist.

References

1. Simons A, Robins LJ, Hooghoudt TE, et al. Pseudonormalisation of the T wave: old wine?: A fresh look at a 25-year-old observation. *Neth Heart J* 2007;15: 257–259.
2. de Zwaan C, Bar FW, Wellens HJ. Characteristic electrocardiographic pattern indicating a critical stenosis high in left anterior descending coronary artery in patients admitted because of impending myocardial infarction. *Am Heart J* 1982;103:730–736.
3. Wehrens XH, Doevendans PA, Ophuis TJ, et al. A comparison of electrocardiographic changes during reperfusion of acute myocardial infarction by thrombolysis or percutaneous transluminal coronary angioplasty. *Am Heart J* 2000;139:430–436.
4. Hayden GE, Brady WJ, Perron AD, et al. Electrocardiographic T wave inversion: differential diagnosis in the chest pain patient. *Am J Emerg Med* 2002;20: 252–262.
5. Rudehill A, Olsson GL, Sundqvist K, et al. ECG abnormalities in patients with subarachnoid haemorrhage and intracranial tumours. *J Neurol Neurosurg Psychiatry* 1987;50:1375–1381.
6. Di Pasquale G, Pinelli G, Andreoli A, et al. Holter detection of cardiac arrhythmias in intracranial subarachnoid hemorrhage. *Am J Cardiol* 1987;59:596–600.

CHAPTER 8

QT Abnormalities and Electrolyte Disturbances

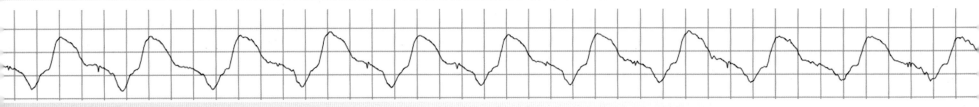

The QT Interval

The QT interval represents ventricular depolarization and repolarization (phases 0–3 of the action potential, Fig. 8.1).

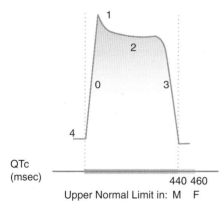

FIGURE 8.1 Relationship between action potential and QTc interval. The upper normal limit differs between men and women.

Acquired Causes

Pharmacologic There are numerous drugs that have been associated with prolonging the QT interval, most often by blocking the potassium rectifier channel (I_{Kr}). They fall under the following general categories:

- **Antipsychotics** Haloperidol, Chlorpromazine, Thioridazine
- **Antidepressants** Fluoxetine, Paroxetine, Tricyclic Antidepressants
- **Antiarrhythmics** Sotalol, Amiodarone, Quinidine, Procainamide, Disopyramide, Flecainide
- **Antibiotics/Antifungals/ Antimalarials** Macrolides, Azoles
- **Antihistamines** Loratidine
- **Antimigraine Drugs** Sumatriptan
- **Methadone**[1]

A more complete list of QT-prolonging drugs can be found at *www.torsades.org* or *www.qtdrugs.org*.

The QT interval is measured from the beginning of the QRS complex to the end of the T wave.

The length of the QT interval is dependent on heart rate. Typically, the QT interval lengthens when the heart rate slows and shortens when the heart rate increases. The QTc measurement corrects for heart rate. To calculate the QTc, look for the lead displaying the longest discernible QT length and plug this length into the Bazett formula.

Calculating the QTc:

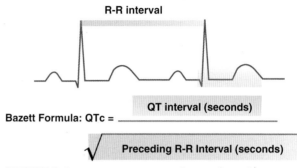

Bazett Formula: $QTc = \dfrac{QT\ interval\ (seconds)}{\sqrt{Preceding\ R\text{-}R\ Interval\ (seconds)}}$

FIGURE 8.2 ECG representation of Bazett formula components.

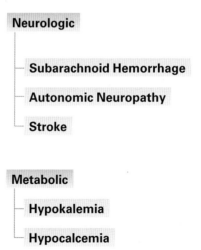

Neurologic
- **Subarachnoid Hemorrhage**
- **Autonomic Neuropathy**
- **Stroke**

Metabolic
- **Hypokalemia**
- **Hypocalcemia**

Congenital Long QT Syndrome

Congenital QT syndrome is a potentially fatal autosomal dominant genetic disorder caused by a mutation in any of several cardiac ion channels involved in ventricular repolarization. Patients with this syndrome are at increased risk of torsades de pointes (TdP) and present with syncope or sudden cardiac death.

Mutations and Channels Several syndromes (and hundreds of mutations in 12 susceptibility genes) have been identified. Many patients with congenital long QT have not been linked to any of these genotypes. There is a wide range in QTc length within genotypes and families. Two named syndromes have been described.

Table 8.1 Different Long QT Syndromes

	Syndrome	Channel	Trigger for TdP	Comment
Mean QTc = 0.49	LQT1	I_{Ks}	Exercise or emotional stress; Diving, swimming	Most common genotype. QT interval becomes longer with exercise.
	LQT2	I_{Kr}	Emotional stress, Sudden loud noise (alarm clock)	Second most common genotype
Mean QTc = 0.51	LQT3	I_{Na}	Sleep	Prone to bradycardia
	LQT4	*		* Involves structure that supports the Na+ channel. Sinus node dysfunction is common.
	LQT5	I_{Ks}	Exercise or emotional stress	Rare genotype
	LQT6	I_{Kr}		Rare genotype
	LQT7	I_{Ks}		Andersen syndrome:Associated with facial abnormalities and periodic paralysis.
	LQT8	L-type Calcium Channel		Timothy syndrome: syndactyly, cognitive defects, ventricular arrhythmias

This is not a complete list.

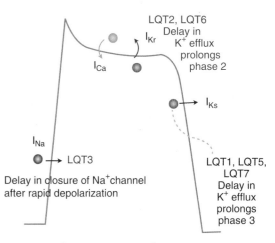

I_{Kr}: rapid potassium rectifier current
I_{Ks}: slow potassium rectifier current

FIGURE 8.3 Sites where long QT mutations prolong the action potential. The action potential also represents the myocardial cell membrane.

ECG Features

QT Prolongation Despite QT prolongation being characteristic of these mutations, the QT interval may be borderline or normal at any given point in time.

QT Dispersion There is greater lead-to-lead variability in QT lengths in patients with congenital prolonged QT syndrome. This may reflect regional variation in ventricular repolarization times that increases the risk for reentry.[2]

Treatment The standard treatment is beta-blocker therapy. Competitive sports are contraindicated. High-risk patients may be selected for ICD placement. Pacemaker therapy may be recommended for patients with bradycardia-associated QT prolongation or those who have failed medical therapy. For asymptomatic patients with no history of syncope, no family history of sudden cardiac death, and who have never demonstrated QTc > 500 msec, therapy may not be indicated.

Short QT Syndrome

This is an inherited syndrome that puts patients with structurally normal hearts at increased risk of syncope and sudden cardiac death from ventricular fibrillation. Inheritance is autosomal dominant. Before this syndrome was identified, many patients were classified as having idiopathic ventricular fibrillation.

Mutations   Mutations in the same genes implicated in long QT syndrome have been identified as the underlying cause for short QT syndrome. Some of these mutations result in a gain of function in potassium channels.

Differential Diagnosis   Hypercalcemia, hyperkalemia, and digitalis effect are all causes of a short QT that should be excluded.

ECG Appearance

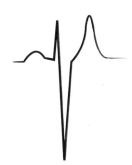

Short QTc   A QTc less than 350 msec when the heart rate is slower than 100 bpm is abnormally short.[3]

Short ST Segment   The ST segment may be absent or extremely short.

Peaked T Waves   The appearance of T waves may vary among different genotypes.

FIGURE 8.4 Appearance of short QT with peaked T wave.

Arrhythmias

Atrial Fibrillation   Patients with this syndrome are also predisposed to paroxysmal atrial fibrillation.

Ventricular Fibrillation

Management   Placement of an ICD is indicated in symptomatic patients.

Hypocalcemia

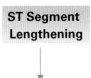

When the level of extracellular calcium is low, less calcium enters the myocardial cell during phase 2 of the action potential and phase 2 becomes prolonged. This phase of the action potential corresponds to the ST segment on the ECG. QT prolongation from hypocalcemia results from prolongation of the ST segment.

Heart block and ventricular dysrhythmias are rare.

Hypercalcemia

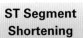

Hypercalcemia shortens the duration of phase 2 of the action potential. This typically occurs with serum calcium levels greater than 13 mg/dL. The corresponding ST segment is shortened, accounting for the shortened QT interval.

ST Elevation   ST elevation occurs in patients with significant hypercalcemia and these changes may be mistaken for acute myocardial infarction (MI).[4] It is possible that ST elevation reflects an ST segment that is shortened enough to make the upright T wave appear joined to the QRS wave. These elevations disappear with correction of the serum calcium level. (Fig. 8.5D)

AV Block   At extremely high calcium levels (>15 mg/dL) varying degrees of AV block may progress to complete heart block.

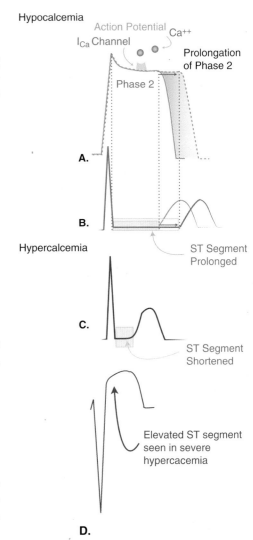

FIGURE 8.5 **A.** Action potential affected by hypocalcemia. **B.** Corresponding change in ECG appearance. **C.** ECG appearance in hypercalcemia. **D.** ST elevation in setting of hypercalcemia.

Hyperkalemia

While the serum level of potassium cannot predict the appearance of an ECG in a single individual and vice versa, the ECG changes associated with hyperkalemia progress in a typical fashion.

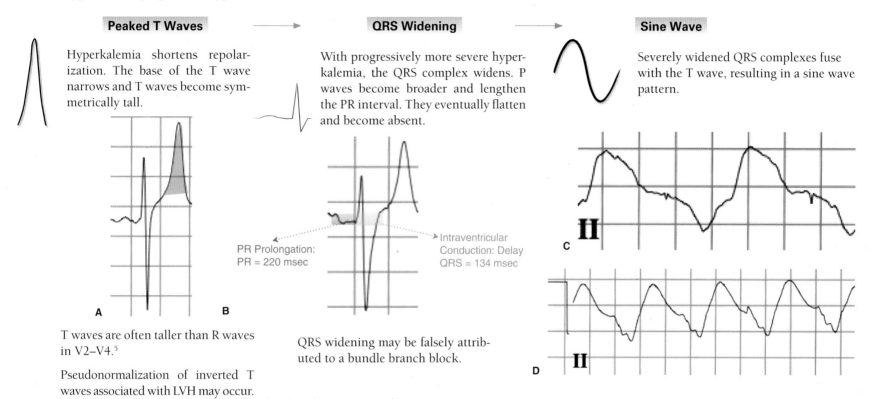

Peaked T Waves →

Hyperkalemia shortens repolarization. The base of the T wave narrows and T waves become symmetrically tall.

QRS Widening →

With progressively more severe hyperkalemia, the QRS complex widens. P waves become broader and lengthen the PR interval. They eventually flatten and become absent.

Sine Wave

Severely widened QRS complexes fuse with the T wave, resulting in a sine wave pattern.

PR Prolongation:
PR = 220 msec

Intraventricular
Conduction: Delay
QRS = 134 msec

C

II

A   B

T waves are often taller than R waves in V2–V4.[5]

Pseudonormalization of inverted T waves associated with LVH may occur.

QRS widening may be falsely attributed to a bundle branch block.

D   II

FIGURE 8.6 ECG appearance of different stages of hyperkalemia. **A.** Peaked T wave. **B.** QRS widening and PR prolongation. **C and D.** Sine waves from two different patients.

Mimics ST elevation (often in leads V1 and V2) can accompany hyperkalemia leading to mistaking this electrolyte disturbance for an ST-elevation MI. ST elevation improves with treatment.[6] Sinus tachycardia with sine wave morphology from severe hyperkalemia can be mistaken for ventricular tachycardia.

ECG Changes Can Be Masked by:

Other Electrolyte Abnormalities Concomitant electrolyte disturbances can mask the ECG changes typical of hyperkalemia.

Chronic Renal Failure In some patients, particularly in those with chronic renal failure, ECG changes may be absent, even in moderate to severe hyperkalemia.

Arrhythmia and Conduction Block Severe hyperkalemia can produce severe bradycardia and AV block. Marked bradycardia with wide QRS complexes should make one suspect severe hyperkalemia. This rhythm can degenerate into asystole or ventricular fibrillation.

Hypokalemia

ECG Features

T Wave Flattening In hypokalemia, the amplitude of the T wave decreases.

ST Depression and T Wave Inversion[7] These changes may mimic subendocardial ischemia.

U Waves As hypokalemia becomes more severe, U waves become more prominent, and their amplitude exceeds that of the T wave. U waves can best be seen in leads V2–V4. With even more severe hypokalemia, the prominent U waves combine with the T waves. (Fig. 8.7C-D)

Prolonged QT Interval The presence of a pathologic U wave is thought to be secondary to a splitting of the T wave. Measurement of the true QT interval should include the U wave (QU interval). Prolongation of the QU interval is considered clinically significant.

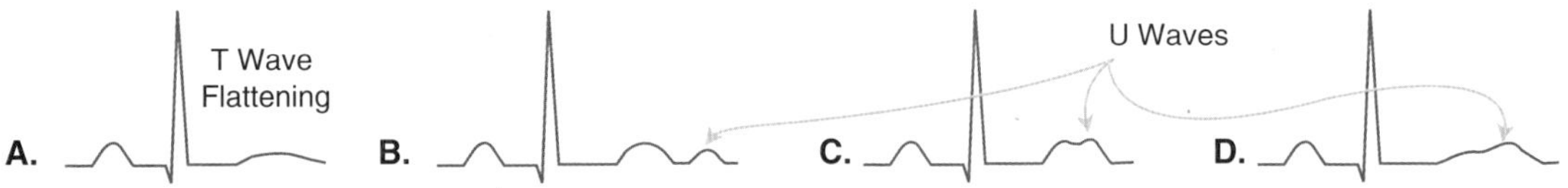

FIGURE 8.7 ECG appearances of different stages of hypokalemia. **A.** T wave flattening. **B.** Appearance of pathologic U wave. **C.** "Camel-hump" appearance of T wave representing T-U wave fusion. **D.** U wave more prominent than T wave.

Mechanism The resting potential of cardiac myocytes is based on the potassium gradient across the cell membrane. When the extracellular potassium concentration drops, the cell loses positive ions and becomes hyperpolarized. Phase 3 repolarization also becomes prolonged. The overall effect is prolongation of the action potential (Fig. 8.8).

Arrhythmias Prolongation of the QU interval predisposes patients to ventricular arrhythmias.

Torsades de Pointes

Ventricular Tachycardia

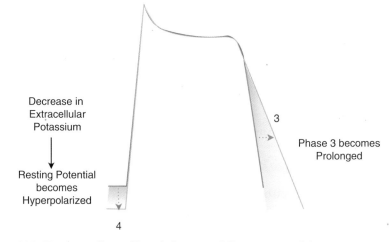

FIGURE 8.8 Effects of hypokalemia on different stages of the action potential.

ECG 8.1a A 70-year-old female complains of numbness and tingling in her hands and feet for 4 days.

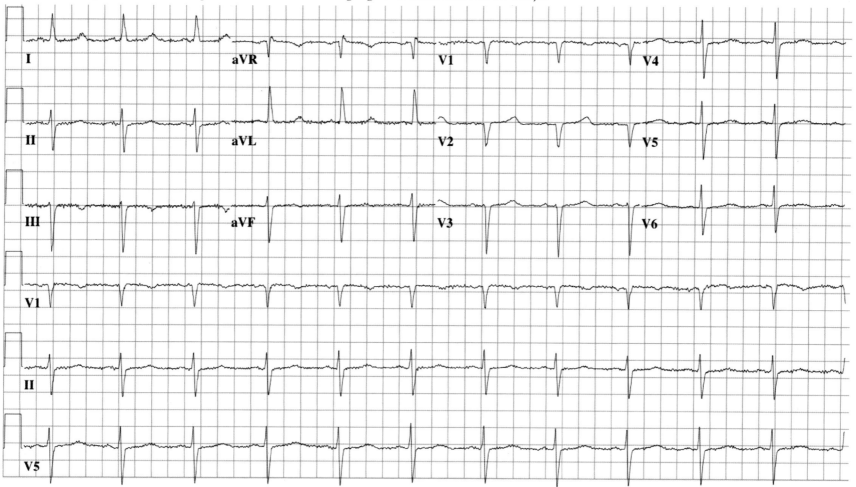

ECG 8.1b A 70-year-old female complains of numbness and tingling in her hands and feet for 4 days.

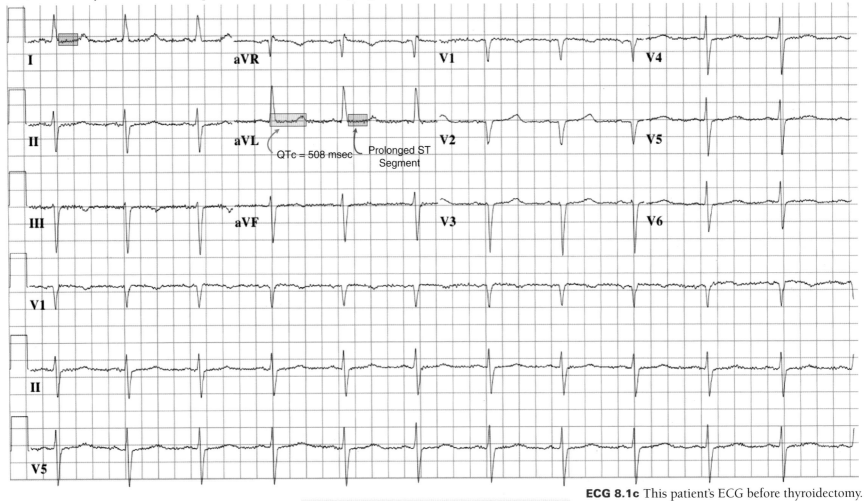

QT Prolongation Secondary to Hypocalcemia

ECG 8.1c This patient's ECG before thyroidectomy.

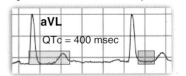

She also complained of perioral tingling. This patient underwent a thyroidectomy 8 days prior to this presentation. Her calcium level was 5.7 mg/dL. An ECG obtained prior to her thyroidectomy demonstrated a normal ST segment and QT interval length.

ECG 8.2a A 55-year-old man is found laying supine on a sidewalk.

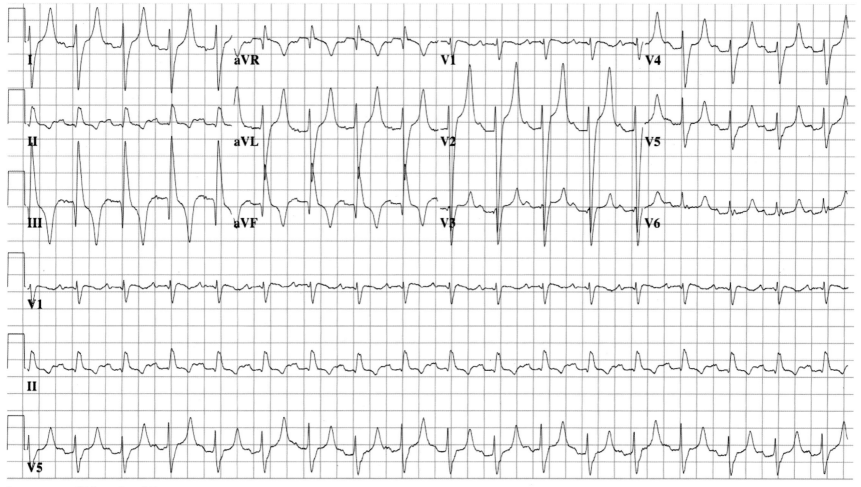

Image courtesy of Roberta Capp, MD.

ECG 8.2b A 55-year-old man is found laying supine on a sidewalk.

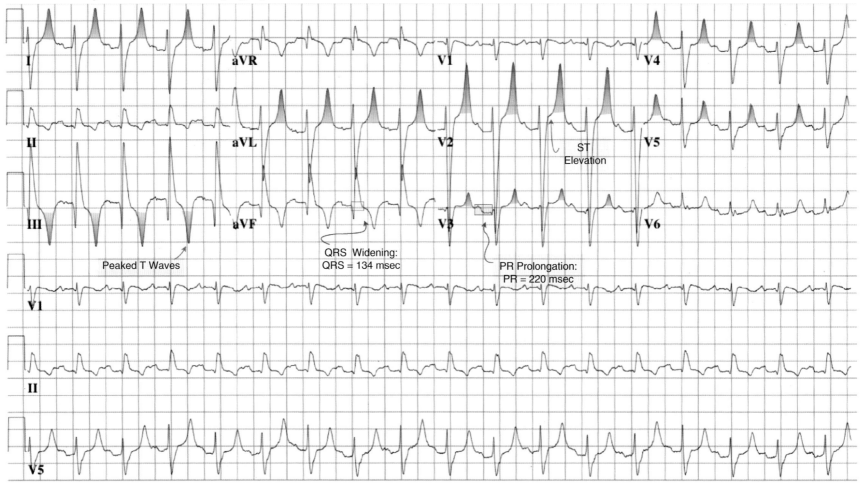

Hyperkalemia: K=7.3 mg/dL

This is an alarming ECG. Not only are the T waves significantly peaked, but the PR interval is prolonged and the QRS wave is widened. The combination of peaked T waves with QRS widening should alert you that the hyperkalemia in this patient is clinically significant.
ST segments can become elevated in hyperkalemia. They are elevated here in V2–V5, I, and aVL. The ECG could be mistaken for an ST-elevation MI with hyperacute T waves. However, the T waves in this ECG are narrower and more diffuse than ischemic T waves.

ECG 8.3a A 60-year-old male presents with weakness.

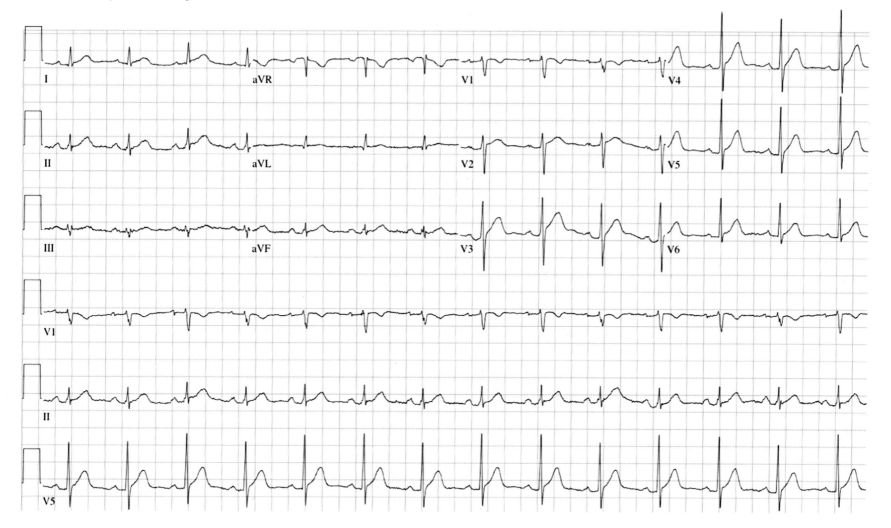

ECG 8.3b A 60-year-old male presents with weakness.

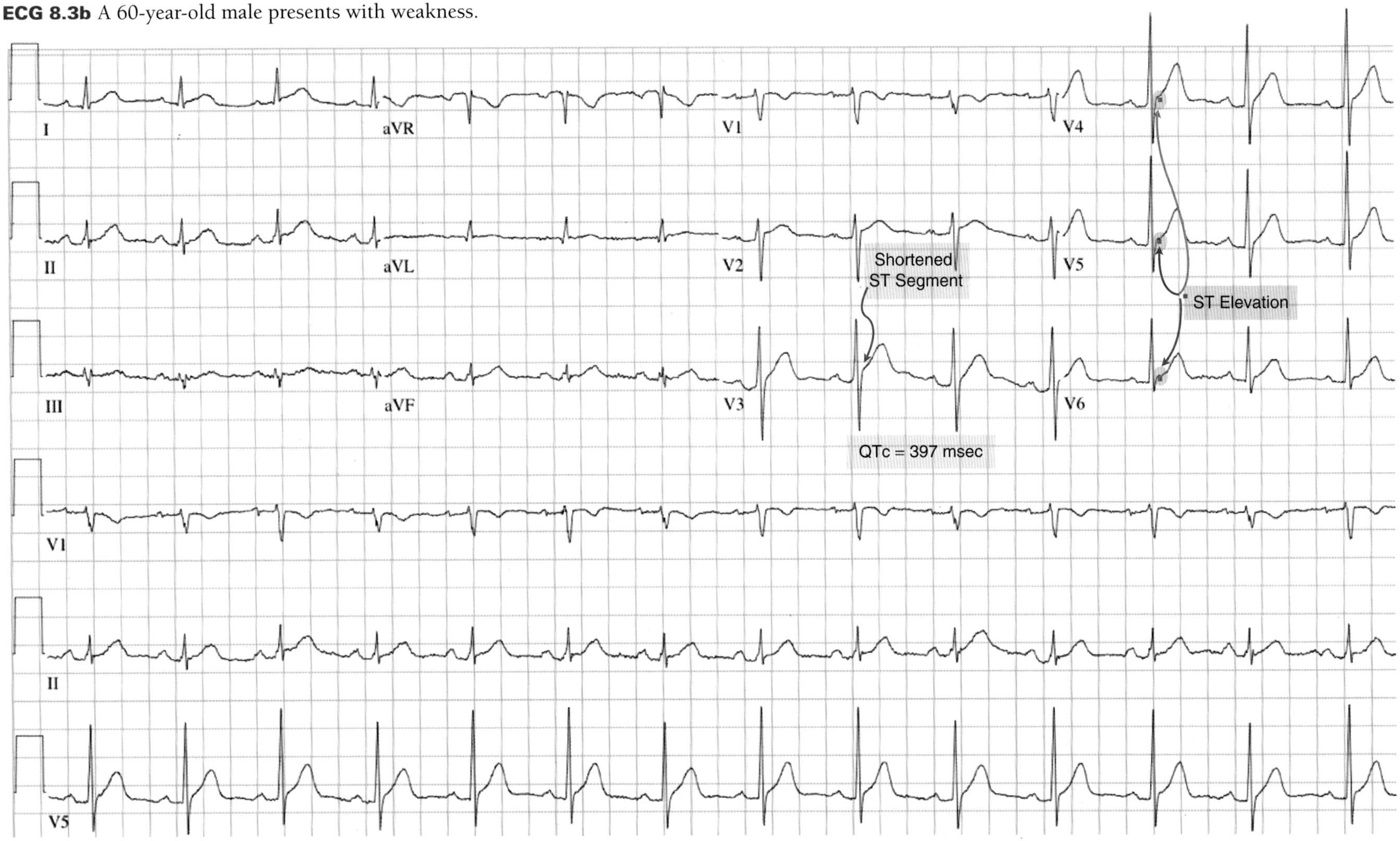
I
aVR
V1
V4
II
aVL
V2
V5
Shortened ST Segment
ST Elevation
III
aVF
V3
V6
QTc = 397 msec
V1
II
V5

Hypercalcemia: Calcium = 13.4 mg/dL

ECG 8.4a

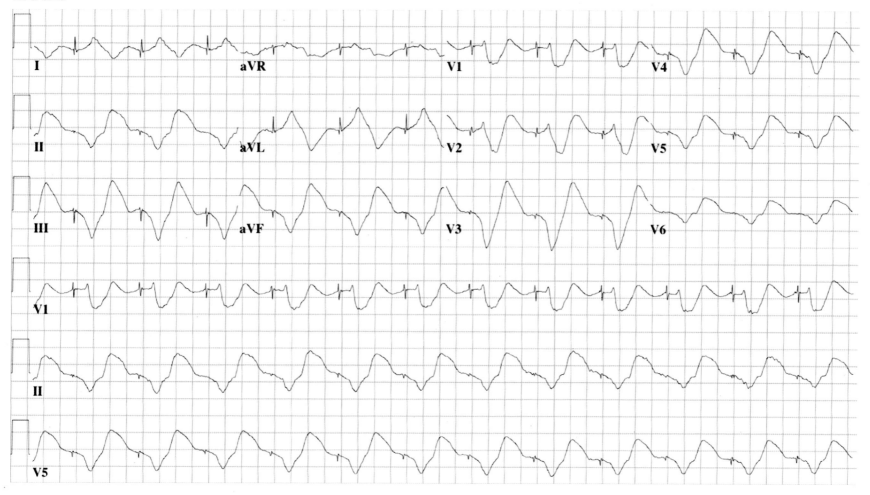

Image courtesy of James Takayesu, MD.

ECG 8.4b

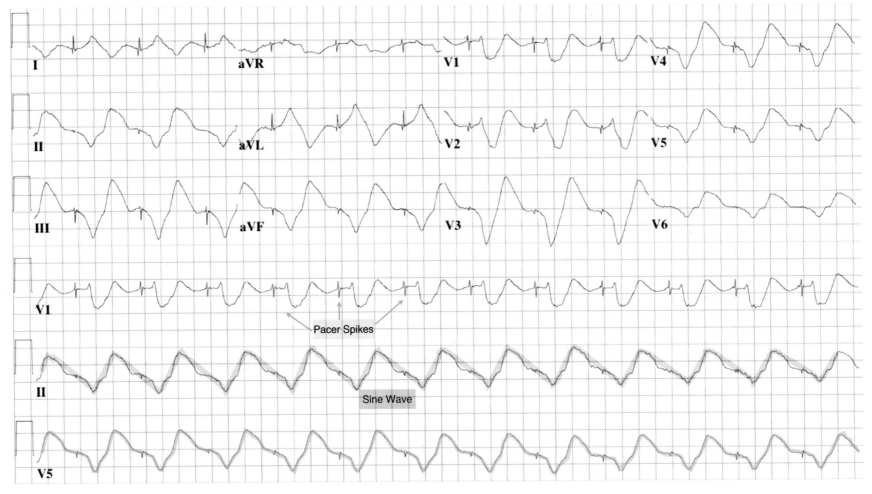

Severe Hyperkalemia: K = 8.7 mg/dL

This is a near-terminal rhythm. The sine wave results from widening of the QRS complex, shortening of the ST segment and fusion of the S and T waves. In severe hyperkalemia, the P waves decrease in amplitude until they become absent. The underlying rhythm can still be controlled by the sinus node (referred to as sinoventricular rhythm) despite there being no detectable P waves. The disappearance of P waves is thought to result from slowing of the sinus impulse across the atria.

ECG 8.5a An asymptomatic 27-year-old male.

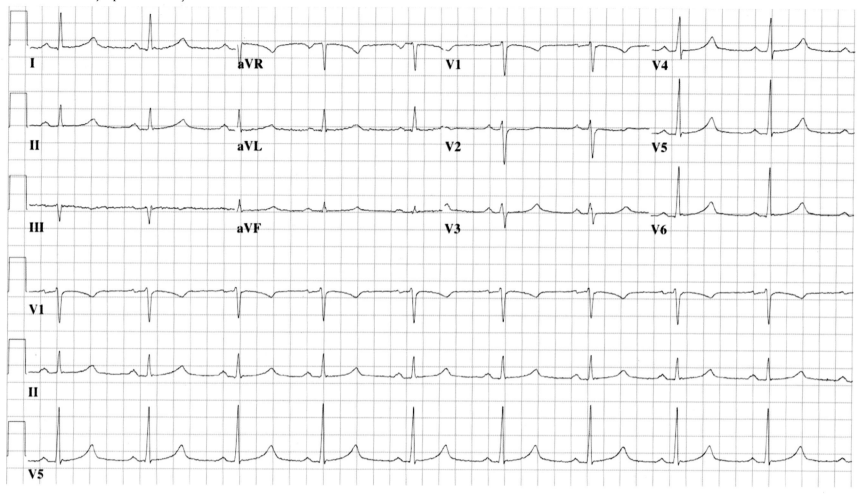

ECG 8.5b An asymptomatic 27-year-old male.

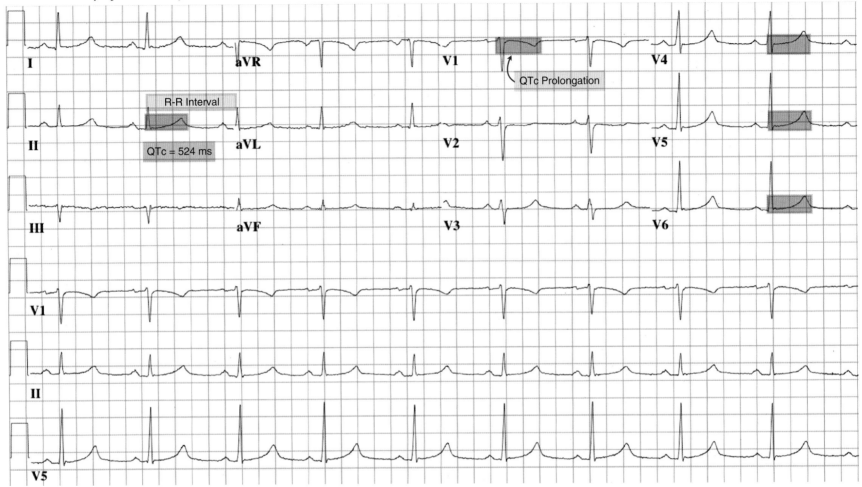

Congenital Prolonged QT Syndrome

Both this patient and his brother have a mutation in the potassium ion channel, resulting in delayed repolarization. Both are on beta-blocker therapy and have AICDs.

ECG 8.6a

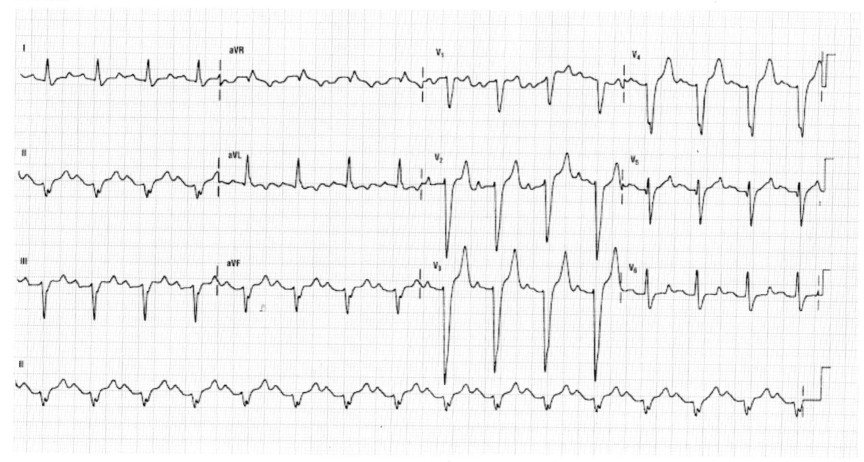

Image courtesy of Josh Kosowsky, MD.

ECG 8.6b

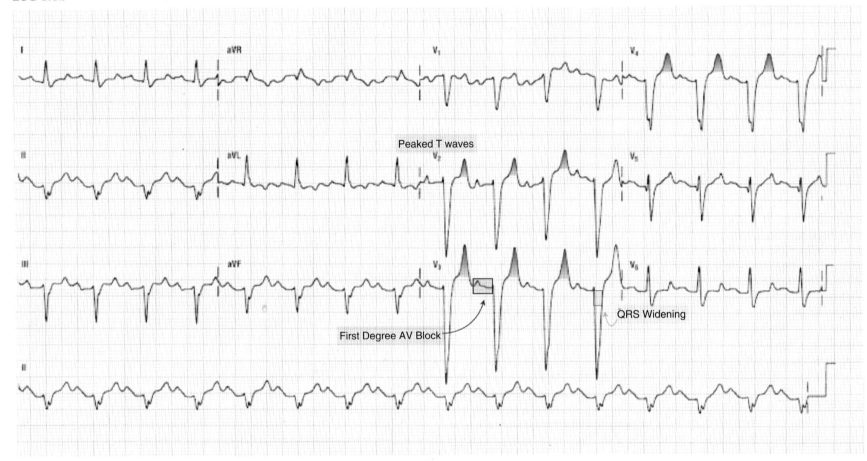

Hyperkalemia

ECG 8.7a A 44-year-old with severe cirrhosis complains of a decreased appetite for the past several days.

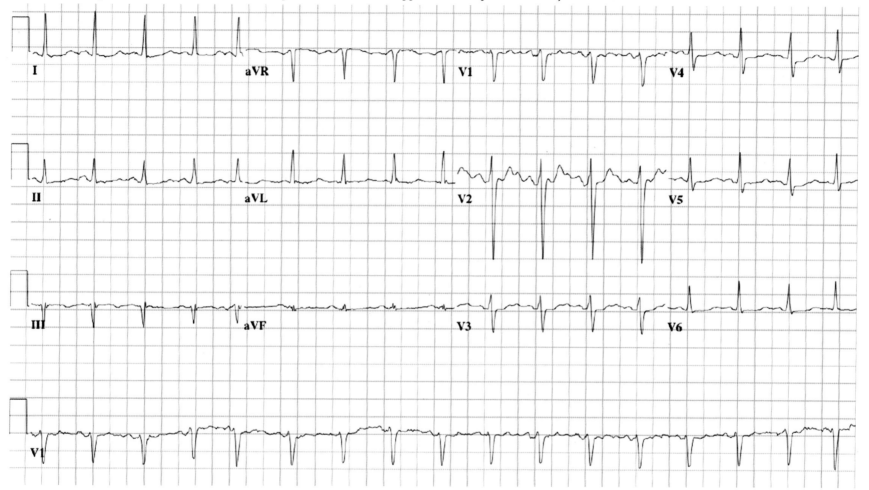

ECG 8.7b A 44-year-old with severe cirrhosis complains of a decreased appetite for the past several days.

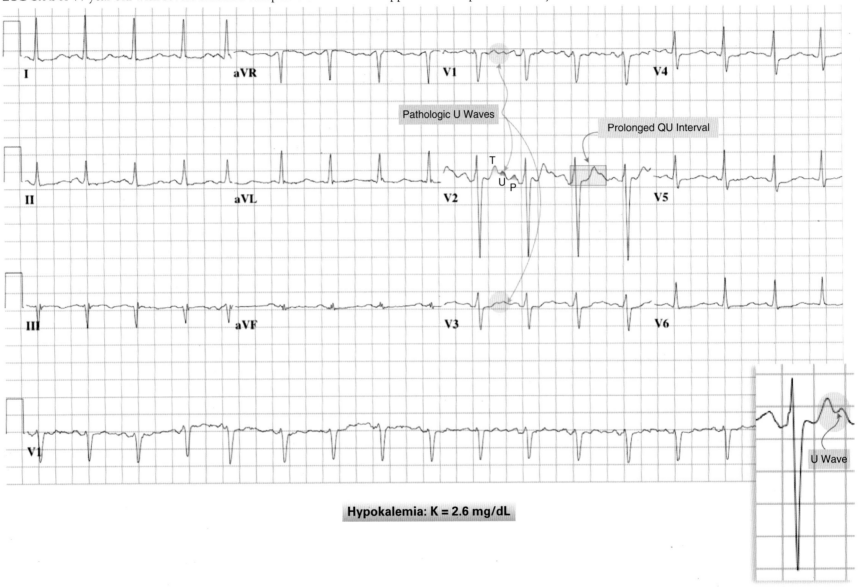

Pathologic U Waves

Prolonged QU Interval

T

U P

U Wave

Hypokalemia: K = 2.6 mg/dL

ECG 8.8a A 75-year-old female with coronary artery disease, hypertension, and end-stage renal disease requiring hemodialysis was minimally responsive at a rehabilitation facility.

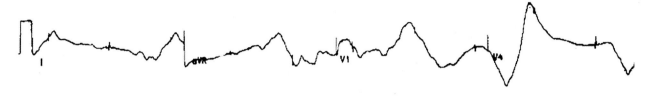

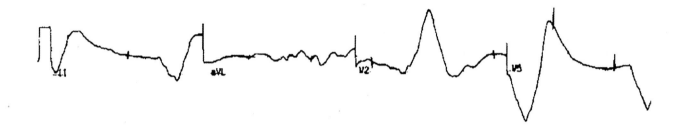

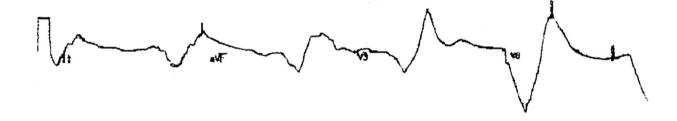

ECG 8.8b A 75-year-old female with coronary artery disease, hypertension, and end-stage renal disease requiring hemodialysis was minimally responsive at a rehabilitation facility.

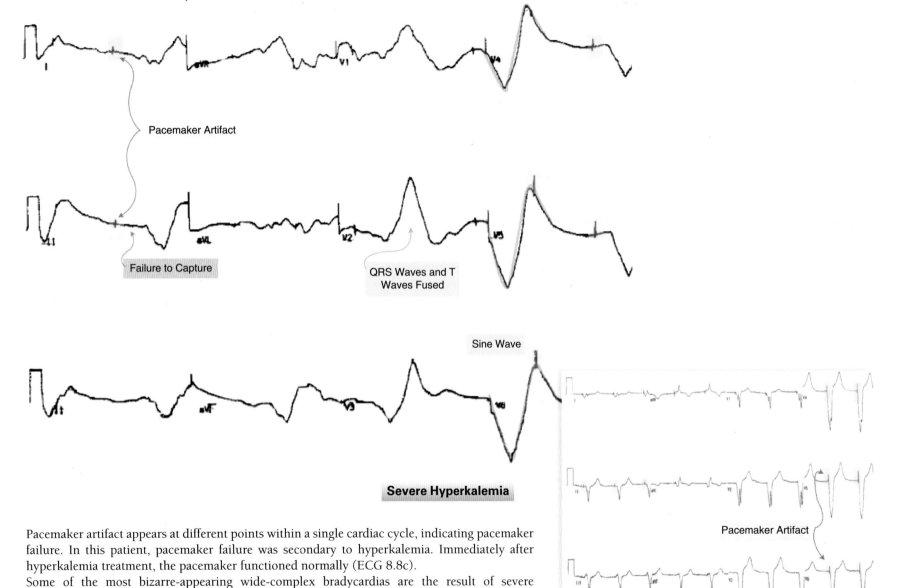

Pacemaker Artifact

Failure to Capture

QRS Waves and T Waves Fused

Sine Wave

Severe Hyperkalemia

Pacemaker Artifact

Pacemaker artifact appears at different points within a single cardiac cycle, indicating pacemaker failure. In this patient, pacemaker failure was secondary to hyperkalemia. Immediately after hyperkalemia treatment, the pacemaker functioned normally (ECG 8.8c).

Some of the most bizarre-appearing wide-complex bradycardias are the result of severe hyperkalemia.

ECG 8.8c After treatment with calcium chloride.

ECG 8.9a A 36-year-old woman with alcohol abuse presents with nausea, vomiting, and generalized weakness.

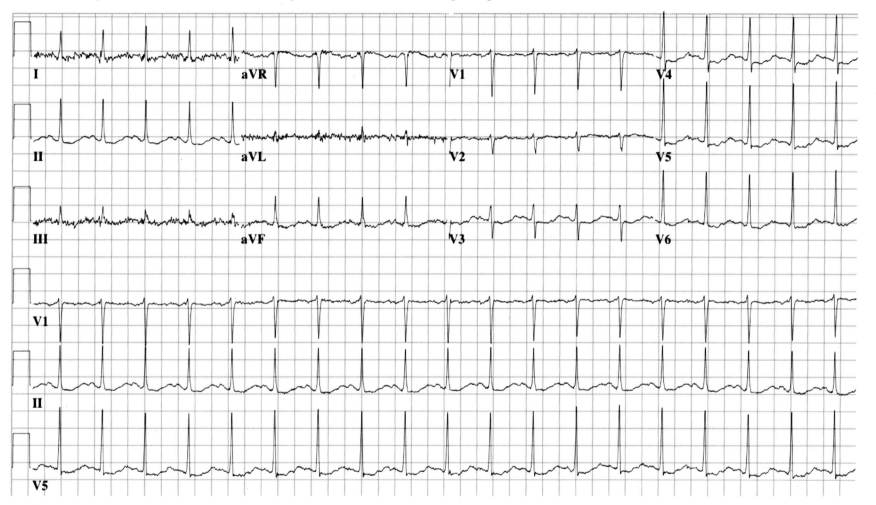

ECG 8.9b A 36-year-old woman with alcohol abuse presents with nausea, vomiting, and generalized weakness.

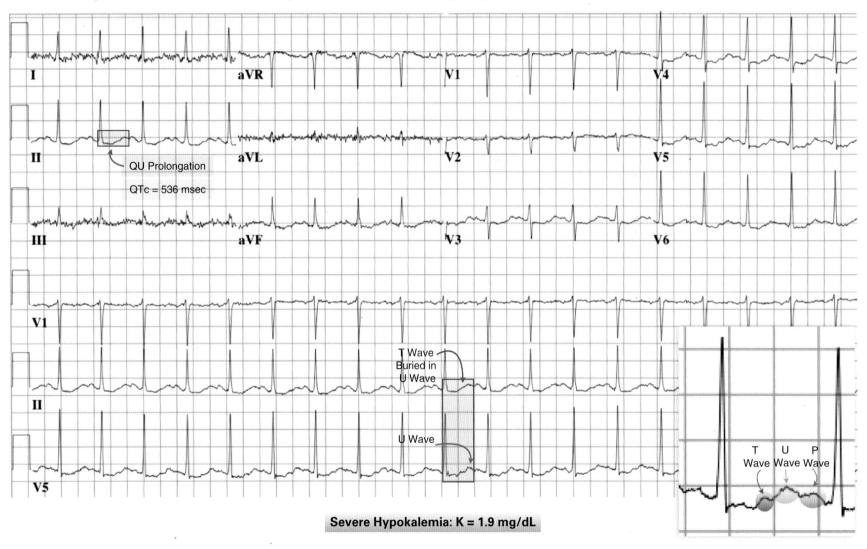

QU Prolongation

QTc = 536 msec

T Wave Buried in U Wave

U Wave

T U P
Wave Wave Wave

Severe Hypokalemia: K = 1.9 mg/dL

Pathologic U waves are most apparent in leads V4–V6. In other leads, the T wave is buried in U wave.

ECG 8.10a A 66-year-old man with diabetes complains of generalized weakness and malaise. His triage vital signs are significant for a systolic blood pressure of 77 mm Hg and a heart rate of 40 bpm.

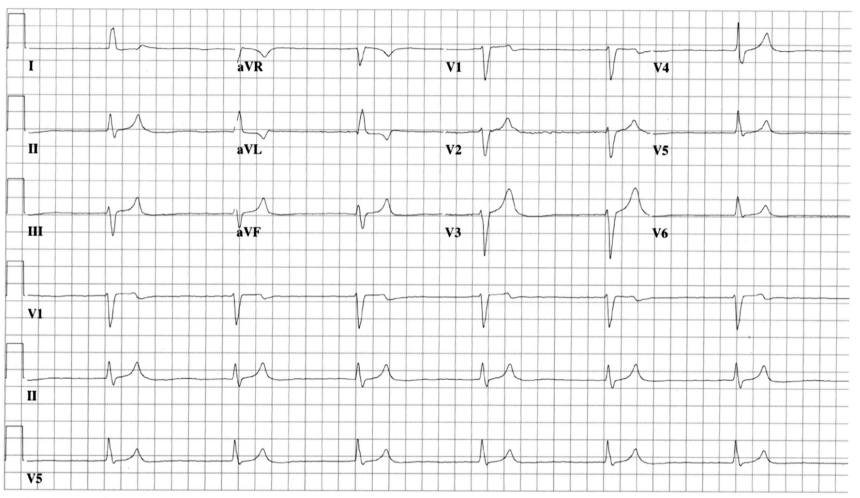

ECG 8.10b A 66-year-old man with diabetes complains of generalized weakness and malaise. His triage vital signs are significant for a systolic blood pressure of 77 mm Hg and a heart rate of 40 bpm.

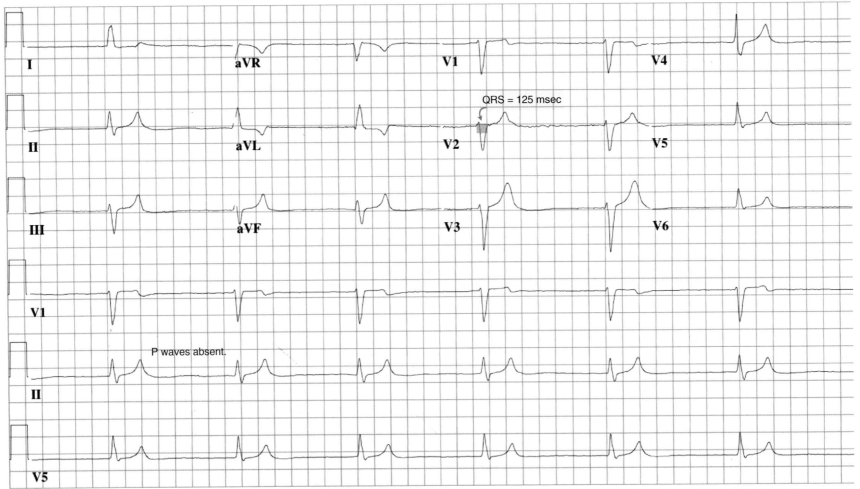

Severe Hyperkalemia: K = 9.4 mg/dL

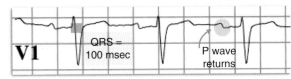

ECG 8.10c 1 hour later when K = 7.8 mg/dL

This patient was found to have renal failure secondary to renal tubular acidosis. This rhythm appears to be junctional bradycardia. However, P waves may have flattened enough to make sinus node conduction to the AV node undetectable. This may actually be a sinoventricular rhythm. After 1 hour of treatment, the patient's potassium decreased to 7.8 mg/dL and the ECG obtained at that time demonstrated narrowing of the QRS and reappearance of P waves (ECG 8.10c).

ECG 8.11a An asymptomatic 58-year-old male.

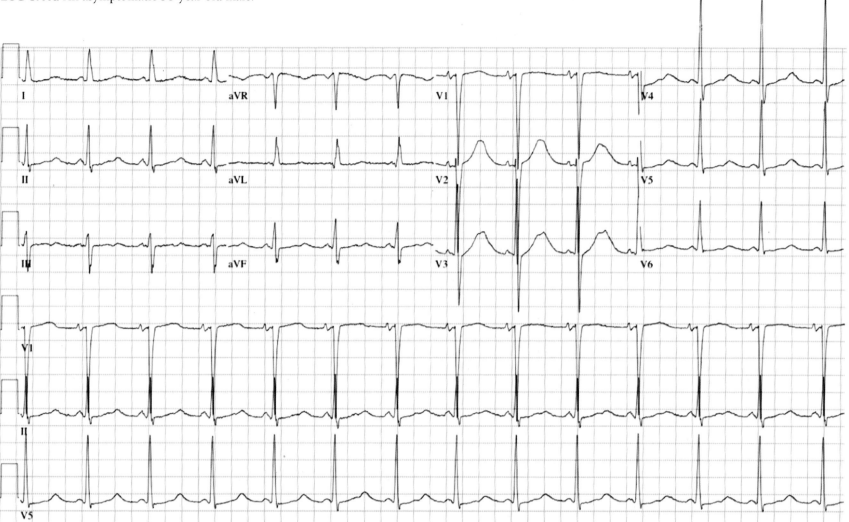

ECG 8.11b An asymptomatic 58-year-old male.

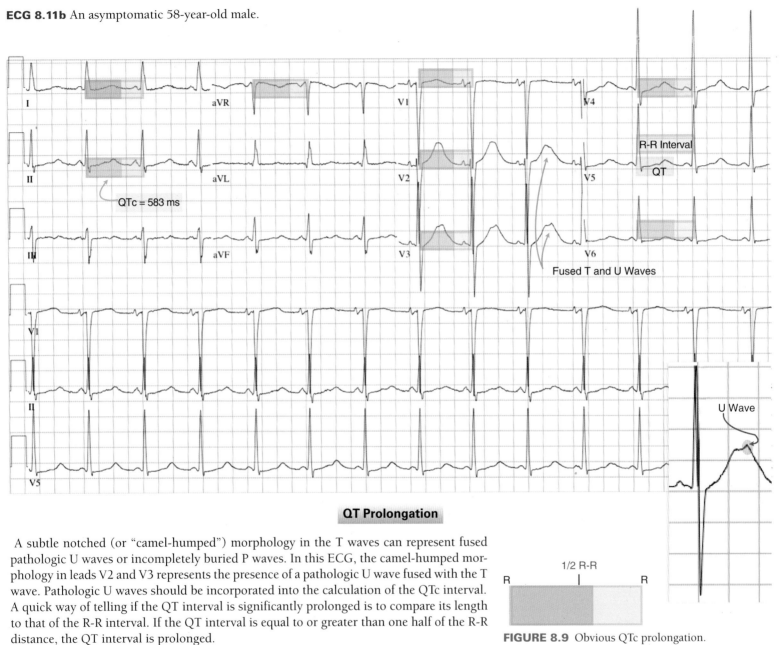

QT Prolongation

A subtle notched (or "camel-humped") morphology in the T waves can represent fused pathologic U waves or incompletely buried P waves. In this ECG, the camel-humped morphology in leads V2 and V3 represents the presence of a pathologic U wave fused with the T wave. Pathologic U waves should be incorporated into the calculation of the QTc interval. A quick way of telling if the QT interval is significantly prolonged is to compare its length to that of the R-R interval. If the QT interval is equal to or greater than one half of the R-R distance, the QT interval is prolonged.

FIGURE 8.9 Obvious QTc prolongation.

ECG 8.12a

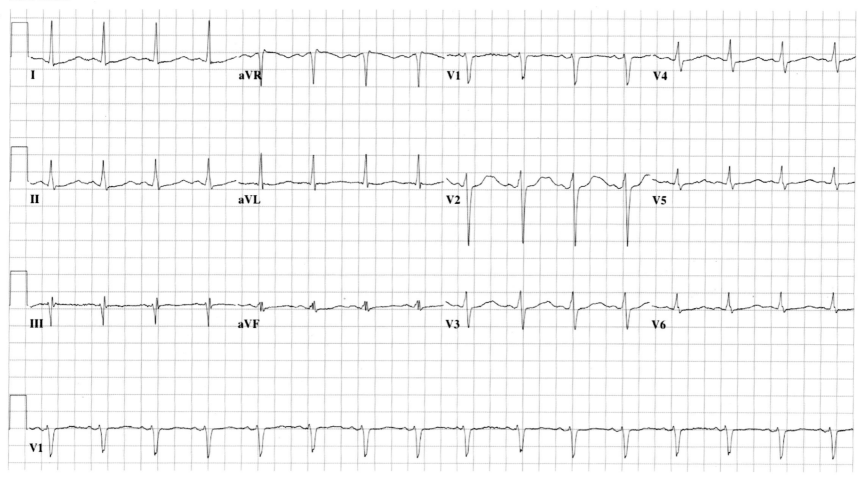

ECG 8.12b

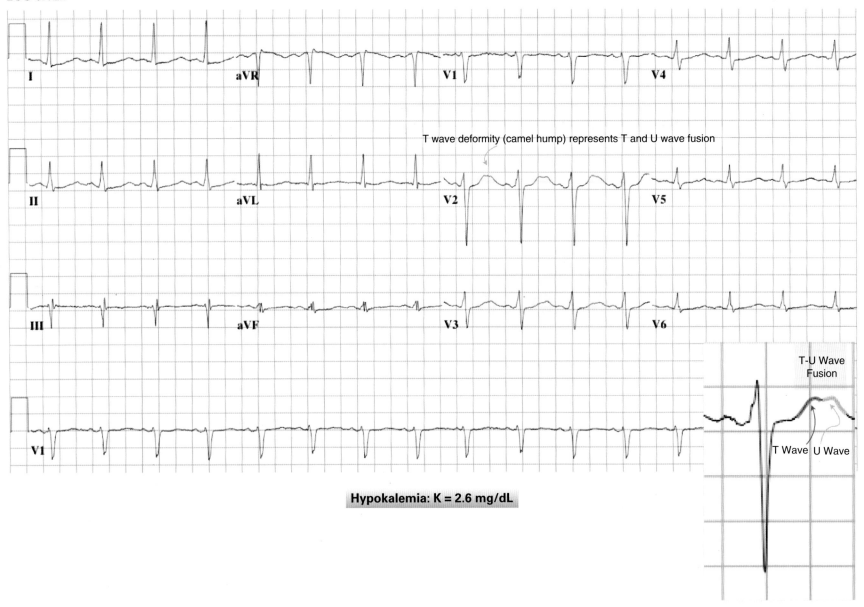

T wave deformity (camel hump) represents T and U wave fusion

T-U Wave Fusion

T Wave   U Wave

Hypokalemia: K = 2.6 mg/dL

ECG 8.13a A 67-year-old male is found on the floor beside his bed, unable to move his left side.

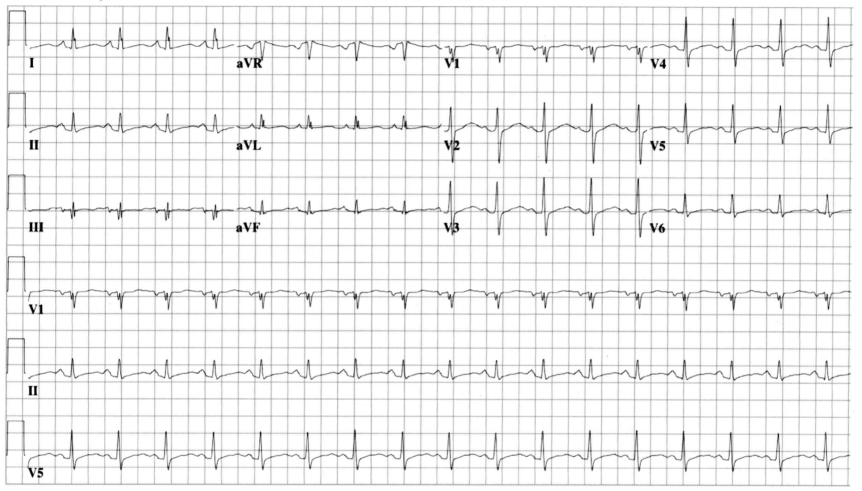

ECG 8.13b A 67-year-old male is found on the floor beside his bed, unable to move his left side.

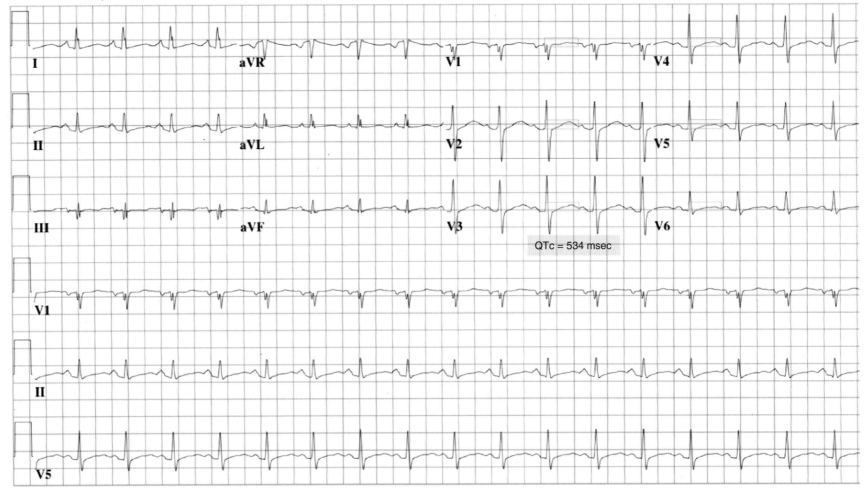

QTc = 534 msec

Prolonged QTc Interval

This patient was found to have a large right parietal-occipital intraparenchymal hemorrhage. QT prolongation can occur in the setting of acute intracranial events.

ECG 8.14a A 90-year-old male presents with bradycardia, hypotension, and lethargy. He has been bed-bound for 3 days.

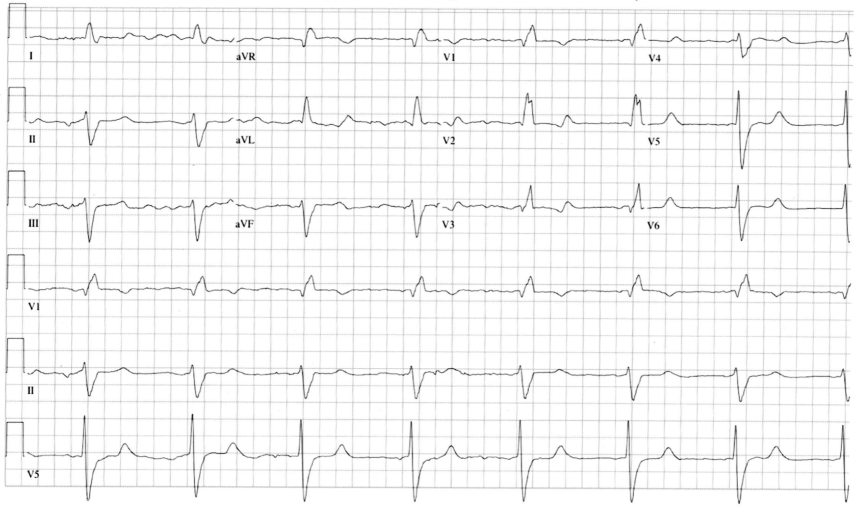

Image courtesy of Roberta Capp, MD

ECG 8.14b A 90-year-old male presents with bradycardia, hypotension, and lethargy. He has been bed-bound for 3 days.

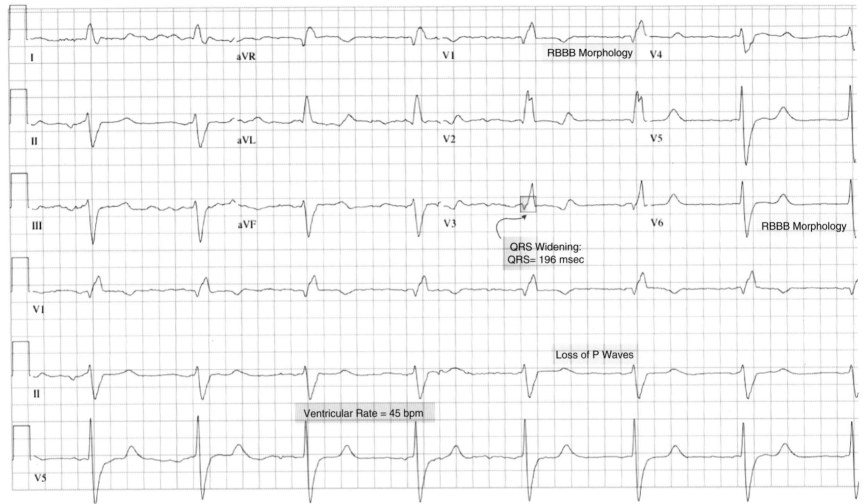

Hyperkalemia: K = 7.0 mg/dL

One might attribute this patient's QRS widening to a preexisting right bundle branch block (RBBB) (this patient had no prior ECGs for comparison). Loss of P waves and significant bradycardia are clues in this ECG that hyperkalemia might be the underlying cause of the QRS widening. This patient was found to have acute renal failure of unclear etiology. He had a profound lactic acidosis.

References

1. Krantz MJ, Kutinsky IB, Robertson AD, et al. Dose-related effects of methadone on QT prolongation in a series of patients with torsade de pointes. *Pharmacotherapy* 2003;23(6):802–805.

2. Linker NJ, Colonna P, Kekwick CA, et al. Assessment of QT dispersion in symptomatic patients with congenital long QT syndromes. *Am J Cardiol* 1992;69(6): 634–638.

3. Olgin JaZD. In: Bonow R, Zipes D, Libby P, eds. *Braunwald's Heart Disease: A Textbook of Cardiovascular Medicine*. 9th ed. Philadelphia, PA: Elsevier; 2011: 771–824.

4. Littmann L, Taylor L III, Brearley WD Jr. ST-segment elevation: a common finding in severe hypercalcemia. *J Electrocardiol* 2007;40(1):60–62.

5. Baltazar R. *Electrolyte Abnormalities. Basic and Bedside Electrocardiography*. Philadelphia, PA: Wolters Kluwer/Lippincott Williams & Wilkins; 2009:396–413.

6. Wang K, Asinger RW, Marriott HJ. ST-segment elevation in conditions other than acute myocardial infarction. *N Engl J Med* 2003;349(22):2128–2135.

7. Diercks DB, Shumaik GM, Harrigan RA, et al. Electrocardiographic manifestations: electrolyte abnormalities. *J Emerg Med* 2004;27(2):153–160.

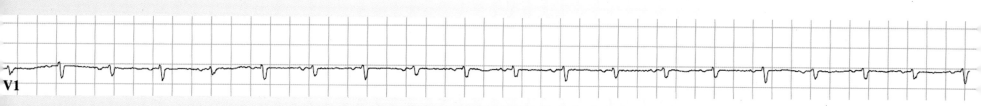

V1

Left Ventricular Hypertrophy

ECG Features

Increased Voltage

Leftward ventricular forces largely outweigh rightward forces and become unopposed briefly after right ventricular activation is completed. The resultant QRS complexes are exaggerated forms of those in a normal ECG (deeper S waves in V1 and taller R waves in V5–V6). There are a number of different sets of criteria for left ventricular hypertrophy (LVH) based on voltage. These criteria overall lack sensitivity, making the ECG a poor screening tool for LVH.[1] A few are presented in Fig. 9.1.

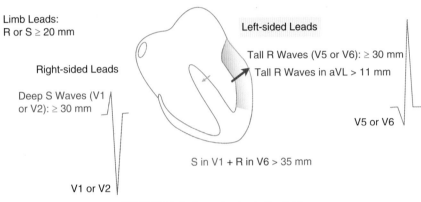

Limb Leads:
R or S ≥ 20 mm

Right-sided Leads

Deep S Waves (V1 or V2): ≥ 30 mm

V1 or V2

Left-sided Leads

Tall R Waves (V5 or V6): ≥ 30 mm
Tall R Waves in aVL > 11 mm

V5 or V6

S in V1 + R in V6 > 35 mm

FIGURE 9.1 Several criteria for LVH.

QRS Widening > 90 msec It takes longer for activation to spread from the endocardium to the epicardium in the thicker left ventricle. The QRS complex becomes slightly widened.

Left Axis Deviation Left axis deviation is associated with LVH.

ST Depression and T Wave Inversion Repolarization can occur before the entire left ventricular myocardium has depolarized. This can result in a downward shift of the ST segment in leads with tall R waves. Earlier repolarization of the endocardium allows repolarization to proceed from the endocardium to the epicardium and result in T wave inversion (TWI). TWI may also result from subendocardial ischemia.

Causes to Consider

Pressure Overload

Systemic Hypertension

Aortic Stenosis

Volume Overload

Aortic Regurgitation

Congestive Heart Failure

Hypertrophic Cardiomyopathy

Hypertrophic cardiomyopathy is an autosomal dominant genetic disorder known to cause sudden cardiac death in young people. Mutations affect the myocardial sarcomere.

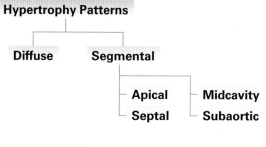

Hypertrophy Patterns
- Diffuse
- Segmental
  - Apical
  - Septal
  - Midcavity
  - Subaortic

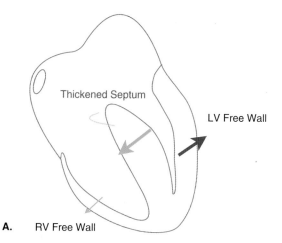

Thickened Septum

LV Free Wall

A.   RV Free Wall

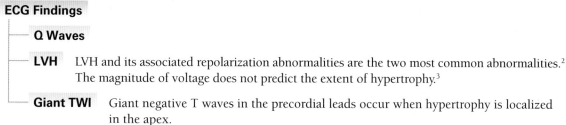

ECG Findings

- **Q Waves**
- **LVH**   LVH and its associated repolarization abnormalities are the two most common abnormalities.[2] The magnitude of voltage does not predict the extent of hypertrophy.[3]
- **Giant TWI**   Giant negative T waves in the precordial leads occur when hypertrophy is localized in the apex.

Clinical Presentations

Patients may complain of dyspnea on exertion, angina, presyncope, or syncope. Syncope may result from outflow tract obstruction or dysrhythmias.

Clinical Complications

- Atrial Fibrillation
- Ventricular Dysrhythmias
- Outflow Tract Obstruction
- Diastolic Dysfunction
- Infective Endocarditis
- Sudden Cardiac Death

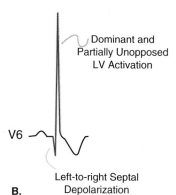

Dominant and Partially Unopposed LV Activation

V6

Left-to-right Septal Depolarization

B.

FIGURE 9.2 A. Vector forces in hypertrophic cardiomyopathy. **B.** Resultant QRS morphology.

Right Ventricular Hypertrophy

The ECG is fairly insensitive for demonstrating right ventricular hypertrophy (RVH) due to the opposing forces of the thicker left ventricle. The mass of the left ventricle is still greater than that of the right ventricle in patients with RVH. The presence of several ECG features, however, can be helpful in cases of significant RVH.

ECG Features

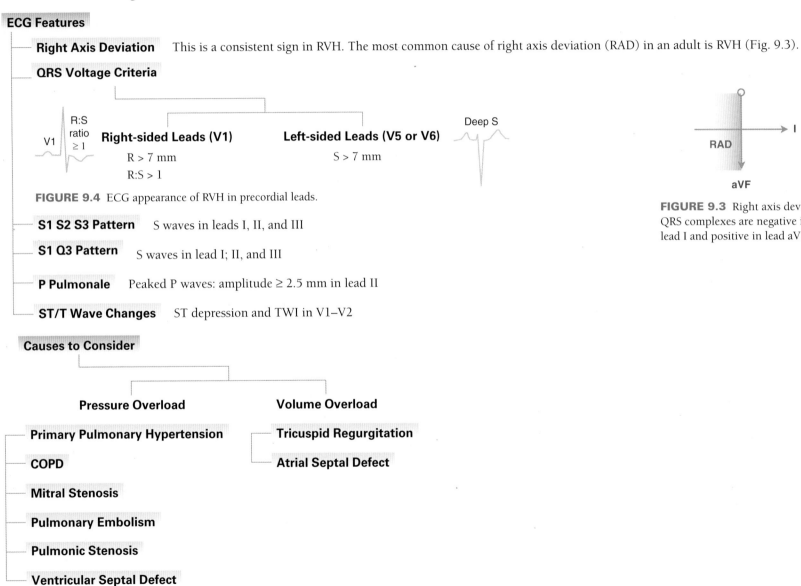

Right Axis Deviation   This is a consistent sign in RVH. The most common cause of right axis deviation (RAD) in an adult is RVH (Fig. 9.3).

QRS Voltage Criteria

V1 | R:S ratio ≥ 1

Right-sided Leads (V1)
R > 7 mm
R:S > 1

Left-sided Leads (V5 or V6)
S > 7 mm

Deep S

FIGURE 9.4 ECG appearance of RVH in precordial leads.

S1 S2 S3 Pattern   S waves in leads I, II, and III

S1 Q3 Pattern   S waves in lead I; II, and III

P Pulmonale   Peaked P waves: amplitude ≥ 2.5 mm in lead II

ST/T Wave Changes   ST depression and TWI in V1–V2

FIGURE 9.3 Right axis deviation. QRS complexes are negative in lead I and positive in lead aVF.

Causes to Consider

Pressure Overload

- **Primary Pulmonary Hypertension**
- **COPD**
- **Mitral Stenosis**
- **Pulmonary Embolism**
- **Pulmonic Stenosis**
- **Ventricular Septal Defect**

Volume Overload

- **Tricuspid Regurgitation**
- **Atrial Septal Defect**

COPD

ECG Findings

Lung Hyperinflation

Low Voltage   Air can dampen the ECG signal.

Vertical Heart Position   Lowered diaphragms cause the heart to be positioned more vertically.

Right Axis Deviation

Poor R-Wave Progression   Results from clockwise rotation of the vertical heart.

RVH in COPD   Deep S waves in V5 and V6
S1 Q3 T3 Pattern: S wave in lead I, abnormal Q wave in III, and TWI in III

The Lead I Sign   The P, QRS, and T wave vectors are all almost perpendicular to lead I. These waves in lead I have low amplitudes.

Pulmonary Embolism

The ECG may be normal or show only minor, nonspecific abnormalities even in the patient with significant pulmonary artery obstruction from pulmonary embolism.

ECG Findings

Rhythm   Normal sinus rhythm is more common than sinus tachycardia in acute submassive PE.[4]

Voltage   Low voltage in the limb leads has been reported in a significant minority of patients with PE.[5]

Signs of RV Strain

Right Bundle Branch Block   Incomplete or complete right bundle branch block (RBBB)

ST/TW Changes   ST depressions and TWIs in the anterior precordial leads are signs of anterior ischemia, which may correlate with severity of pulmonary embolism.[6] Normalization of inverted T waves can be a sign of decreased clot burden after thrombolysis.

P Pulmonale   Peaked P waves in II, III, and aVF reflect increased right atrial pressure, a down stream effect from increased pulmonary artery pressures. This sign has poor sensitivity.

S1 Q3 T3

A prominent S wave in lead I and a Q wave with inverted T wave in lead III has been described as a classic finding in a series of patients with PE. This sign has been shown to be equally prevalent in control groups[7] and occurs only in a minority (approximately 10%)[1] of patients with PE.

Right Axis Deviation

This has been taught as the classic axis associated with pulmonary embolism. Left axis, right axis, and indeterminate axis have all been described in the setting of PE. Several studies have reported that left axis deviation occurs as commonly as, or more commonly than, RAD in PE.[8]

The Low Voltage ECG

Criteria

Table 9.1 Low Voltage Criteria in Limb and Precordial Leads

Leads	Average QRS Height
Limb	<5 mm
Precordial	<10 mm

The Differential Diagnosis Low voltage can result from cardiac causes in which the myocardium fails to generate significant voltage. Low voltage can also result when sufficient voltage signal is attenuated by extracardiac factors. Some of these decrease the signal by increasing the distance from the heart to the chest wall.

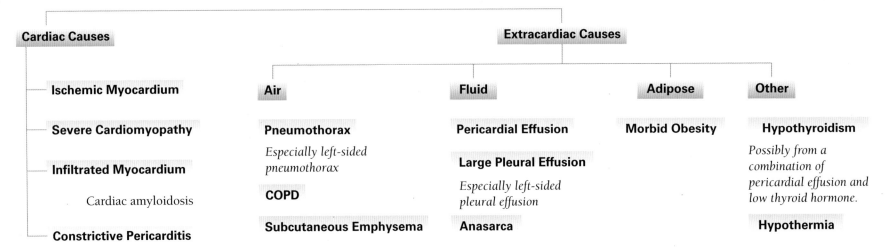

Cardiac Causes

— Ischemic Myocardium

— Severe Cardiomyopathy

— Infiltrated Myocardium

  Cardiac amyloidosis

— Constrictive Pericarditis

Extracardiac Causes

Air

Pneumothorax

Especially left-sided pneumothorax

COPD

Subcutaneous Emphysema

Fluid

Pericardial Effusion

Large Pleural Effusion

Especially left-sided pleural effusion

Anasarca

Adipose

Morbid Obesity

Other

Hypothyroidism

Possibly from a combination of pericardial effusion and low thyroid hormone.

Hypothermia

Electrical Alternans

QRS Wave Alternans

Pericardial Effusion   Alternating voltage of the QRS complex results from the pendular motion of the heart within a fluid-filled pericardial space.

SVT   Alternans can also occur at very high heart rates seen in re-entrant supraventricular tachycardias.

ECG 9.1a A 54-year-old woman presents with dyspnea.

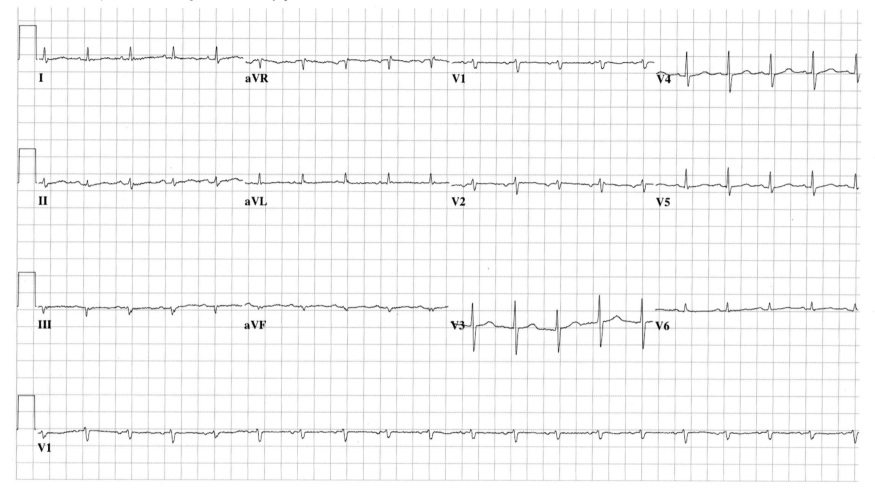

ECG 9.1b A 54-year-old woman presents with dyspnea.

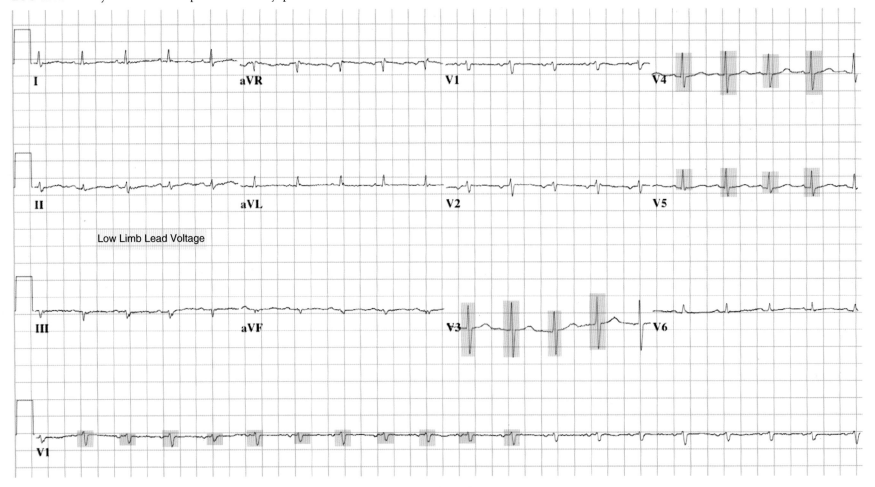

Electrical Alternans

The low voltage is most profound in the limb leads and right precordial leads. Subtle changes in QRS amplitude suggestive of pericardial effusion can be appreciated even in these low-voltage leads.

ECG 9.2a An asymptomatic 9-year-old boy with Friedreich's ataxia.

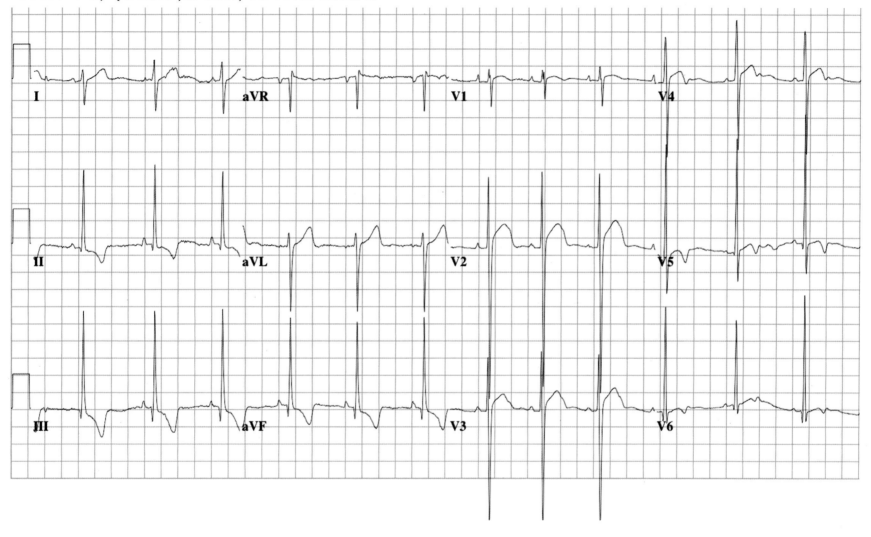

ECG 9.2b An asymptomatic 9-year-old boy with Friedreich's ataxia.

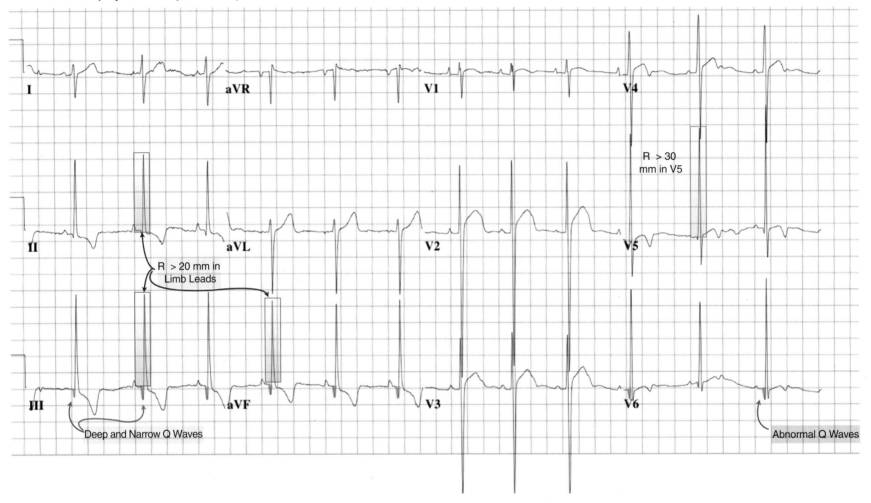

Hypertrophic Cardiomyopathy

Hypertrophic cardiomyopathy is associated with a number of syndromes (Friedreich's ataxia, Noonan syndrome, Lentiginosis), metabolic disorders (Hunter syndrome, Hurler syndrome, Fabry disease), and mitochondrial diseases.

ECG 9.3a A 33-year-old male presents with shortness of breath for 4 days and intermittent chest pain.

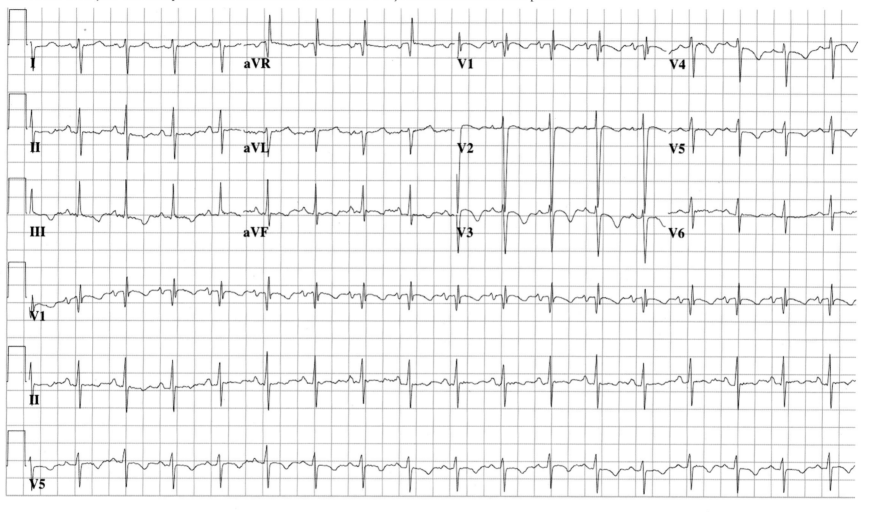

ECG 9.3b A 33-year old-male presents with shortness of breath for 4 days and intermittent chest pain.

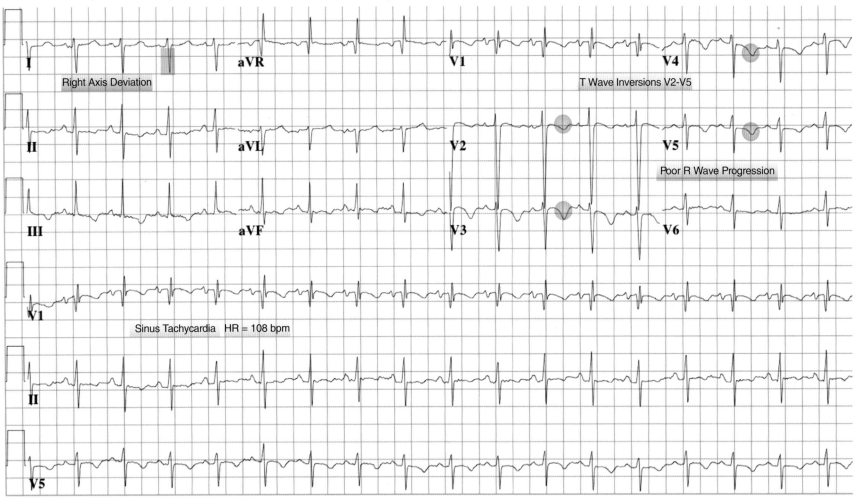

Massive Pulmonary Embolism

The poor R-wave progression and rS pattern throughout the precordial leads reflect RVH. This pattern can be seen in acute pulmonary embolism and chronic obstructive pulmonary disease (COPD). Note the T wave inversions present in the precordial and inferior limb leads. T wave inversions in the precordial leads are common in massive PE.[6] This patient was taken to the operating room where he underwent pulmonary embolectomy, closure of an atrial septal defect and removal of thrombus from the left atrium. He was noted to have significant pulmonary hypertension for several days following the surgery.

ECG 9.4a A 48-year-old woman complains of dyspnea on exertion.

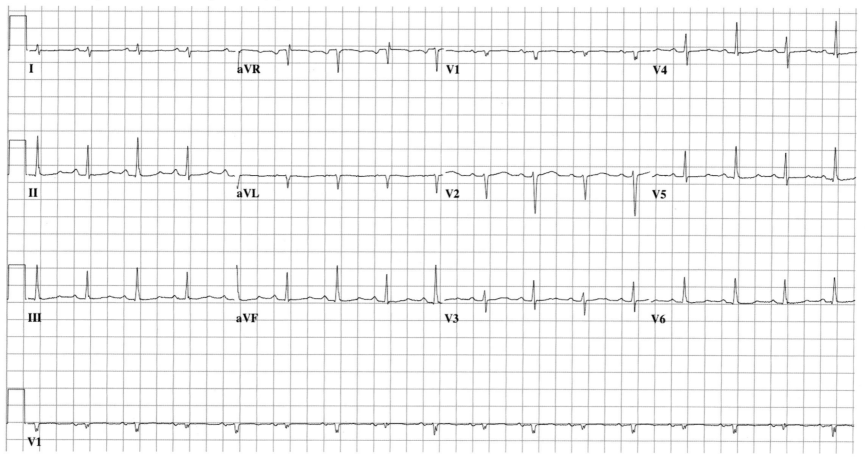

ECG 9.4b A 48-year-old woman complains of dyspnea on exertion.

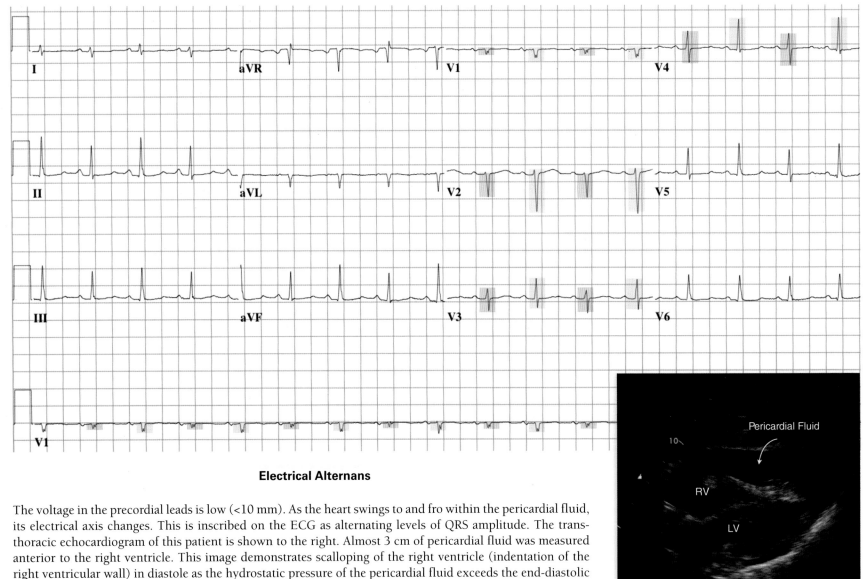

Electrical Alternans

The voltage in the precordial leads is low (<10 mm). As the heart swings to and fro within the pericardial fluid, its electrical axis changes. This is inscribed on the ECG as alternating levels of QRS amplitude. The transthoracic echocardiogram of this patient is shown to the right. Almost 3 cm of pericardial fluid was measured anterior to the right ventricle. This image demonstrates scalloping of the right ventricle (indentation of the right ventricular wall) in diastole as the hydrostatic pressure of the pericardial fluid exceeds the end-diastolic pressure of the right ventricle. This patient had 610 mL of fluid drained from the pericardial space.

FIGURE 9.5 Image from this patient's echocardiogram.

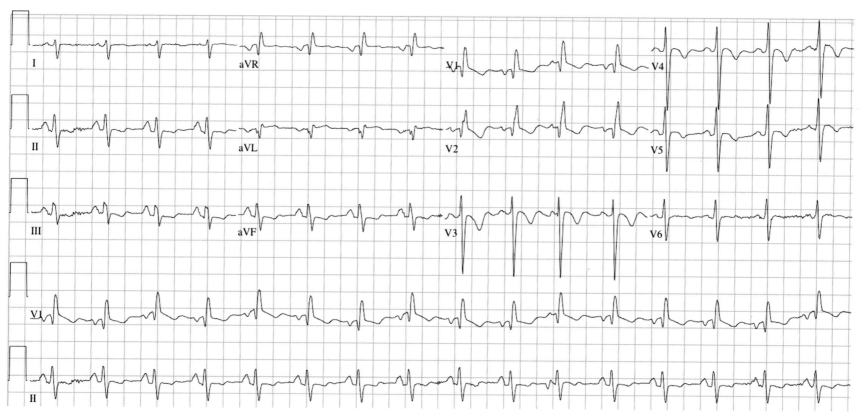

ECG 9.5a A 59-year-old presents with dyspnea and hypoxia (oxygen saturation 72% on room air).

ECG 9.5b A 59-year-old presents with dyspnea and hypoxia (oxygen saturation 72% on room air).

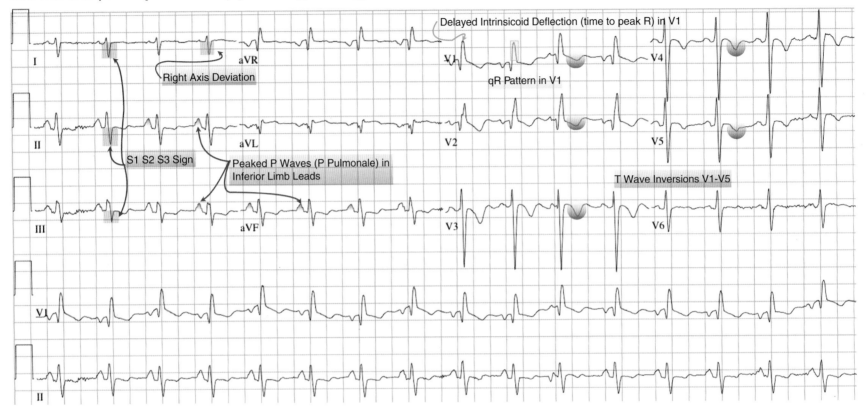

Right Ventricular Hypertrophy

A chest CT revealed centrilobular emphysema and dilated pulmonary arteries. There was no evidence of pulmonary embolism. RVH in this patient is secondary to COPD and pulmonary hypertension.

ECG 9.6a A 63-year-old male presents with lethargy and confusion.

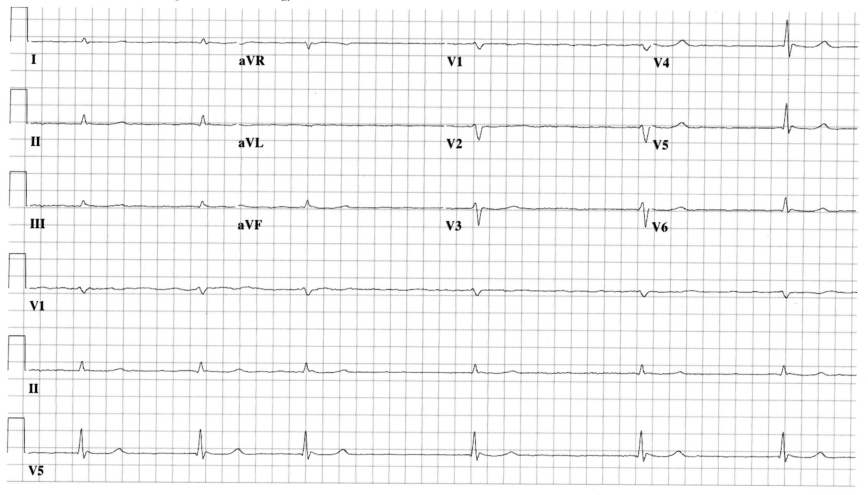

Reprinted from Martindale JL, et al. Altered mental status and hypothermia. *J Emerg Med* 2010;39(4):491–496, with permission from Elsevier.

ECG 9.6b A 63-year-old male presents with lethargy and confusion.

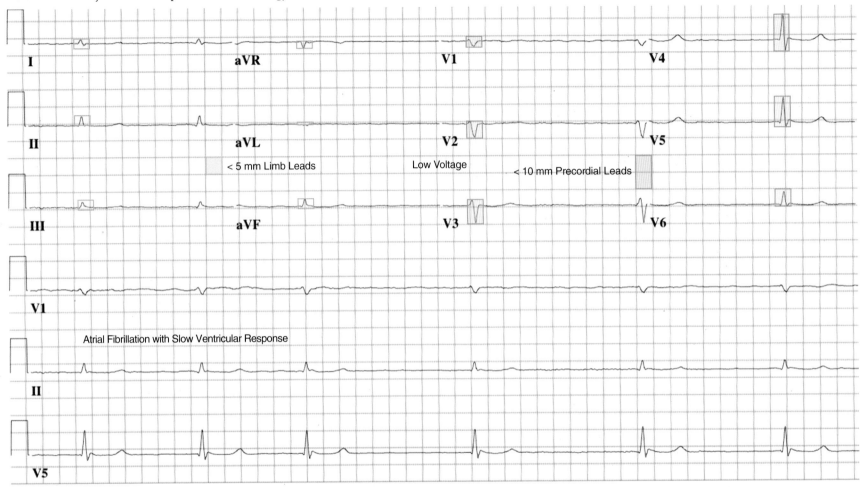

Hypothermia and Myxedema Coma

This patient's rectal temperature was 31°C (87.8°F). His serum TSH was 216.9 microunits/mL. Atrial fibrillation with slow ventricular response is a common arrhythmia in hypothermic patients.

ECG 9.7a A 67-year-old male presents with shortness of breath.

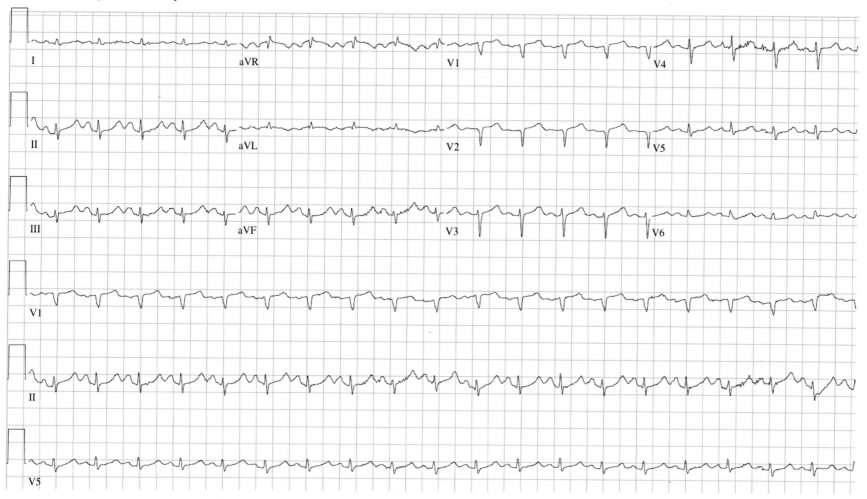

ECG 9.7b A 67-year-old male presents with shortness of breath.

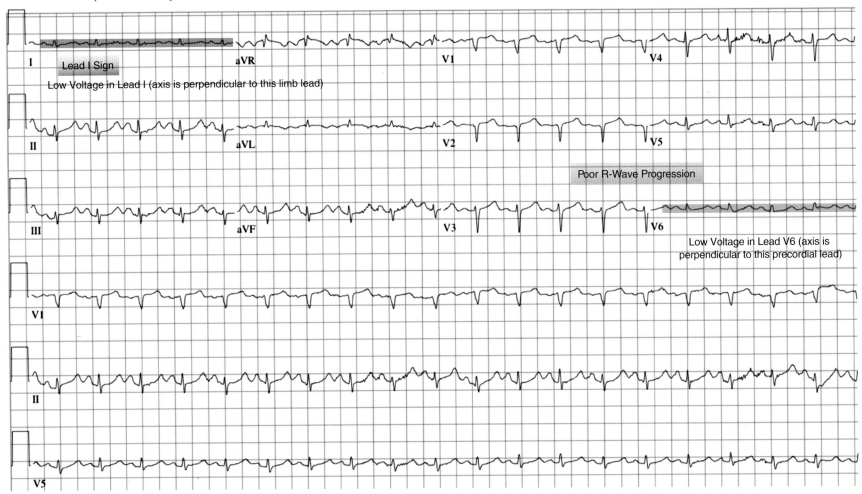

Chronic Obstructive Pulmonary Disease

ECG 9.8a A 46-year-old male is sent from his doctor's office for having a blood pressure of 230/110.

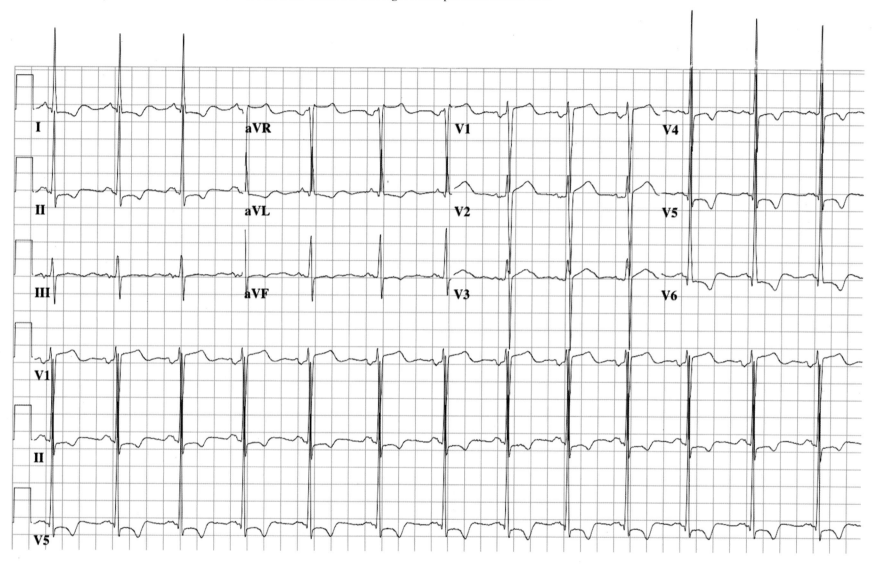

ECG 9.8b A 46-year-old male is sent from his doctor's office for having a blood pressure of 230/110.

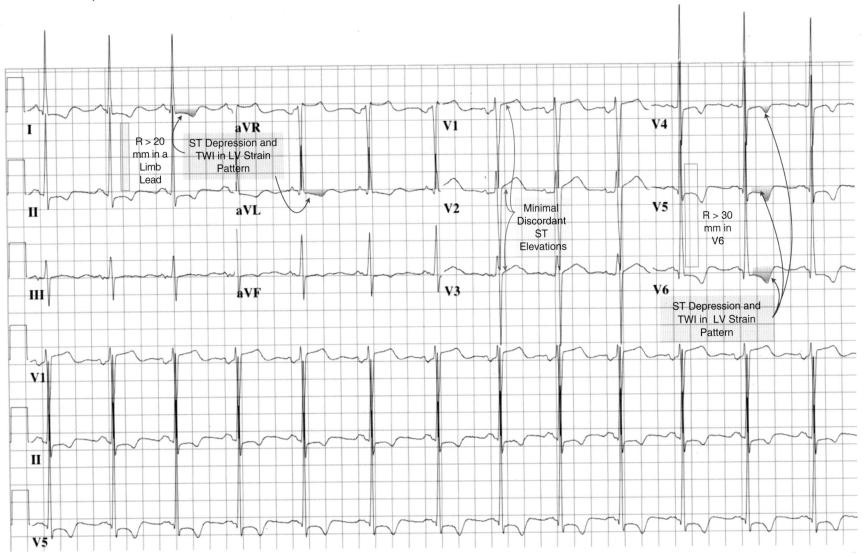

Left Ventricular Hypertrophy

ECG 9.9a An 83-year-old male on amiodarone presents with bradycardia, hypotension, and altered mental status.

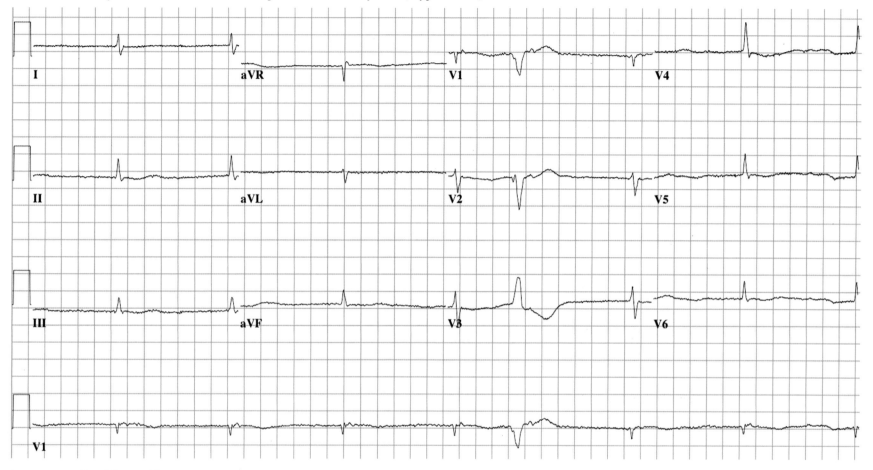

Image courtesy of Sarah Frasure, MD.

ECG 9.9b An 83-year-old male on amiodarone presents with bradycardia, hypotension, and altered mental status.

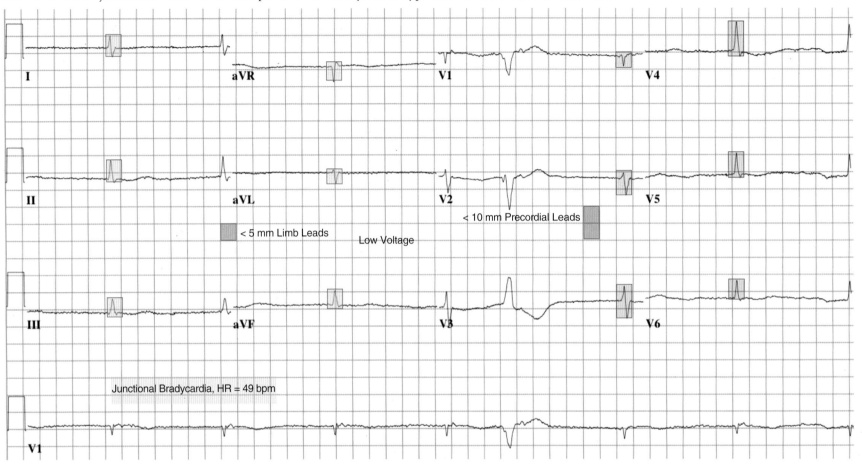

Mild Hypothermia and Myxedema Coma

This patient's rectal temperature was 92.9°F.

ECG 9.10a A 76-year-old with chronic atrial fibrillation and morbid obesity.

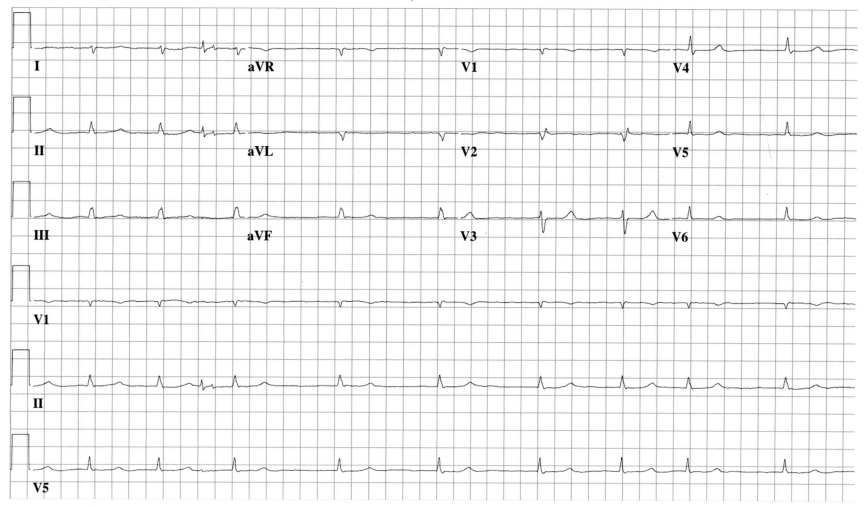

ECG 9.10b A 76-year-old with chronic atrial fibrillation and morbid obesity.

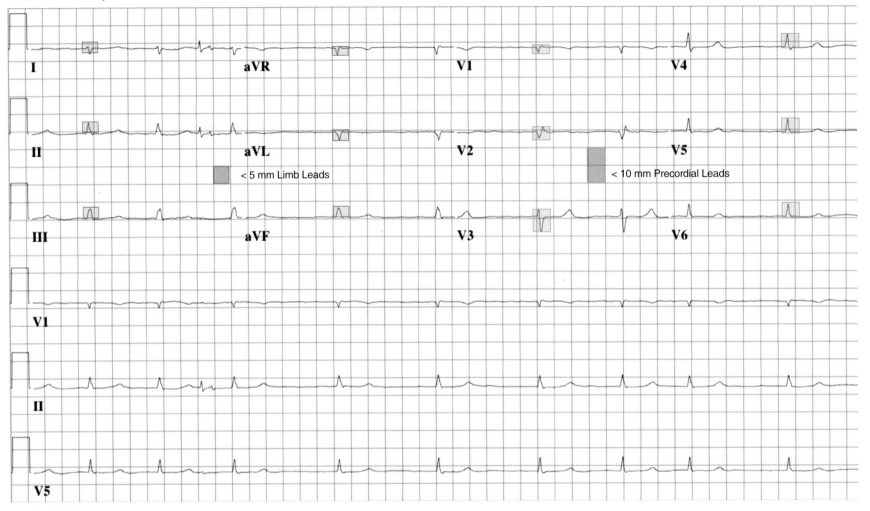

< 5 mm Limb Leads

< 10 mm Precordial Leads

Low Voltage

Fluid, air, and adipose tissue can all dampen ECG signal and result in low-voltage waveforms.

ECG 9.11a A 58-year-old man complains of dyspnea.

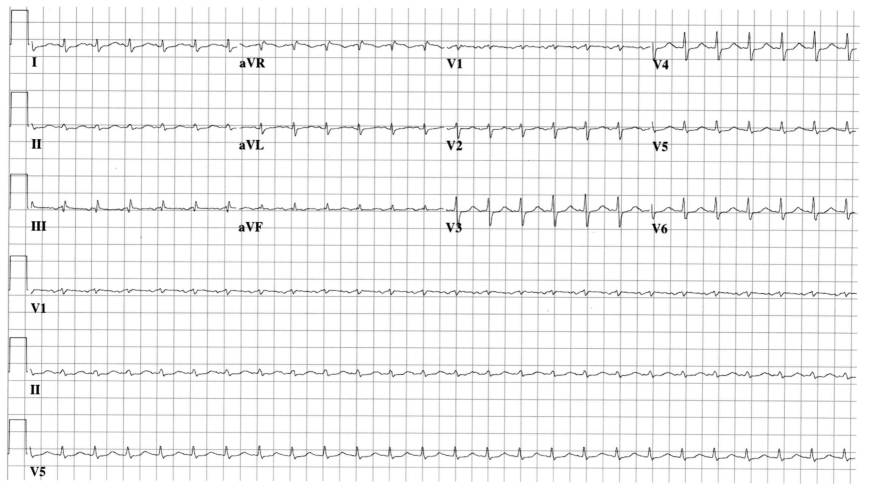

ECG 9.11b A 58-year-old man complains of dyspnea.

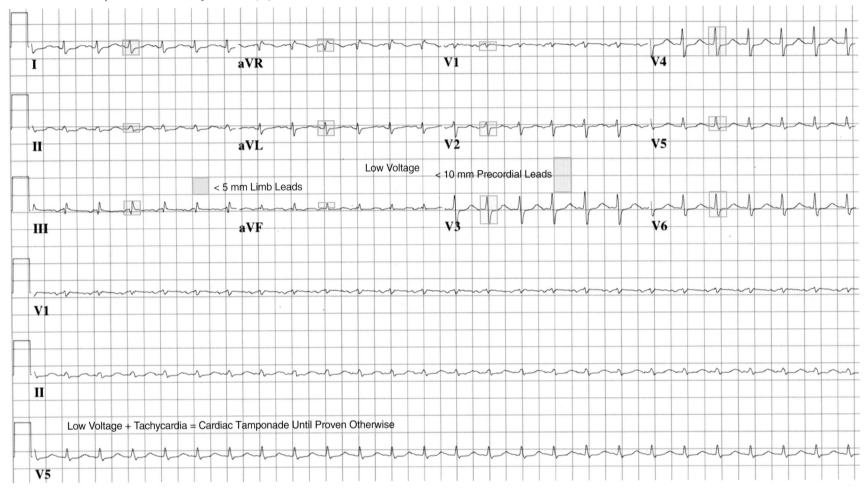

Cardiac Tamponade

This patient was taken urgently to the cath lab, where 1,250 mL of sanguinous pericardial fluid was drained. Cytology demonstrated high-grade large B-cell lymphoma.

ECG 9.12a

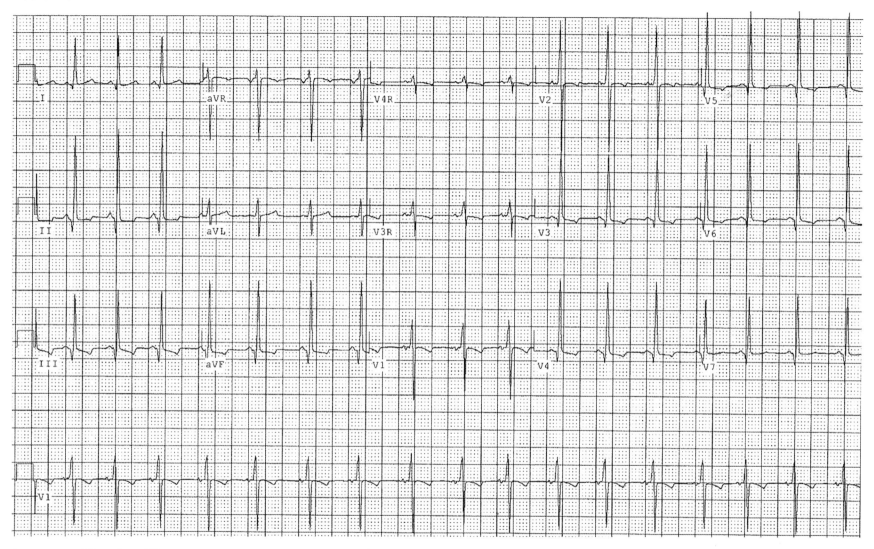

Image courtesy of Henry Cheng, MD.

ECG 9.12b

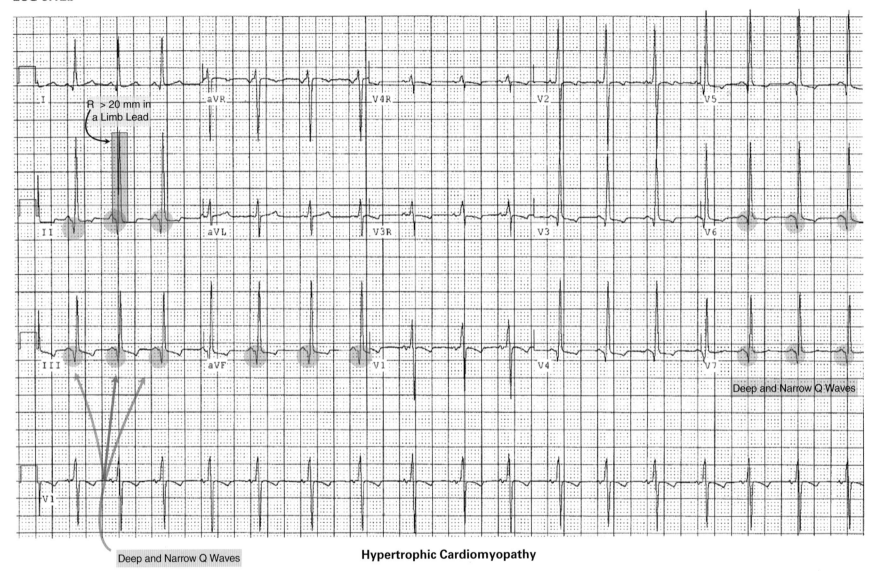

R > 20 mm in a Limb Lead

Deep and Narrow Q Waves

Deep and Narrow Q Waves

Hypertrophic Cardiomyopathy

ECG 9.13a A 60-year-old male complains of having to stop every 30 feet to catch his breath.

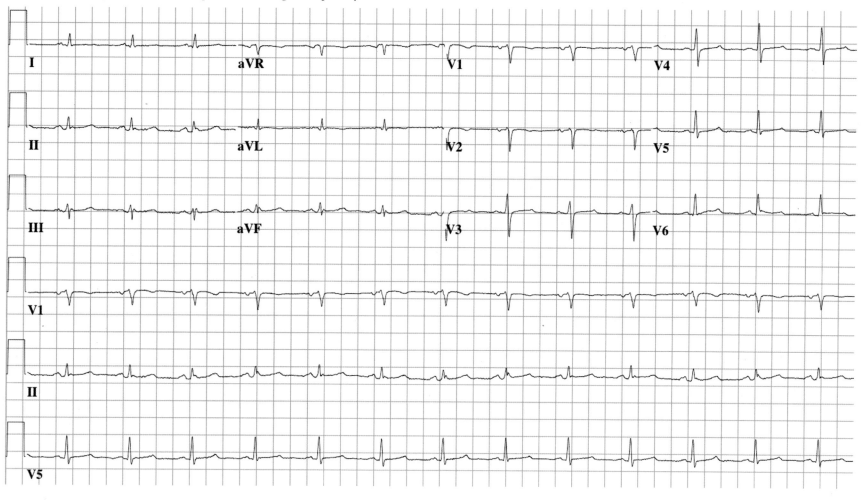

ECG 9.13b His ECG 1 year prior.

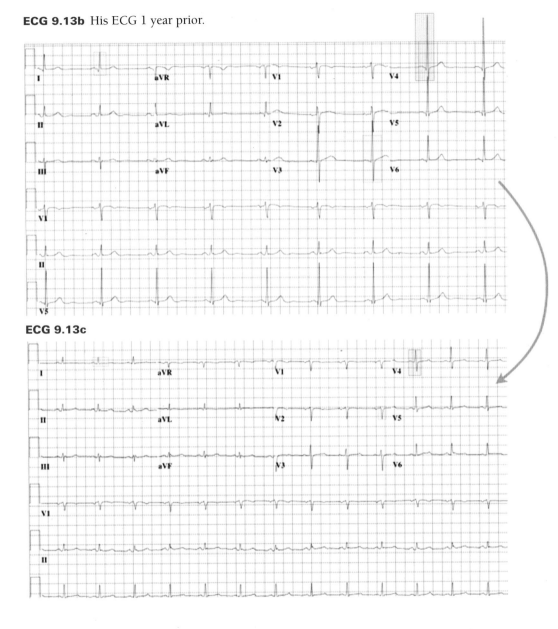

ECG 9.13c

FIGURE 9.6 This patient's echocardiogram.

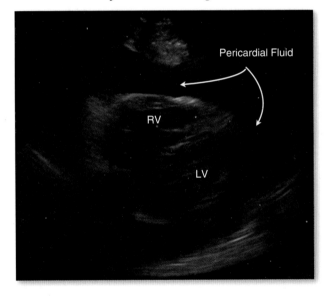

Cardiac Tamponade

The voltage of this patient's more recent ECG is notably less than the one obtained 1 year prior. Even if an ECG does not satisfy low voltage criteria, a significant decrease in voltage from a prior study can be clinically significant. This patient's transthoracic echocardiogram is shown to the right (Fig. 9.6). A total of 1,200 mL of fluid was drained during this patient's pericardiocentesis. The cytology obtained from this pericardial fluid demonstrated non-small cell lung cancer.

ECG 9.14a A 47-year-old male presents with chest pain.

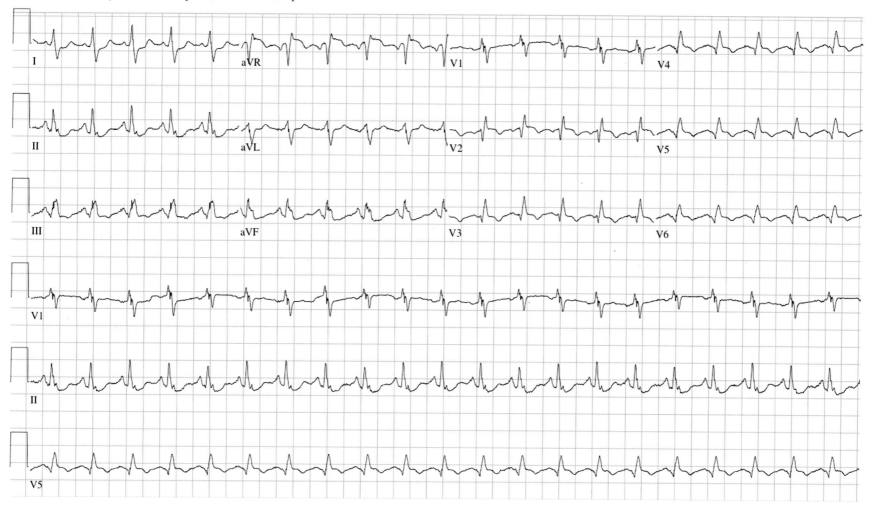

ECG 9.14b A 47-year-old male presents with chest pain.

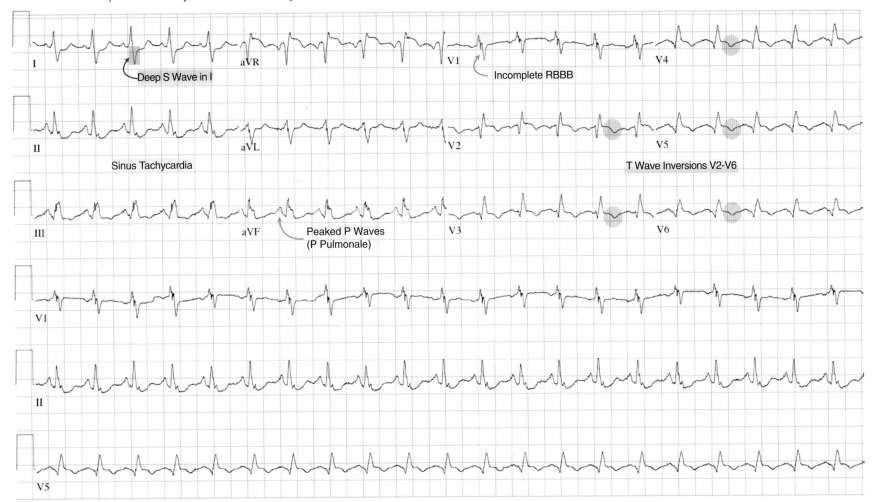

Saddle Pulmonary Embolism

References

1. Mirvis DaG A. Electrocardiography. In: Bonow RMD, Zipes D, Libby P, eds. *Braunwald's Heart Disease: A Textbook of Cardiovascular Medicine*. 9th ed. Philadelphia, PA: Elsevier; 2011.
2. Savage DD, Seides SF, Clark CE, et al. Electrocardiographic findings in patients with obstructive and nonobstructive hypertrophic cardiomyopathy. *Circulation* 1978;58:402–408.
3. Montgomery JV, Harris KM, Casey SA, et al. Relation of electrocardiographic patterns to phenotypic expression and clinical outcome in hypertrophic cardiomyopathy. *Am J Cardiol* 2005;96:270–275.
4. Richman PB, Loutfi H, Lester SJ, et al. Electrocardiographic findings in Emergency Department patients with pulmonary embolism. *J Emerg Med* 2004;27:121–126.
5. Stein PD, Dalen JE, McIntyre KM, et al. The electrocardiogram in acute pulmonary embolism. *Prog Cardiovasc Dis* 1975;17:247–257.
6. Ferrari E, Imbert A, Chevalier T, et al. The ECG in pulmonary embolism. Predictive value of negative T waves in precordial leads–80 case reports. *Chest* 1997;111:537–543.
7. Rodger M, Makropoulos D, Turek M, et al. Diagnostic value of the electrocardiogram in suspected pulmonary embolism. *Am J Cardiol* 2000;86:807–809, A10.
8. Lynch RE, Stein PD, Bruce TA. Leftward shift of frontal plane QRS axis as a frequent manifestation of acute pulmonary embolism. *Chest* 1972;61:443–446.
9. Tajiri J, Morita M, Higashi K, et al. The cause of low voltage QRS complex in primary hypothyroidism. Pericardial effusion or thyroid hormone deficiency? *Jpn Heart J* 1985;26:539–547.

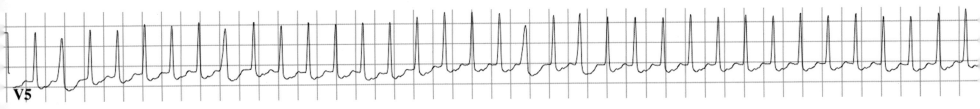

V5

Mechanisms Underlying Supraventricular Tachyarrhythmias

Reentry

Reentry occurs when the refractory periods and conduction speeds of two separate pathways differ. The initial impulse (marked by blue star) is often a premature complex. It encounters the anterograde limb in a state that can be depolarized while it encounters the other limb in its refractory period.

Increased Automaticity

Cells with pacemaker ability spontaneously depolarize. The speed of spontaneous depolarization is represented by the slope of phase 4 of the action potential. The steeper the slope, the faster the heart rate. The initial stimulus for these rhythms may be elevated adrenergic tone or toxicity from digitalis.

Triggered Activity

Afterdepolarizations are triggered by the depolarization in the previous action potential. They can occur during phase 2 or 3 (early after depolarizations) or during phase 4 of the action potential (late afterdepolarizations).

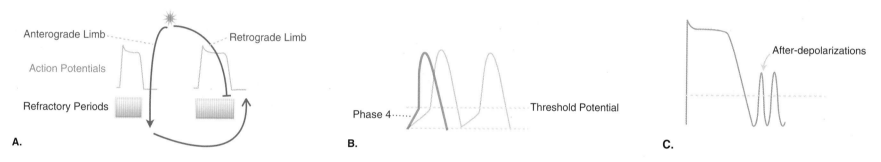

FIGURE 10.1 Schematic of A. reentry mechanism. B. Increased automaticity. C. Triggered mechanism.

Table 10.1 Comparison of reentry mechamisms

	Reentry	Increased Automaticity	Triggered Activity
Initial Event	Premature impulse	Increased adrenergic tone, digitalis toxicity	Digitalis toxicity
Onset	Sudden, abrupt	Gradual	

Narrow Complex Tachycardias Classified

There are a number of ways to classify supraventricular tachyarrythmias. A common way to separate them is by the underlying mechanisms: reentry, increased automaticity, and triggered activity. "Supraventricular" includes all territory above the bifurcation of the bundle of His (Fig. 10.2A,B).

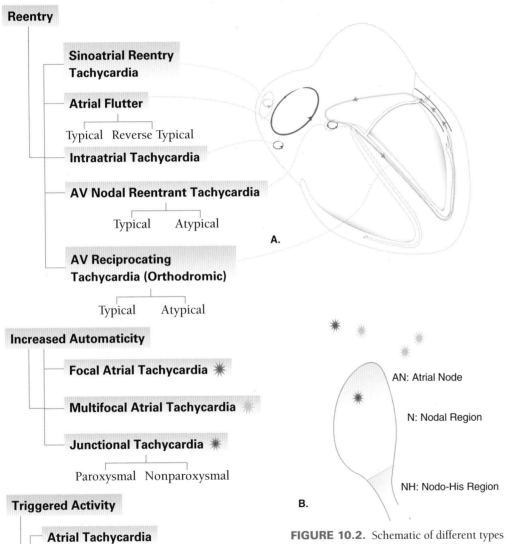

Reentry

- **Sinoatrial Reentry Tachycardia**
- **Atrial Flutter**
  - Typical   Reverse Typical
- **Intraatrial Tachycardia**
- **AV Nodal Reentrant Tachycardia**
  - Typical   Atypical
- **AV Reciprocating Tachycardia (Orthodromic)**
  - Typical   Atypical

Increased Automaticity

- **Focal Atrial Tachycardia**
- **Multifocal Atrial Tachycardia**
- **Junctional Tachycardia**
  - Paroxysmal   Nonparoxysmal

Triggered Activity

- **Atrial Tachycardia**
- **Nonparoxysmal Junctional Tachycardia**

A.

AN: Atrial Node

N: Nodal Region

NH: Nodo-His Region

B.

FIGURE 10.2. Schematic of different types of supraventricular rhythms resulting in narrow complex tachycardias. A. Reentry can occur within the sinus node or atrium, but most often involves the AV node. B. Foci capable of taking over a rhythm by increased automaticity are located within the atria and the AN and NH segments (shaded in) of the AV node. Several foci may be simultaneously in control.

Atrial Fibrillation

Atrial fibrillation (AF) is a common arrhythmia characterized by an irregularly irregular ventricular rhythm and extremely rapid atrial waves, called fibrillatory waves. AF is associated with significant morbidity and mortality related to thromboembolic complications.

Mechanism   AF involves different mechanisms. Independent foci with increased automaticity or triggered activity may simultaneously fire to initiate AF. Reentry in multiple circuits may perpetuate the rhythm. Foci within the pulmonary veins are often the origin of AF. They trigger premature depolarizations that propagate across the left atrium which can then activate several macroreentry circuits in the atria. A critical mass in the atria is required for these reentrant circuits to self-perpetuate. Pulmonary vein isolation is an effective method for treating paroxysmal AF.

In AF, the AV node is bombarded with atrial impulses. The ventricular rate depends on the balance of parasympathetic and sympathetic tone at the AV node.

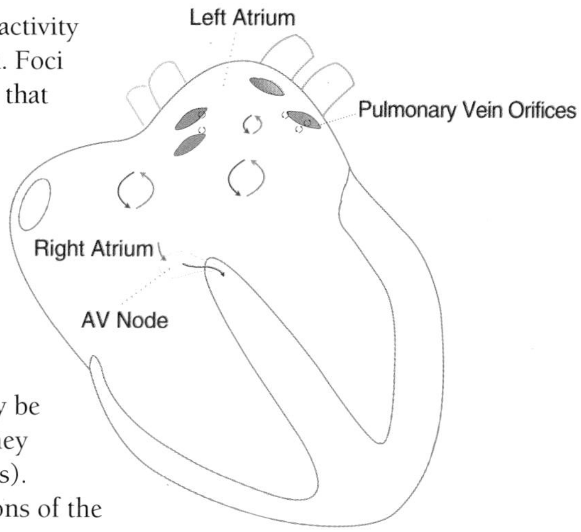

ECG Features

f Waves   Fibrillatory waves (f waves) represent independent reentrant waves within the atria. The rate of these waves is ≥ 350 bpm and they appear as undulations in the baseline. They may be coarse or fine. When very coarse, they may be mistaken for P waves and when very fine they may be imperceptible (diagnosis of AF is then based on the irregularity of the R-R intervals). Fibrillatory waves in V1 may appear uniform like flutter waves, but nonuniform undulations of the baseline present in other leads will help to differentiate AF from atrial flutter.

R-R Intervals   Irregularly irregular.

FIGURE 10.3 Schematic of micro- and macroreentrant circuits in atrial fibrillation.

Notable Ventricular Responses

Rapid Ventricular Response   When the QRS complexes are closer together, they may appear regular at first glance and the rhythm may be mistaken for reentrant supraventricular tachycardia (SVT).

Regularized Ventricular Response   Regular R-R intervals in a patient with AF represents complete AV dissociation. Digitalis toxicity is a notable cause. Regular rhythms may also occur if the patient is in an accelerated junctional rhythm or if the patient is paced.

Classification[1]:

Table 10.2   Classification of Atrial Fibrillation

Classification Term	Description
Paroxysmal	Terminates spontaneously within 7 days
Vagotonic	Afib initiated when vagal tone is higher; occurs in subset of patients with paroxysmal AF
Adrenergic	Afib initiated in setting of increased sympathetic activity; occurs in a subset of patients with paroxysmal AF
Persistent	Continuous for more than 7 days
Longstanding	Persistent for more than 1 year
Permanent	Longstanding AF refractory to cardioversion
Lone	AF in patients younger than 60 who do not have structural heart disease or hypertension

Atrial Flutter

Atrial flutter is a macroreentrant rhythm most commonly confined to the right atrium. The reentrant rhythm is usually initiated by a premature atrial beat. The atrial rate is regular and typically occurs at 250 to 350 bpm. In patients treated with antiarrhythmic medications, such as amiodarone, sotalol, or quinidine, the atrial rate can be less than 250 bpm. The ventricular rate depends on AV nodal conduction and is regular unless the rhythm is atrial flutter with variable conduction.

Typical Aflutter In typical atrial flutter, the rhythm is conducted counterclockwise up the atrial septal wall and down the free wall of the right atrium. This occurs in 90% of atrial flutter. Flutter waves are usually more obvious in the inferior leads.

Reverse Typical Aflutter In reverse typical atrial flutter, the atrial conduction proceeds down the septal wall and up the free wall of the atrium (clockwise in the frontal plane). Flutter waves are more obvious in the right precordial leads. This occurs in 10% of atrial flutter.

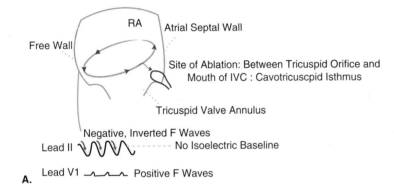

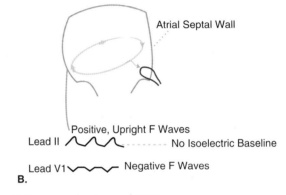

FIGURE 10.4 **A.** Typical atrial flutter mechanism and ECG appearance. **B.** Atypical atrial flutter mechanism and ECG appearance.

The reentrant circuit of atrial flutter can also occur in the left atrium or around surgical scars.
Because atrial conduction follows a single reentrant circuit, the atrial rate in this atrial rhythm is regular. The atrial rate is at least 240 bpm.

Flutter waves can be difficult to recognize, especially when there is 2:1 conduction. They can appear as follows:

S Waves
When they distort the QRS complex.

Buried
Within the QRS complex.

Inverted T Waves
When they are between two QRS complexes.

Mimics

Motion Artifact Motion artifact may appear as coarse P waves with some regularity. This can occur in Parkinson's disease.

Atrial Tachycardia Atrial flutter with 2:1 block and atrial tachycardia with 2:1 block can look similar. The atrial rate of atrial tachycardia (200 +/− 50 bpm) is slower than that of atrial flutter (300 +/− 50 bpm). In atrial tachycardia, the P waves in the inferior limb leads are typically upright with a discernible isoelectric line.

Supraventricular Tachycardia An abrupt cessation of the rhythm to vagal maneuvers or AV nodal agents is diagnostic of SVT. These agents will slow the ventricular response to atrial flutter but not convert flutter into sinus rhythm.

AV Nodal Reentrant Tachycardia (Typical)

AV nodal reentrant tachycardia (AVNRT) is the most common cause of paroxysmal SVT. A reentrant circuit can occur within nodal tissue when there is a difference in *conduction velocity* and *refractory period length* between two groups of cells.

The reentrant pathway is triggered by a premature atrial beat that encounters the fast AV nodal pathway in its refractory period. By default, the impulse is conducted down the available slow pathway. If anterograde conduction down the slow pathway is slow enough, it will encounter a fast pathway that is no longer in its refractory period. The impulse then conducts in a retrograde fashion up this fast pathway (Fig. 10.5).

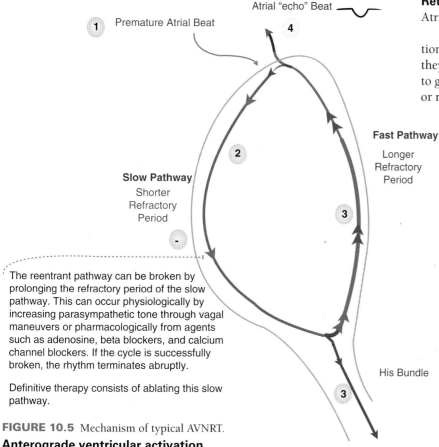

The reentrant pathway can be broken by prolonging the refractory period of the slow pathway. This can occur physiologically by increasing parasympathetic tone through vagal maneuvers or pharmacologically from agents such as adenosine, beta blockers, and calcium channel blockers. If the cycle is successfully broken, the rhythm terminates abruptly.

Definitive therapy consists of ablating this slow pathway.

FIGURE 10.5 Mechanism of typical AVNRT.

Anterograde ventricular activation

The resulting QRS is narrow and normal-appearing since activation of ventricular tissue occurs along the normal pathway from the AV node to the His Bundle and down both bundle branches. An abnormal QRS morphology results only if the patient has preexisting bundle branch or fascicular blocks.

The ventricular rate is typically between 150 and 250 bpm.

Retrograde Atrial Activation

Atrial conduction occurs in a retrograde fashion.

The P wave is often obscured by the QRS because ventricular and atrial activation from this reentry circuit occur nearly simultaneously. If P waves are visible, they are located very close to the QRS waveform. The P wave may be close enough to give the appearance of a pseudo-q wave if it occurs before the QRS or a pseudo-s or r wave if it occurs after the QRS complex.

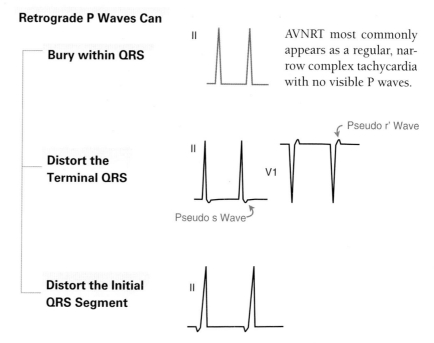

AVNRT most commonly appears as a regular, narrow complex tachycardia with no visible P waves.

FIGURE 10.6 Relationship of P waves to QRS complexes in typical AVNRT.

AV Nodal Reentrant Tachycardia (Atypical AVNRT)

In atypical AVNRT, the impulse conducts retrogradely to the atria through the slow pathway and anterograde down the fast pathway to the ventricles. The reentrant rhythm is initiated by an ectopic ventricular impulse.

ECG Features The ECG will appear as a regular, narrow complex tachycardia. Retrograde P waves will precede QRS complexes (Fig. 10.7).

FIGURE 10.7 Schematic of ECG in atypical AVNRT.

Mimics Atrial Tachycardia: A more common cause of inverted P waves preceding QRS waves is atrial tachycardia.

Treatment Maneuvers and medications that prolong the refractory period of the anterograde-conducting pathway within the AV node are used for acute treatment of the AVNRT. DC cardioversion is recommended for the hemodynamically unstable patient (Figs. 10.8 and 10.9).

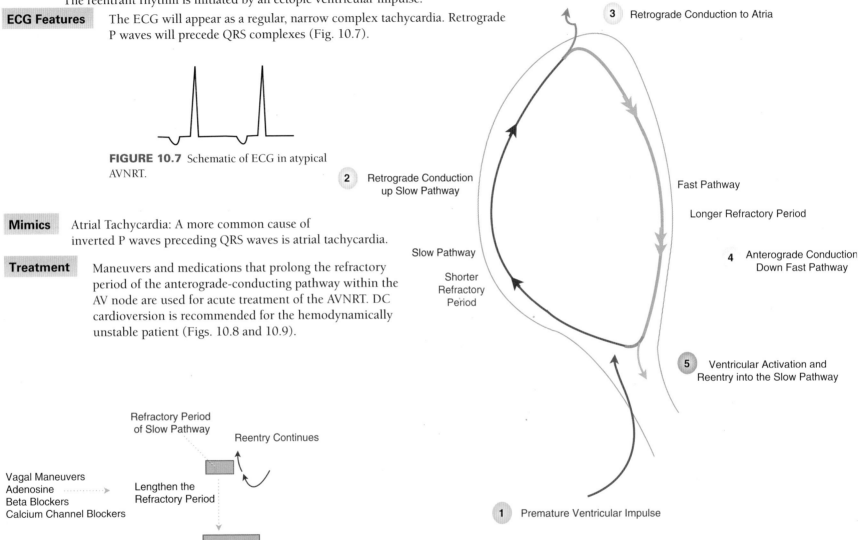

Vagal Maneuvers
Adenosine
Beta Blockers
Calcium Channel Blockers

Refractory Period of Slow Pathway

Reentry Continues

Lengthen the Refractory Period

Reentry Abruptly Stopped

FIGURE 10.8 Illustration of treatment mechanism in AVNRT.

3 Retrograde Conduction to Atria

2 Retrograde Conduction up Slow Pathway

Fast Pathway

Longer Refractory Period

Slow Pathway

Shorter Refractory Period

4 Anterograde Conduction Down Fast Pathway

5 Ventricular Activation and Reentry into the Slow Pathway

1 Premature Ventricular Impulse

FIGURE 10.9 Mechanism of atypical AVNRT.

Orthodromic Atrioventricular Reciprocating Tachycardia

This is a regular, narrow complex tachycardia, with a bypass tract that connects the atrium to the ventricle.

Mechanism

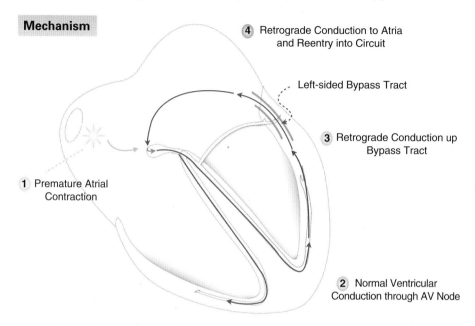

FIGURE 10.10 Schematic of AVRT involving a left-sided bypass tract and initiated by a PAC.

ECG Features Retrograde P waves typically appear separated from QRS complexes because ventricular and atrial impulses in orthodromic atrioventricular reciprocating tachycardia (AVRT) often occur at distinct times.

QRS complexes are narrow since both ventricles are activated simultaneously through the AV node.

Typically, the bypass tract conducts faster than the AV-nodal pathway. After ventricular activation through the AV node-His-Purkinje system, retrograde conduction via the bypass tract to the atria occurs relatively quickly. Inverted P waves in the inferior leads thus follow the QRS complex closely (short RP interval). When the bypass tract conducts slowly relative to the normal conduction system, the retrograde P wave appears farther from the preceding QRS complex (long RP interval). (Fig. 10.12)

Concealed Bypass Tract

When the bypass pact is capable of retrograde conduction only (from ventricle to atrium), the QRS complexes during normal sinus rhythm show no evidence of preexcitation. A concealed bypass tract can still function as part of a macroreentrant loop involved in AVRT and is responsible for approximately 30% of patients with SVT.[2] A bypass tract is considered *manifest* if it is capable of conducting in anterograde fashion, thereby causing ventricular preexcitation.

AVRT can be triggered by an ectopic atrial impulse. This impulse encounters an AV node no longer in its refractory state and a bypass tract that is still in its refractory period.

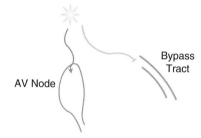

FIGURE 10.11 Initial event of reentrant tachycardia.

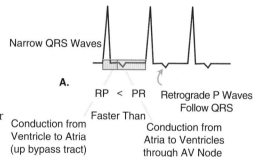

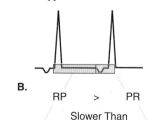

FIGURE 10.12 EKG appearance of A. typical and B. atypical AVRT.

Focal Atrial Tachycardia

Atrial tachycardia, an uncommon form of SVT, is generated from a single ectopic focus in the atria.

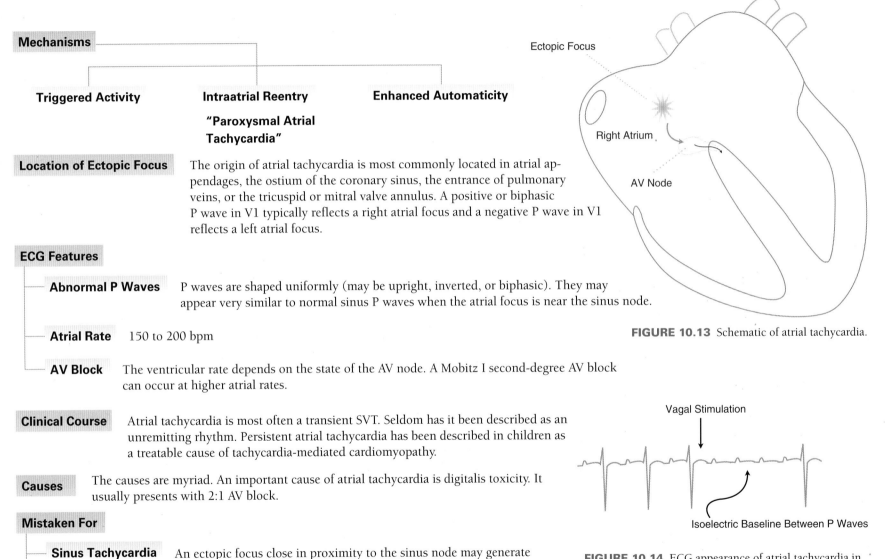

Mechanisms

Triggered Activity   **Intraatrial Reentry**   **Enhanced Automaticity**

"Paroxysmal Atrial Tachycardia"

Location of Ectopic Focus   The origin of atrial tachycardia is most commonly located in atrial appendages, the ostium of the coronary sinus, the entrance of pulmonary veins, or the tricuspid or mitral valve annulus. A positive or biphasic P wave in V1 typically reflects a right atrial focus and a negative P wave in V1 reflects a left atrial focus.

ECG Features

Abnormal P Waves   P waves are shaped uniformly (may be upright, inverted, or biphasic). They may appear very similar to normal sinus P waves when the atrial focus is near the sinus node.

Atrial Rate   150 to 200 bpm

AV Block   The ventricular rate depends on the state of the AV node. A Mobitz I second-degree AV block can occur at higher atrial rates.

Clinical Course   Atrial tachycardia is most often a transient SVT. Seldom has it been described as an unremitting rhythm. Persistent atrial tachycardia has been described in children as a treatable cause of tachycardia-mediated cardiomyopathy.

Causes   The causes are myriad. An important cause of atrial tachycardia is digitalis toxicity. It usually presents with 2:1 AV block.

Mistaken For

Sinus Tachycardia   An ectopic focus close in proximity to the sinus node may generate P waves that appear normal.

Atypical AVNRT   This is another cause of a regular, narrow complex tachycardia in which abnormal-appearing (inverted) P waves precede QRS complexes.

Ectopic Focus

Right Atrium

AV Node

FIGURE 10.13 Schematic of atrial tachycardia.

Vagal Stimulation

Isoelectric Baseline Between P Waves

FIGURE 10.14 ECG appearance of atrial tachycardia in lead V1. Because the ventricular rate depends on conduction through the AV node, slowed conduction from vagal maneuvers results in slowing of the ventricular rate and more distinct appearance of the ectopic P waves.

Junctional Tachycardia

Enhanced automaticity in the AV node or His Bundle can result in a regular, narrow complex tachycardia. Atria are typically activated by retrograde conduction from the AV node (Table 10.3).

Table 10.3 Comparison of the Two Types of Junctional Tachycardia Resulting from Increased Automaticity

	Nonparoxysmal Junctional Tachycardia	Paroxysmal Junctional Tachycardia
Atrial Rate	70–120 bpm	110–250 bpm
Onset/Termination	Gradual	Sudden
Otherwise known as...	Accelerated junctional rhythm	Focal junctional tachycardia

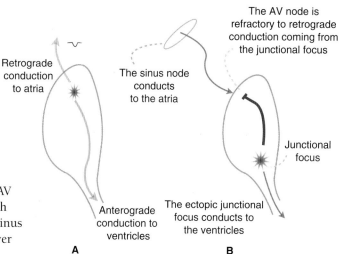

FIGURE 10.15 Diagrams of junctional tachycardia with A. retrograde conduction to the atria and B. blocked retrograde conduction. AV dissociation results when the sinus node controls the atrial rate and the junctional focus controls the ventricular rate. These two rates are very similar.

Mechanism

Accelerated junctional rhythm results from increased automaticity within the AV node. Segments within the AV node (AN and NH) contain pacemaker cells with their own automaticity. These cells have the potential to outpace those in the sinus node and take over ventricular conduction. They may also successfully take over atrial conduction by conducting in a retrograde fashion.

ECG Features

Inverted or Absent P Waves

P waves can occur before or after the QRS complexes. Because the impulse spreads superiorly to the atria, away from the more inferiorly located AV node, P waves are more often inverted in the inferior limb leads II, III, and aVF. Atrial and ventricular conduction can occur near-simultaneously from the junctional focus; P waves can be buried in QRS complexes.

AV Dissociation

The junctional focus may be able to conduct to the ventricles only. Retrograde conduction from this focus may be blocked by another part of the AV node. The sinus node then conducts to and gains control of the atria. This is one type of AV dissociation.

Regular Ventricular Rate

A normal and regular ventricular rate in the presence of atrial fibrillation indicates that the ventricular rate is dissociated from the atrial rate. The ventricular rate is controlled by accelerated automaticity of a pacemaker within the AV node. This form of AV dissociation is most commonly caused by digitalis toxicity.

Mistaken for:

AVNRT

Both junctional tachycardia and AVNRT produce regular, narrow complex tachycardias that lack visible P waves.

Multifocal Atrial Tachycardia

Multifocal atrial tachycardia (MAT) arises from several independent atrial foci competing simultaneously for conduction to the AV node. The resultant ventricular rhythm is irregularly irregular.

Mechanism   Enhanced automaticity.

ECG Features

Variable P waves   There are at least three consecutive P waves with different morphologies. Each morphology represents atrial conduction from a separate ectopic atrial focus (Figs. 10.16 and 10.17).

Rhythm   The PR intervals vary in length and the ventricular rhythm is irregularly irregular.

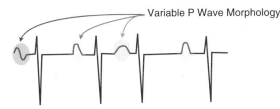

FIGURE 10.16 ECG appearance of MAT.

Causes   MAT is most commonly present in patients with exacerbations of COPD or other chronic lung diseases. Beta agonist therapy and theophylline may also be culprit causes.

Course   This rhythm can progress to AF and atrial flutter. More commonly, this rhythm will resolve when the underlying disease is treated.

Mistaken For   AF with rapid ventricular response.

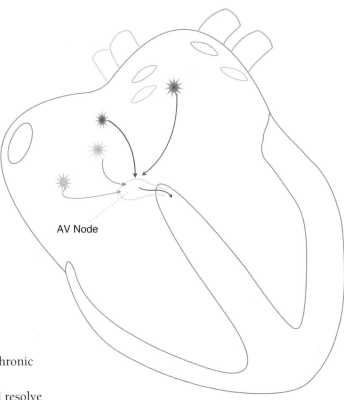

FIGURE 10.17 Schematic of MAT. Each star represents a separate ectopic atrial focus.

Causes of *Irregular* Narrow Complex Tachycardias

MAT   **Atrial Flutter with Variable Block**   **Atrial Fibrillation**

Digitalis Toxicity—Electrophysiology

Digoxin inhibits the Na+/K+ ATPase channel responsible for maintaining the resting membrane potential. Inhibition of this pump leads to an increase in intracellular sodium and a subsequent decrease in the concentration gradient that calcium efflux depends on. Intracellular calcium increases with resultant increase in inotropy.

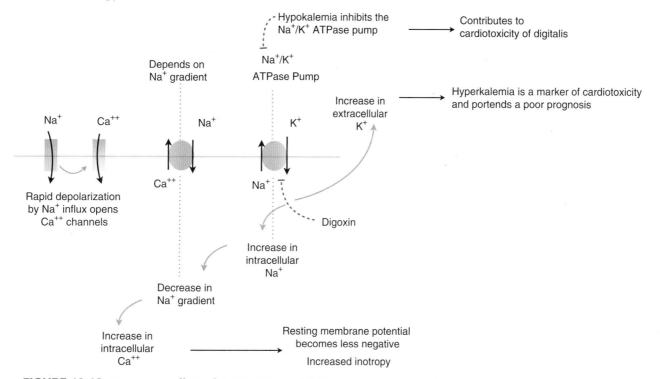

FIGURE 10.18 Downstream effects of Na+/K+ ATPase inhibition.

This type of toxicity is not limited to digitalis. It can result from toxicity of other cardiac glycosides by the same mechanism of sodium/potassium ATPase channel inhibition.

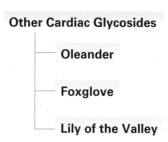

Other Cardiac Glycosides

— **Oleander**

— **Foxglove**

— **Lily of the Valley**

Digitalis Toxicity

There are a number of different ECG abnormalities that result from digitalis toxicity. They result from the drug's dual actions of increasing automaticity and slowing conduction.

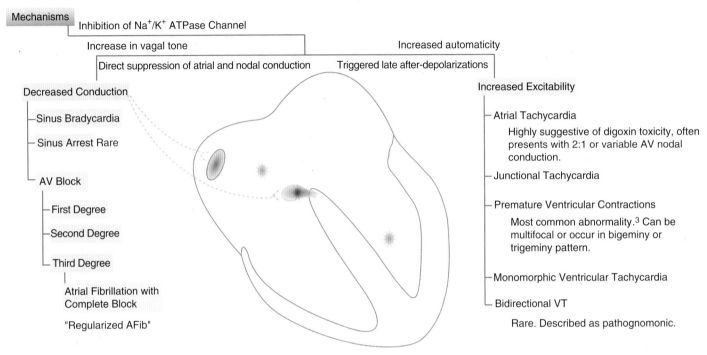

FIGURE 10.19 Schematic of digoxin toxicity. Blue stars indicate sites of increased automaticity, red coloring represents sites of decreased conduction.

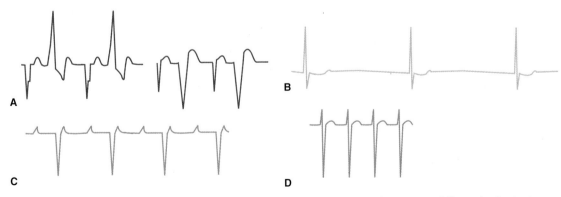

FIGURE 10.20 Four rhythms suggestive of digoxin toxicity. **A.** Bidirectional VT in two different leads. QRS direction may be concordant in some leads while discordant in others. **B.** AF with complete heart block. **C.** Atrial tachycardia with 2:1 or variable block. **D.** Junctional tachycardia.

ECG 10.1a

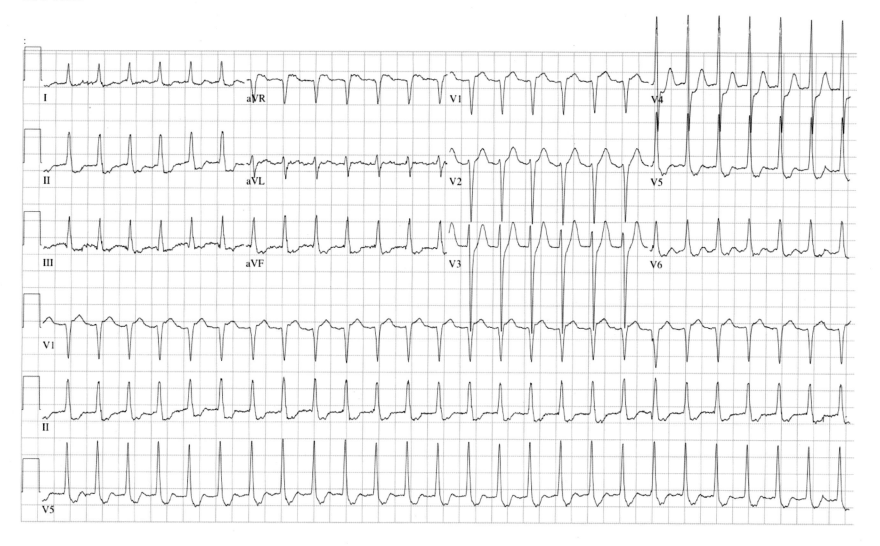

ECG 10.1b

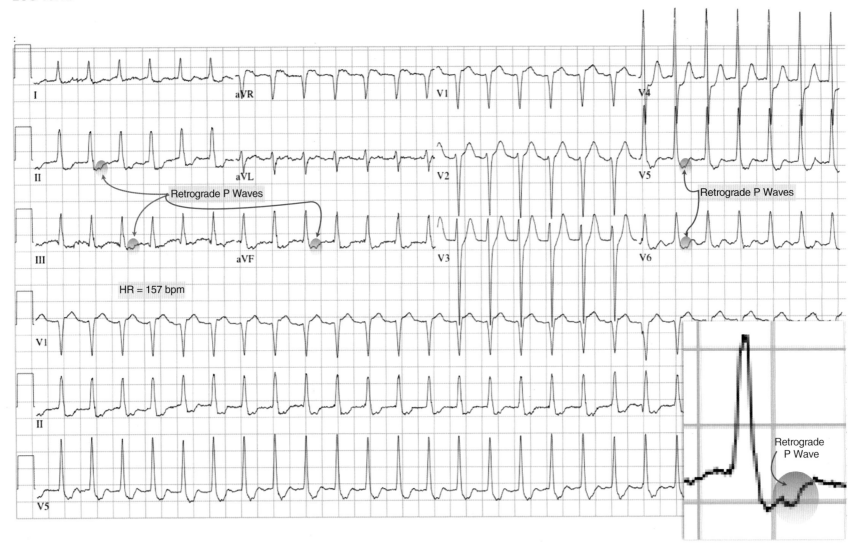

HR = 157 bpm

Reentrant SVT: AVNRT vs. AVRT

This rhythm is narrow, fast, and regular. The retrograde P waves, most notable in the inferior limb leads and lateral precordial leads, suggest a reentrant SVT (either AVNRT or AVRT). Without electrophysiologic studies, it is difficult to definitively classify this rhythm as AVNRT or AVRT.

ECG 10.2a A 74-year-old male complains of chest pain and shortness of breath.

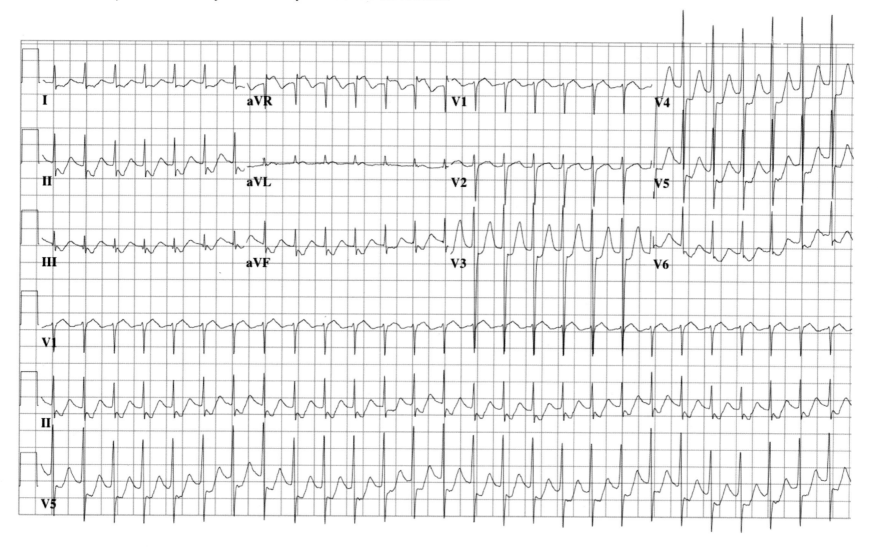

ECG 10.2b A 74-year-old male complains of chest pain and shortness of breath.

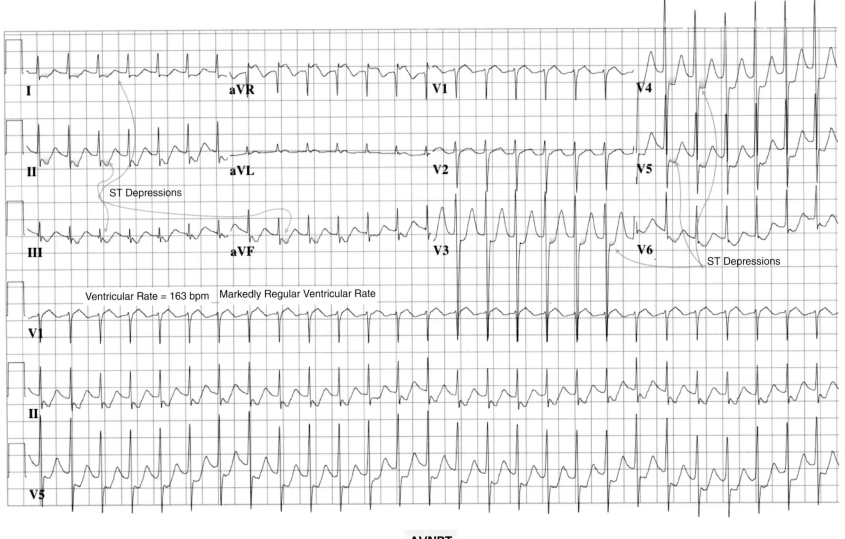

ST Depressions

ST Depressions

Ventricular Rate = 163 bpm   Markedly Regular Ventricular Rate

AVNRT

This is a regular and narrow complex tachycardia in which P waves are difficult to discern. The rhythm could be reentrant tachycardia, atrial tachycardia, or junctional tachycardia. When the focus of the rhythm is within the AV junction, P waves can be buried within the QRS waves because anterograde and retrograde impulses often occur simultaneously. There are diffuse ST depressions in this ECG. They likely reflect rate-related subendocardial ischemia. Cardiac markers in this patient were negative. ST changes disappeared once normal sinus rhythm was restored. In the electrophysiology lab, the patient underwent ablation of the slow pathway within the AV node.

ECG 10.3a A 49-year-old male presents with dyspnea and a sense of his heart racing.

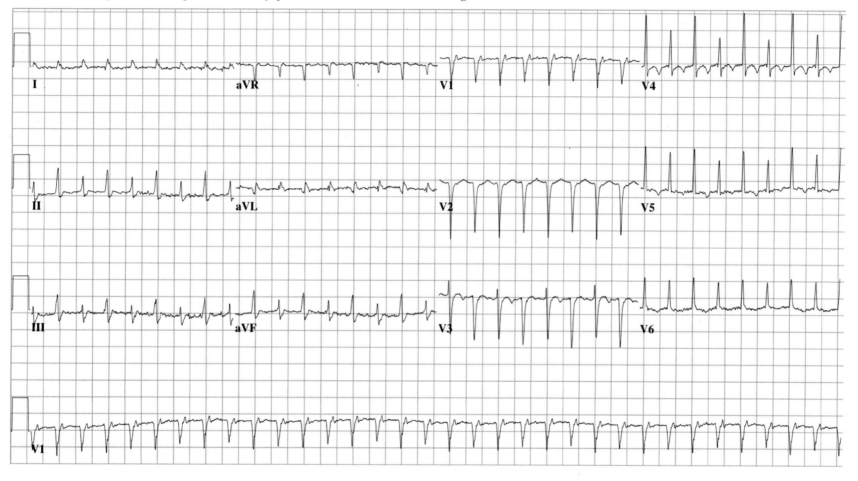

ECG 10.3b A 49-year-old male presents with dyspnea and a sense of his heart racing.

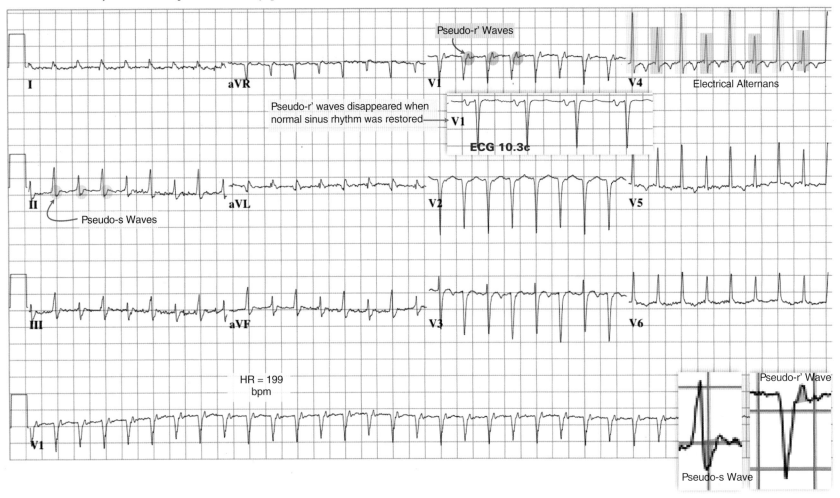

SVT: Likely AVNRT

This converted immediately to sinus tachycardia after a single dose of adenosine.

This ECG represents a reentrant SVT. Findings suggestive of AVNRT in this ECG include regular QRS complexes and distortion of the QRS complexes by retrograde P waves. This creates the appearance of pseudo-s waves in leads with positive QRS complexes and pseudo-r' waves in leads with predominantly negative QRS complexes.

Another notable finding in this ECG is the presence of electrical alternans. This patient did not have a pericardial fluid collection, and the alternans present in this ECG disappeared when he converted to sinus tachycardia at a much slower ventricular rate. Electrical alternans occurs in SVT and may be related to extremely fast heart rates.

ECG 10.4a

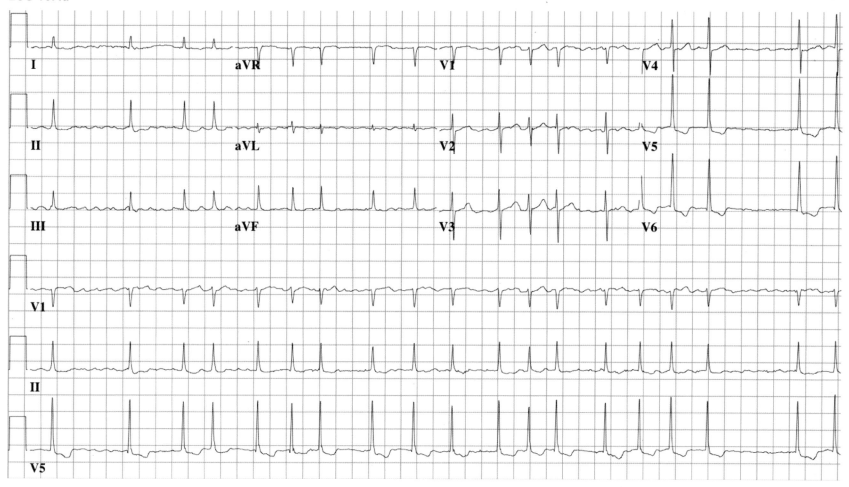

ECG 10.4b

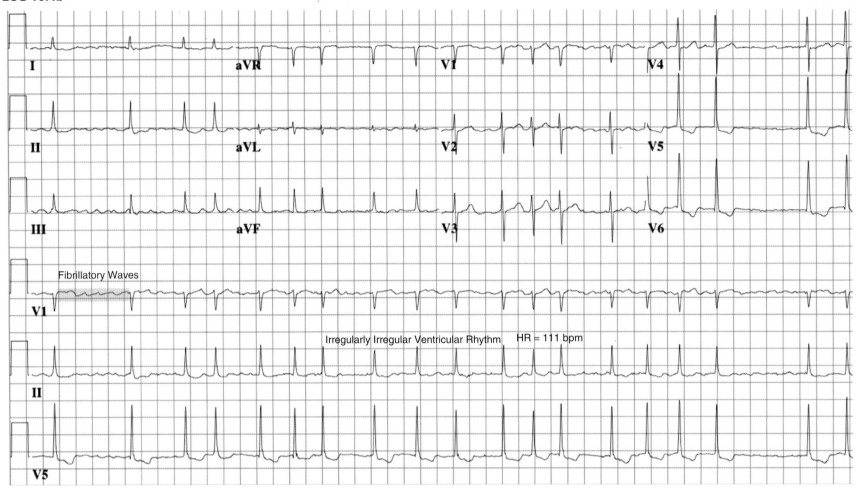

Atrial Fibrillation with Rapid Ventricular Response

Fibrillatory waves in lead V1 can be coarse and mistaken for flutter waves.

ECG 10.5a

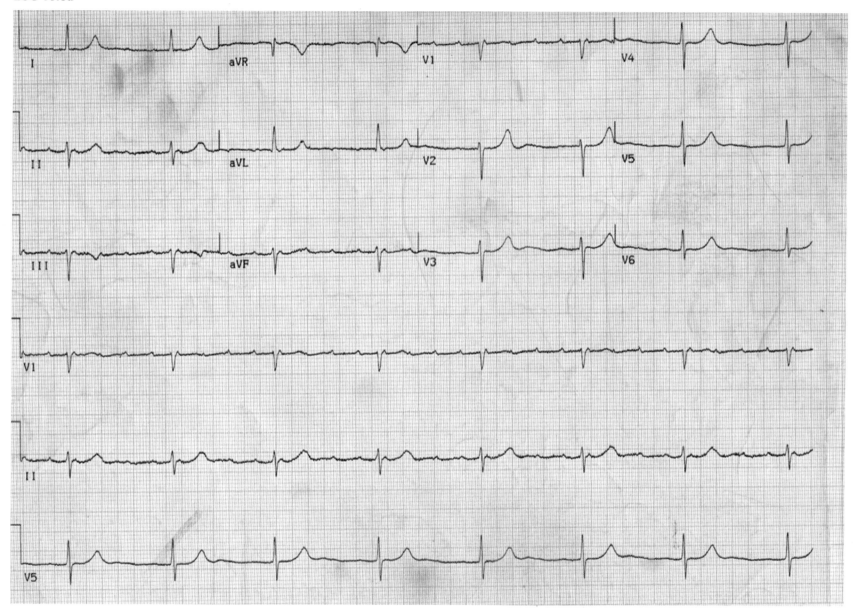

ECG 10.5b

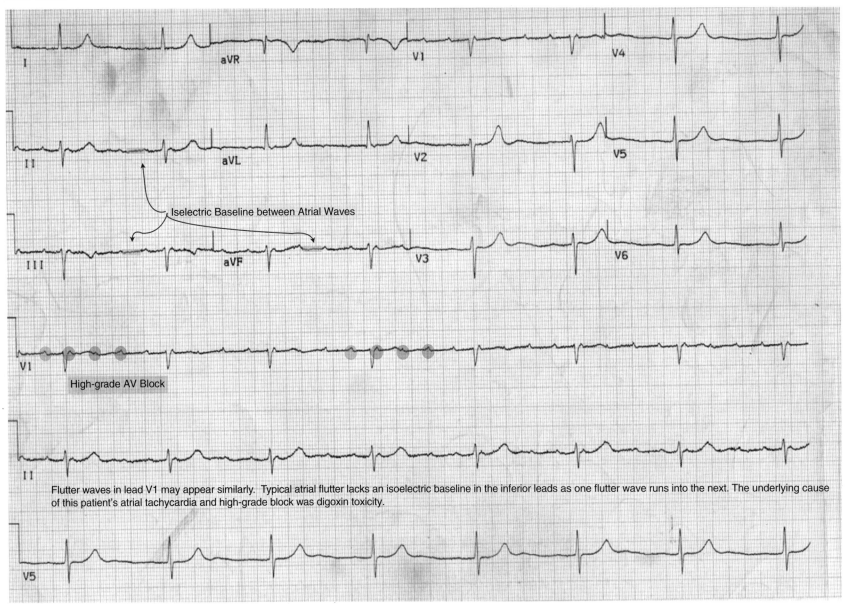

Iselectric Baseline between Atrial Waves

High-grade AV Block

Flutter waves in lead V1 may appear similarly. Typical atrial flutter lacks an isoelectric baseline in the inferior leads as one flutter wave runs into the next. The underlying cause of this patient's atrial tachycardia and high-grade block was digoxin toxicity.

Atrial Tachycardia with 4:1 AV Block

ECG 10.6a

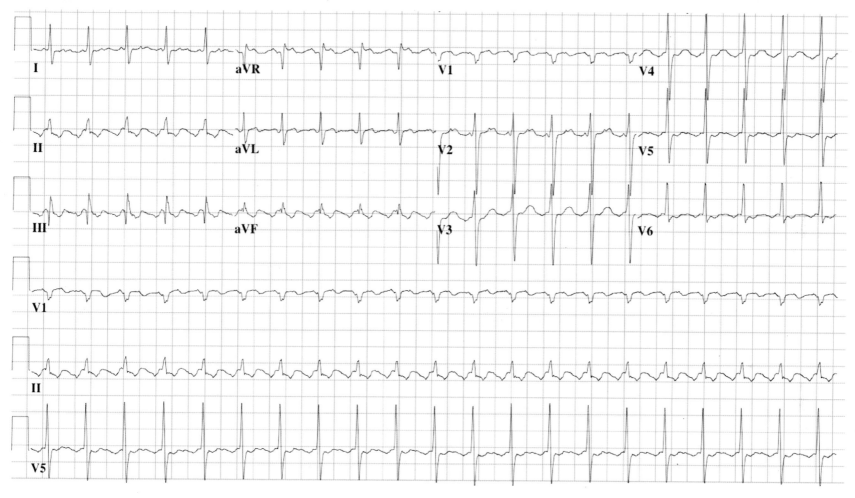

Image courtesy of Maya Yiadom, MD.

ECG 10.6b

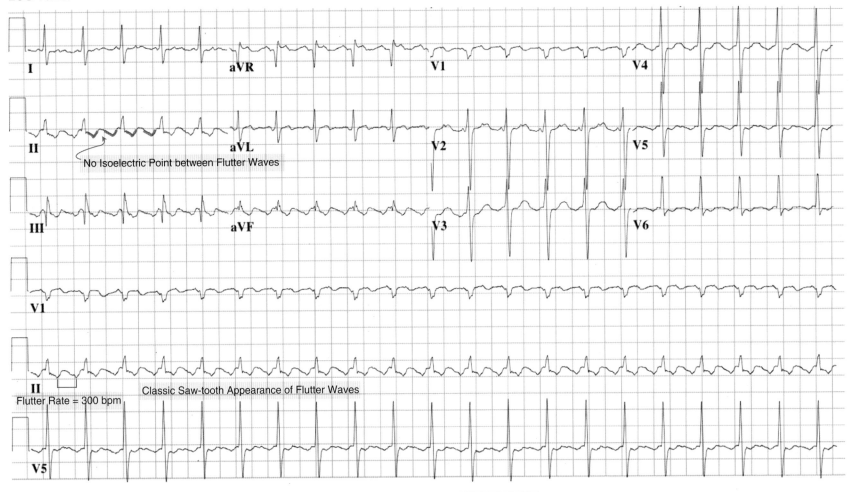

No Isoelectric Point between Flutter Waves

Flutter Rate = 300 bpm

Classic Saw-tooth Appearance of Flutter Waves

Atrial Flutter with 2:1 Conduction

ECG 10.7a A 63-year-old female complains of chest pain, shortness of breath, and fluttering in her chest.

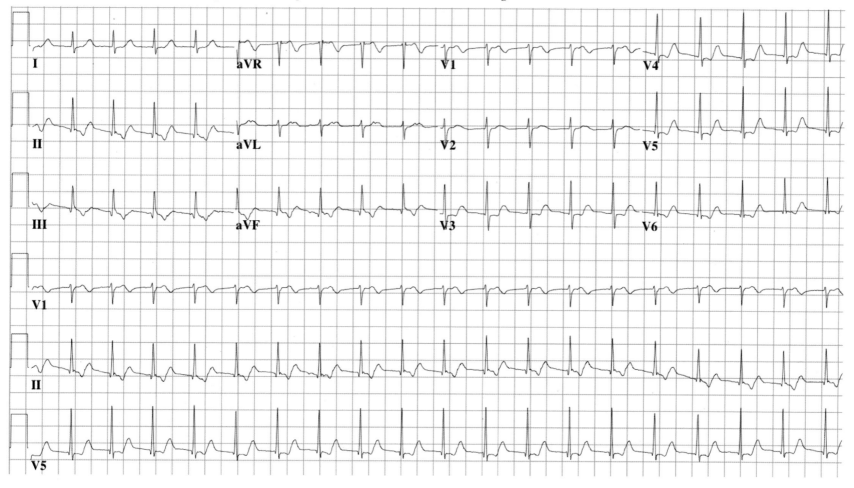

Image courtesy of Chris Kabrhel, MD.

ECG 10.7b A 63-year-old female complains of chest pain, shortness of breath, and fluttering in her chest.

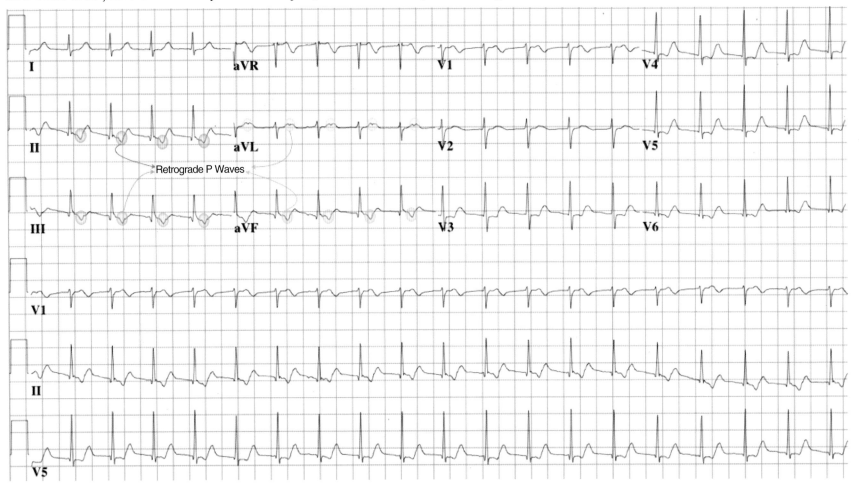

SVT: Likely AVRT

This patient broke into a normal sinus rhythm with Valsalva maneuver (ECG 10.7C). The space that separates QRS complexes and retrograde P waves suggests that AVRT is the underlying rhythm. The inverted P waves in this ECG depress the ST segments. In the absence of other signs of ischemia, these ST depressions are only artifacts from retrograde P waves.

ECG 10.7c This patient in sinus rhythm.

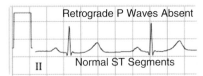

ECG 10.8a A 51-year-old male presents with palpitations, dyspnea, and light-headedness.

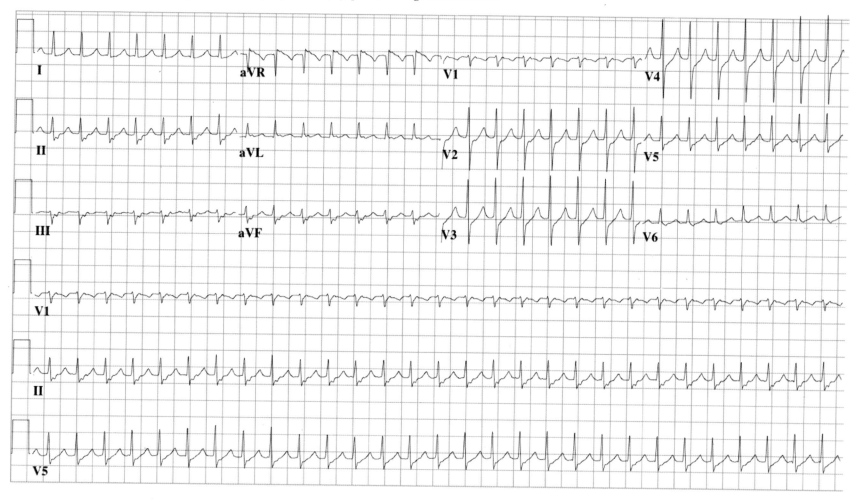

ECG 10.8b A 51-year-old male presents with palpitations, dyspnea, and light-headedness.

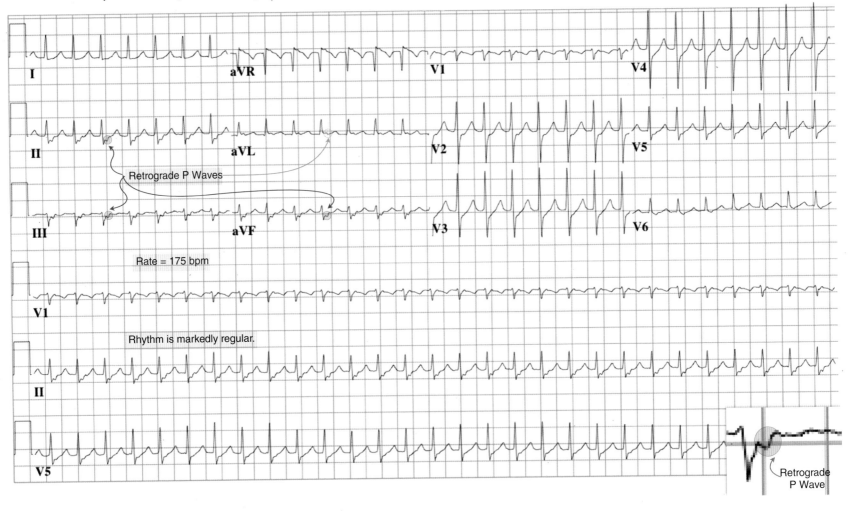

The patient converted to normal sinus rhythm after he received adenosine. This patient had an 11-year history of similar episodes. He underwent ablation of the slow pathway within the AV node.

AVNRT

ECG 10.9a

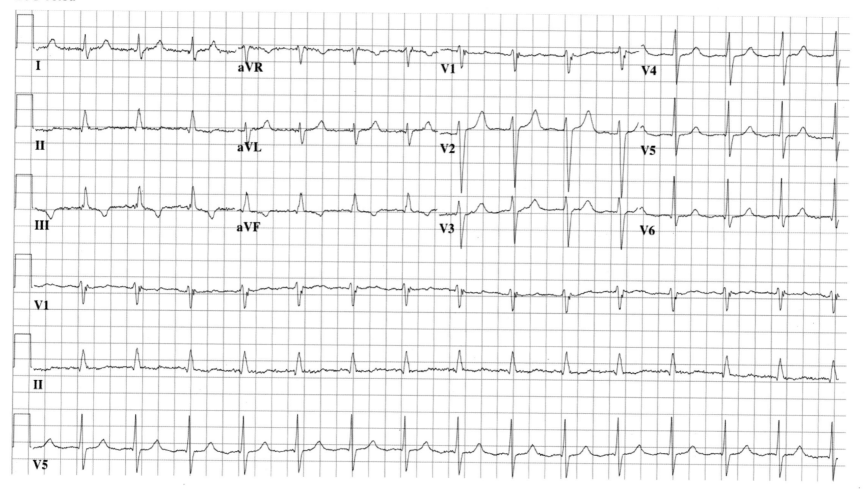

ECG 10.9b

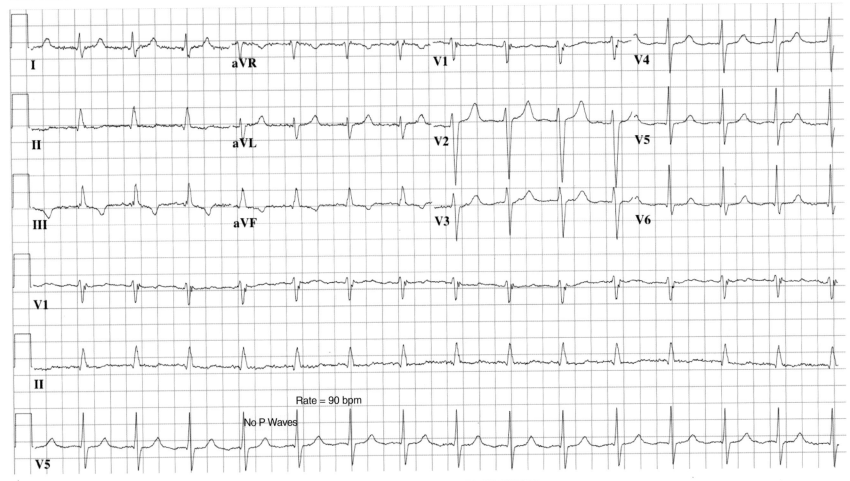

Accelerated Junctional Rhythm

ECG 10.10a

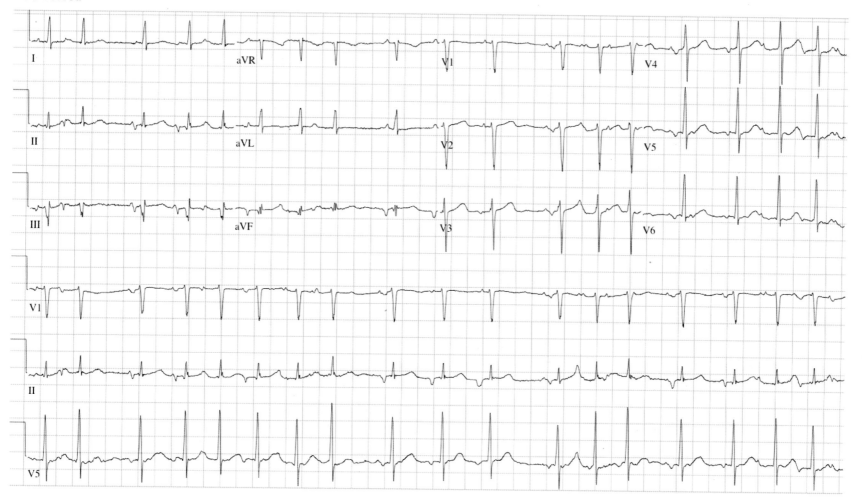

ECG 10.10b

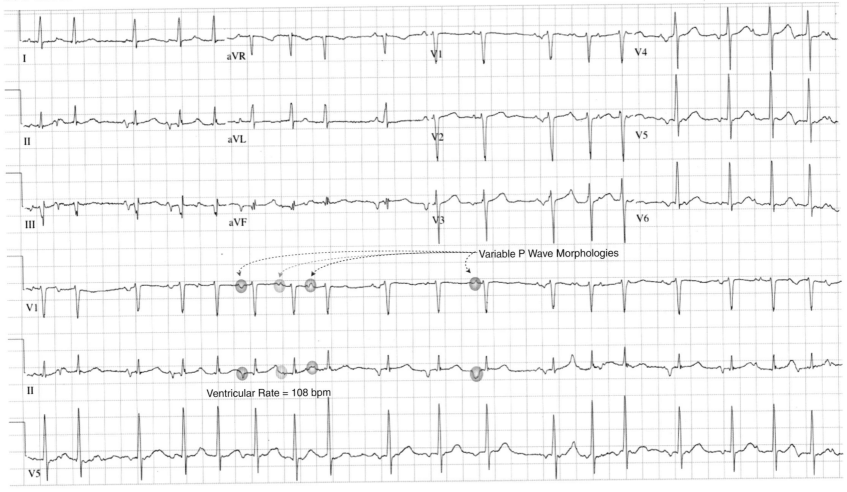

Multifocal Atrial Tachycardia

This rhythm could be mistaken for the more common AF with rapid ventricular response. However, distinct P waves can be appreciated preceding each QRS complex. The baseline between these P waves is isoelectric. The PR intervals in this rhythm vary, reflecting variable distances between these ectopic atrial sites and the AV node.

ECG 10.11a

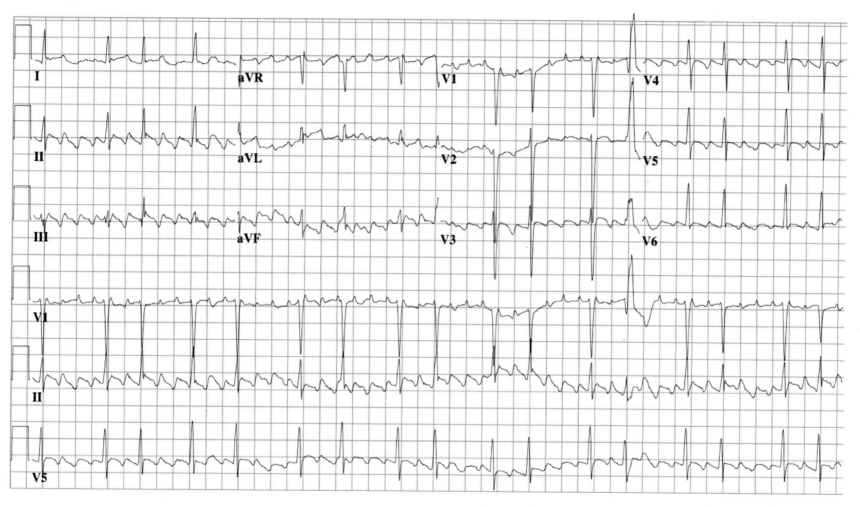

ECG 10.11b

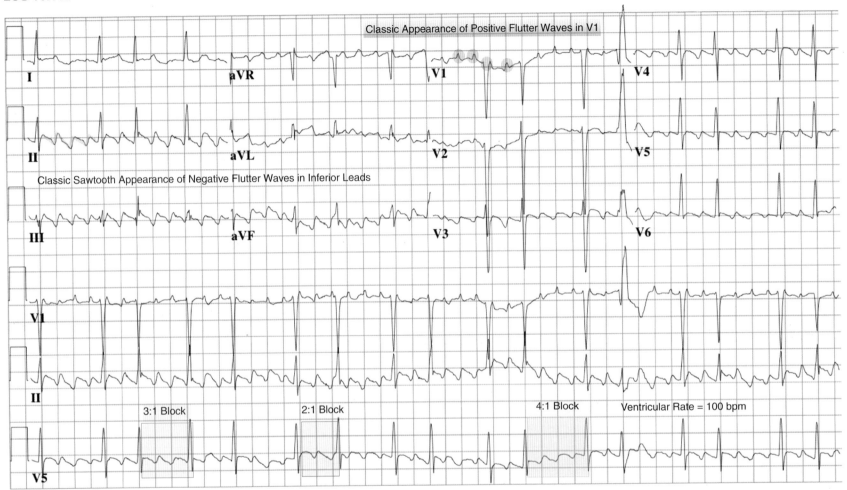

Classic Appearance of Positive Flutter Waves in V1

Classic Sawtooth Appearance of Negative Flutter Waves in Inferior Leads

3:1 Block   2:1 Block   4:1 Block   Ventricular Rate = 100 bpm

Atrial Flutter with Variable Block

ECG 10.12a

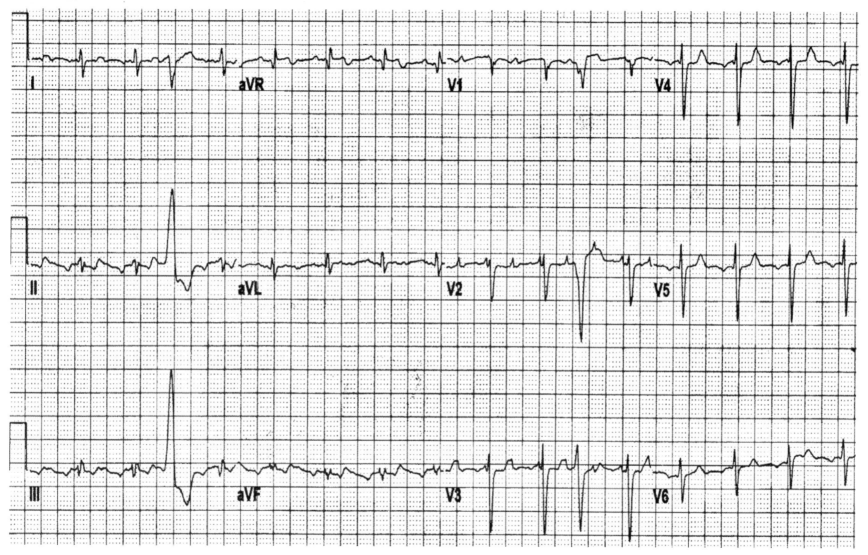

ECG 10.12b

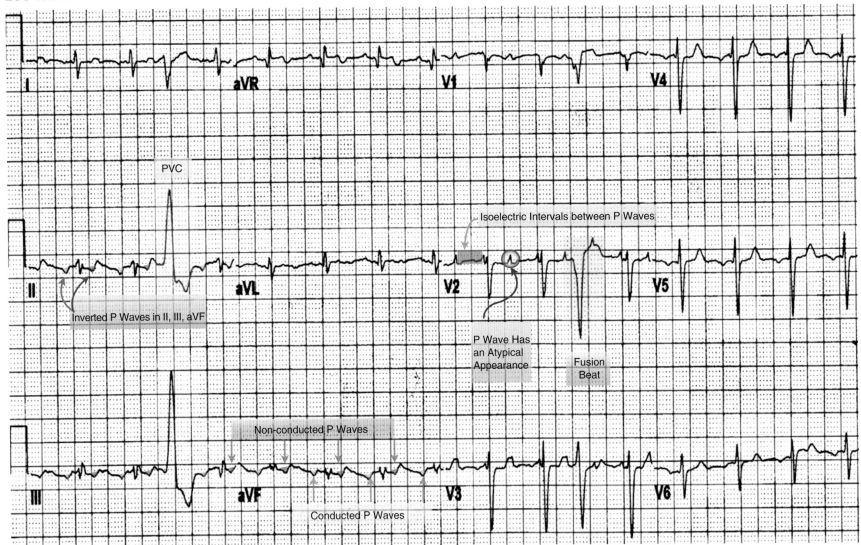

Paroxysmal Atrial Tachycardia with 2:1 Block

This rhythm could easily be mistaken for atrial flutter given the resemblance of the negative atrial waves in the inferior leads to flutter waves. The negative P waves, however, result from the retrograde conduction of atrial impulses from an ectopic location low in the atria. The atrial rate is less than 250 bpm, making atrial flutter less likely. Atrial tachycardia is commonly associated with some form of AV block. Pink arrows point to nonconducted P waves. This most often occurs in the setting of digoxin toxicity. This patient was found to have digoxin toxicity.

ECG 10.13a A 70-year-old female with metastatic melanoma presents with dyspnea.

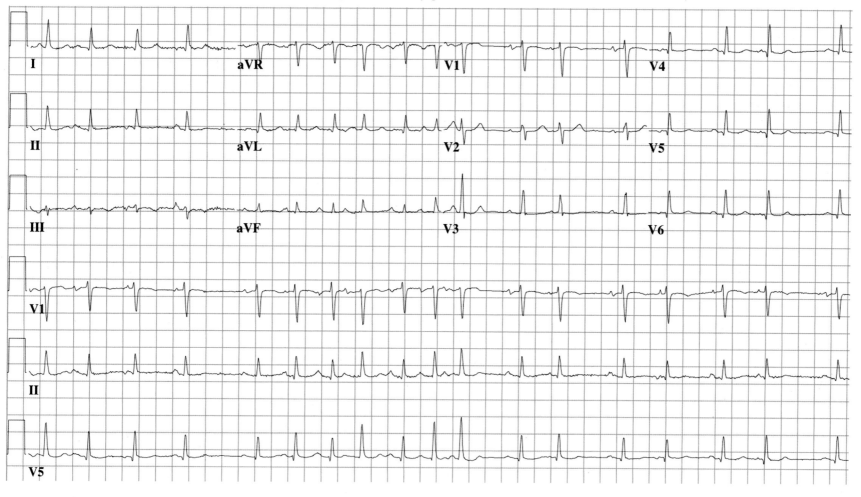

ECG 10.13b A 70-year-old female with metastatic melanoma presents with dyspnea.

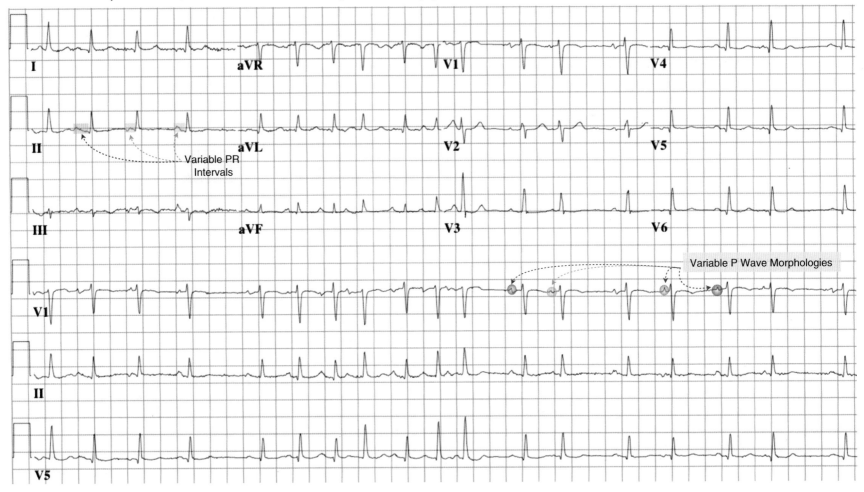

Multifocal Atrial Tachycardia

This patient was found to have multiple lung nodules and large bilateral pleural effusions. This rhythm was initially mistaken for AF and later read as multifocal atrial tachycardia. She was discharged with home oxygen but without the need for anticoagulation.

ECG 10.14a

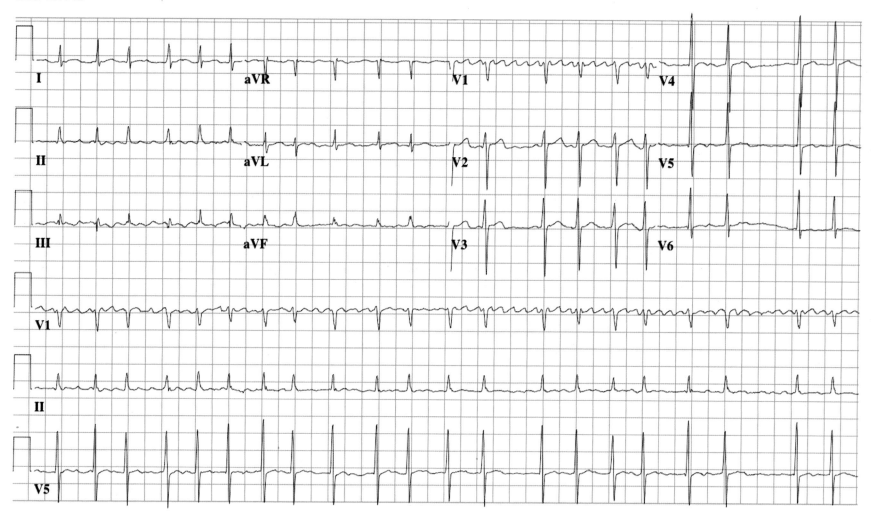

ECG 10.14b

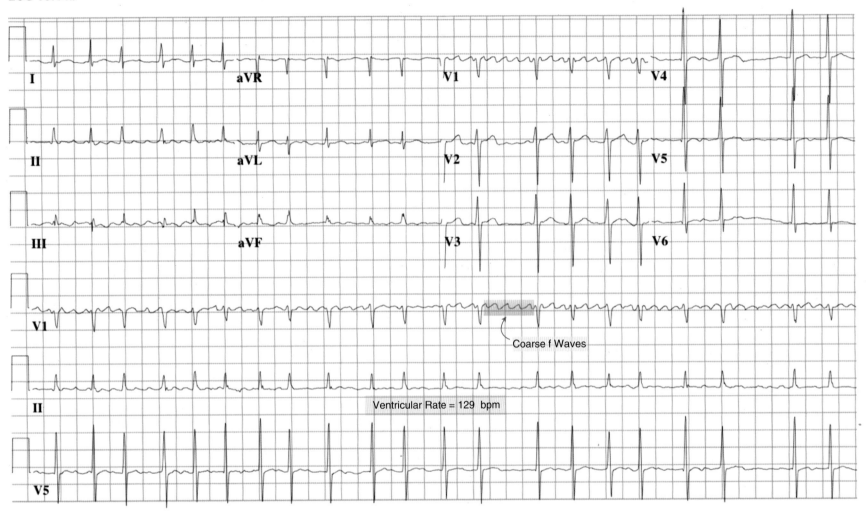

Coarse f Waves

Ventricular Rate = 129 bpm

AF with Rapid Ventricular Response

The coarse fibrillatory waves in V1 could be mistaken for flutter waves. The rhythm, however, is irregularly irregular and the atrial rate is approximately 375 bpm, faster than the rate of atrial flutter.

ECG 10.15a A 62-year-old male presents with light-headedness and palpitations. His rhythm failed to respond to two doses of adenosine.

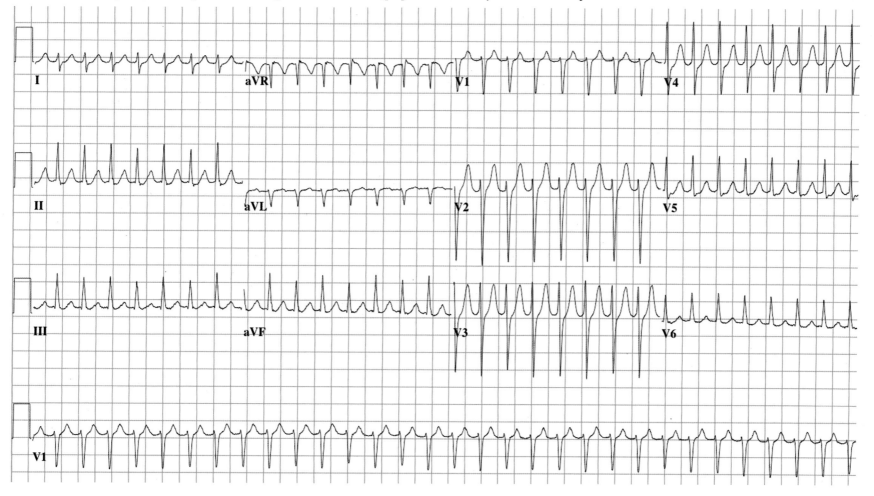

ECG 10.15b A 62-year-old male presents with light-headedness and palpitations. His rhythm failed to respond to two doses of adenosine.

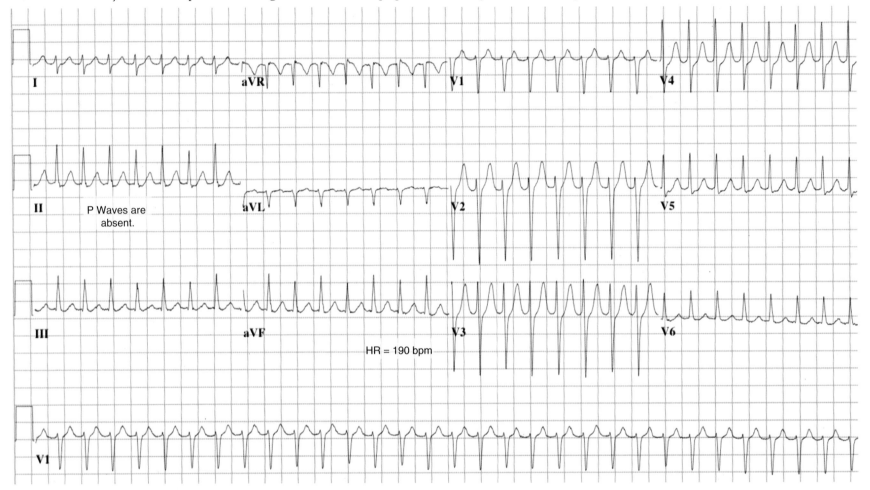

I

aVR

V1

V4

II   P Waves are absent.

aVL

V2

V5

III

aVF

HR = 190 bpm

V3

V6

V1

Atrial Tachycardia

In the electrophysiology lab, this patient was diagnosed with ectopic atrial tachycardia. The ectopic focus was successfully ablated. Ectopic P waves in this ECG are buried in the T waves.

Differential of Buried P Waves in a Narrow Complex Tachyarrhythmia

— AVNRT (Buried in QRS)

— Junctional Tachycardia (Buried in QRS)

— Atrial Tachycardia (Buried in T wave)

ECG 10.16a A 28-year-old female comes to the emergency room for evaluation of upper respiratory symptoms. She feels her heart start to race in the waiting room.

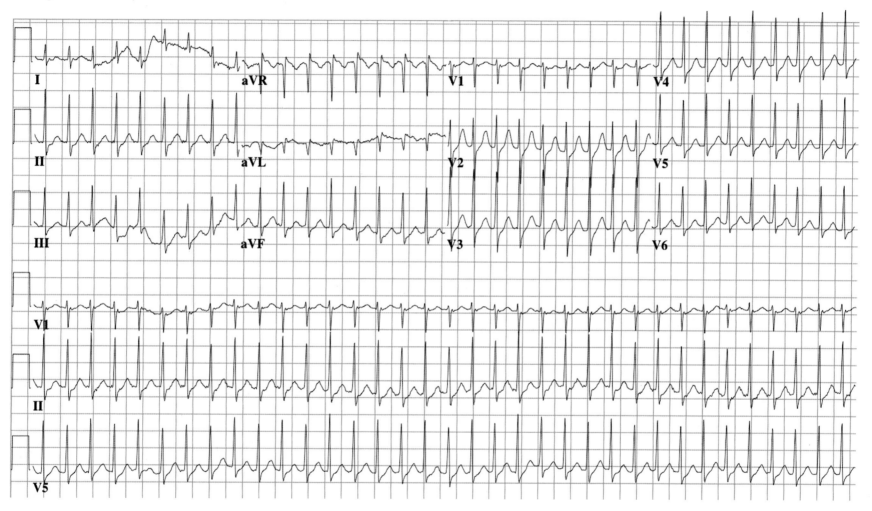

ECG 10.16b A 28-year-old female comes to the emergency room for evaluation of upper respiratory symptoms. She feels her heart start to race in the waiting room.

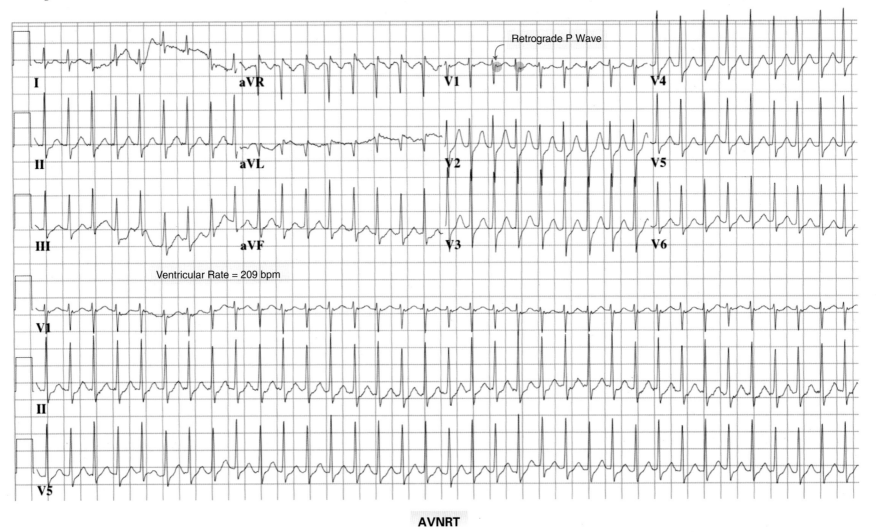

Retrograde P Wave

Ventricular Rate = 209 bpm

AVNRT

This patient had a history of several similar episodes occurring since the age of 13. She has been able to break each episode with Valsalva maneuver. This particular episode broke after several minutes of attempting Valsalva maneuver. She awaits ablation.

ECG 10.17a An 84-year-old male presents with progressive dyspnea for 4 days.

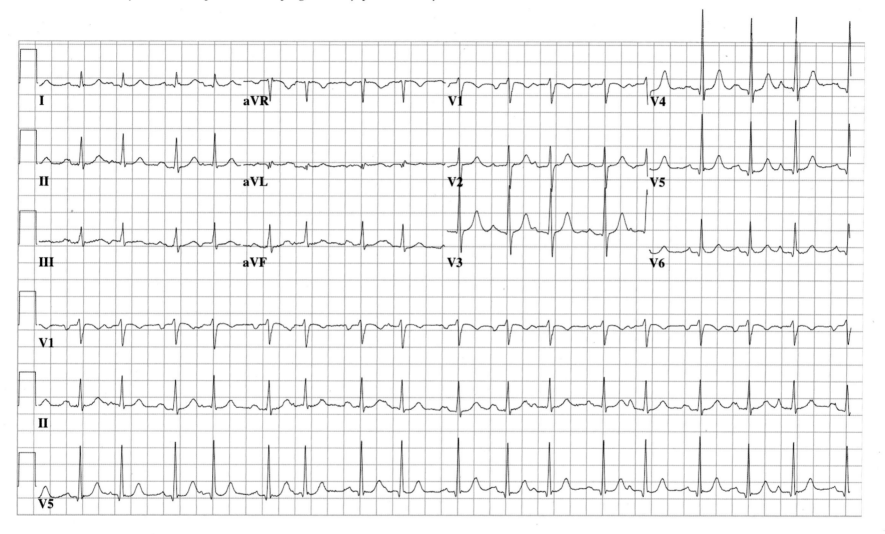

ECG 10.17b An 84-year-old male presents with progressive dyspnea for 4 days.

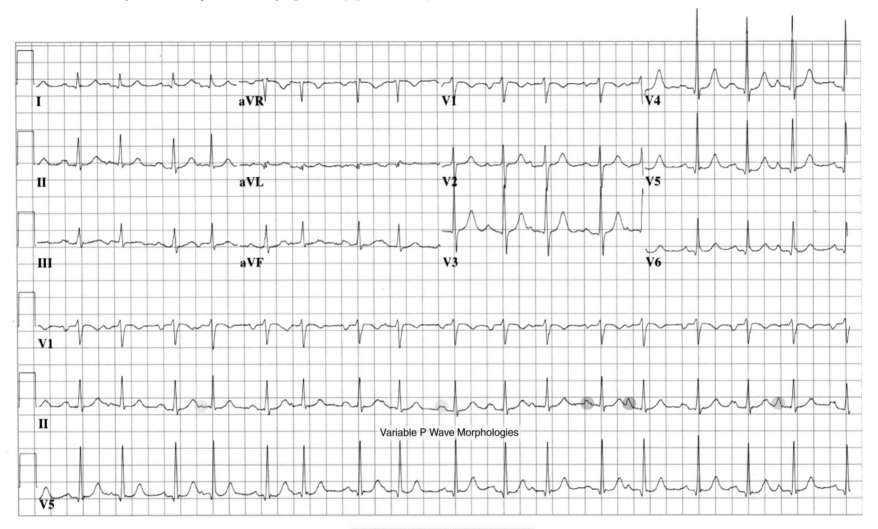

Variable P Wave Morphologies

Multifocal Atrial Tachycardia

References

1. Morady FaZ, D.. Atrial fibrillation: clinical features, mechanisms, and management. In: Bonow R, Zipes D, Libby P, eds. *Braunwald's Heart Disease: A Textbook of Cardiovascular Medicine*. 9th ed. Philadelphia, PA: Elsevier; 2011:825–844.
2. Olgin JaZD. In: Bonow R, Zipes D, Libby P, eds. *Braunwald's Heart Disease: A Textbook of Cardiovascular Medicine*. 9th ed. Philadelphia, PA: Elsevier; 2011:771–824.
3. Irons GV Jr, Orgain ES. Digitalis-induced arrhythmias and their management. *Prog Cardiovasc Dis* 1966;8:539–569.

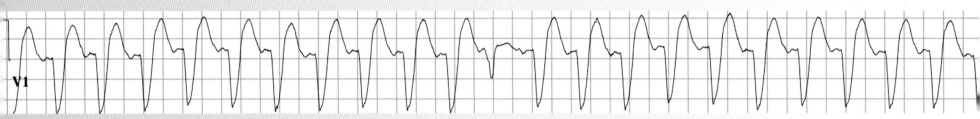

V1

Ventricular Tachycardia

Three or more consecutive QRS complexes originating from the ventricles at a rate greater than 100 bpm constitutes ventricular tachycardia (VT). When the rate is less than 100 bpm, the rhythm is referred to as *accelerated ventricular rhythm*. If the rhythm lasts less than 30 seconds, it is considered *nonsustained*. VT is often classified into the following categories:

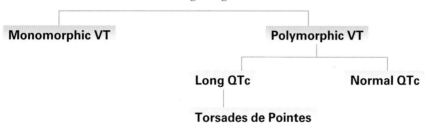

Monomorphic VT

Mechanism

- **Reentry**   This is the most common mechanism.
- **Increased Automaticity**
- **Triggered Activity**

Location   VT can involve myocardium or specialized conduction tissue distal to the bundle of His bifurcation. This includes the outflow tracts of the right and left ventricles. Two specific locations to consider in young, healthy patients unlikely to have coronary artery disease are the right ventricular outflow tract (RVOT) and the fascicles of the left bundle branch.

Causes

- **Acute Myocardial Ischemia**   VT in this setting is very unstable, easily degenerating into ventricular fibrillation.
- **Scarred Myocardium**   A complication of myocardial infarction is VT. This may not occur until decades after the acute infarction.
- **Cardiomyopathy**   Dilated cardiomyopathy, hypertrophic cardiomyopathy, and arrhythmogenic right ventricular dysplasia can all increase the risk of VT.
- **Antiarrhythmic Drugs**   Drugs that prolong the action potential and widen the QRS wave (flecainide) can predispose to sustained VT.
- **Infiltrative Diseases**   Sarcoidosis, Amyloidosis
- **Sympathetic Tone**   Increased adrenergic tone from cocaine, methamphetamine, and caffeine can lead to VT.
- **Inherited Channelopathies**   Long QT Syndrome, Short QT Syndrome, Brugada syndrome
- **Valvular Disease**   This includes mitral valve prolapse.

Origins of Monomorphic VT

Monomorphic VT

Idiopathic

Nonischemic Cardiomyopathies

Ischemic

The prognosis for idiopathic forms of VT is good. They may be effectively treated by medication or ablation.

Outflow Tract Tachycardia

Right Ventricular Outflow Tract Tachycardia

RVOT is the most common cause of idiopathic VT.[1] The mechanism underlying RVOT is thought to be triggered afterdepolarizations. A triggered focus in the right ventricle results in a monomorphic VT with a left bundle branch block (LBBB) morphology. The axis is inferior (either normal or right axis deviation). RVOT can be driven by an increase in catecholamines (exercise, isoproterenol). Acute treatment includes drugs that suppress triggered rhythms such as adenosine and verapamil. Definitive treatment is with radiofrequency catheter ablation.

Arrhythmogenic right ventricular dysplasia can cause RVOT and should be investigated as a cause of RVOT.

Left Ventricular Outflow Tract Tachycardia

A triggered focus in the left ventricle results in a monomorphic VT with a right bundle branch block (RBBB) morphology and inferior axis.

Fascicular VT

Also called idiopathic left ventricular tachycardia. This form of VT arises from the fascicles in the left ventricle. QRS complexes typically have a RBBB morphology and are wide, but QRS duration may only be slightly longer than 120 msec. There are several underlying mechanisms, but reentry is thought to be the most common. This rhythm can often be terminated with verapamil. Ablation is a successful definitive treatment.

Left Anterior Fascicular VT   RBBB morphology and RAD.

Left Posterior Fascicular VT   Most common. RBBB morphology and LAD.

Septal Fascicular VT   Rare. LBBB morphology.

Adrenergic VT

This can present as monomorphic VT with either RBBB or LBBB morphology and as polymorphic VT. It is also referred to as propranolol-sensitive automatic ventricular tachycardia. It is initiated by exercise and terminated by beta blockers.

Annular VT

This can arise from the mitral or tricuspid valve in patients with structurally normal hearts.

Mitral Annulus   QRS complexes display RBBB morphology.

Tricuspid Annulus   QRS complexes display LBBB morphology.

Monomorphic VT: ECG Features

In clinical practice, it is safer to assume that a wide-complex tachycardia is ventricular in origin.

However, aberrant conduction from a supraventricular tachyarryhthmia (SVT) may widen the QRS complexes in a way that makes the rhythm look like VT. Clinical stability has been shown to be an unreliable diagnostic tool (i.e., patients with VT can remain stable, and patients with SVT with aberrancy can become unstable).[2] Several ECG features suggest VT as the underlying rhythm.

QRS Duration   Widening of the QRS complex beyond 160 msec in precordial leads with LBBB morphology or beyond 140 msec in precordial leads with RBBB morphology suggests VT.

Axis   QRS axis more negative than –90° or more positive than +180° (northwest axis) indicates VT. QRS waves are negative in leads I and aVF. This is a form of extreme axis deviation is less likely to occur in SVT.

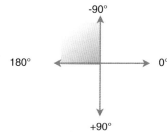

FIGURE 11.1 The hexaxial reference system. Northwest axis is highlighted.

Fusion Beat   This is a hybrid beat that results from a ventricle simultaneously activated by the reentrant circuit of VT and by another focus. This focus can be supraventricular or ventricular. The QRS complex morphology differs from the other QRS complexes in the ECG and the patient's native QRS complex (that which would appear in the patient's normal sinus rhythm).

Capture Beat   In VT, the sinus impulse continues to fire but most often arrives at the ventricles when they are in a refractory state. If properly timed, however, a sinus impulse traveling down the normal conduction system may reach the ventricles no longer in their refractory period. The QRS complex of a capture beat has the same morphology as the patient's native QRS complex.

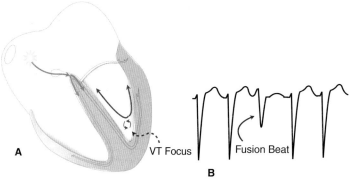

FIGURE 11.2 Mechanism A. and ECG appearance of B. a fusion beat.

AV Dissociation   AV dissociation is an insensitive finding in VT. When atria and ventricles have independent rhythms, P waves are often difficult to discern because they are often buried by T waves or wide QRS complexes. Because AV dissociation can also occur in SVT, this finding is not entirely specific for VT.

During VT, atrial and ventricular conduction can actually be linked through retrograde conduction from the ventricles to the atria. Retrograde P waves are then associated with their preceding QRS complexes.

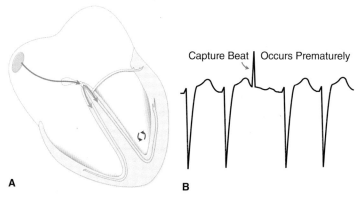

FIGURE 11.3 Mechanism A. and ECG appearance of B. a capture beat.

Monomorphic VT: V1 and V6 Morphologies Suggestive of VT

VT can be classified as having a LBBB or RBBB pattern based on the R:S ratio in V1. Several morphologies associated with each pattern are more likely to occur when the rhythm is VT.[3–5] Some are incorporated into different algorithms for differentiating VT from SVT. The presence of any of these morphologies may favor the diagnosis of VT but is not diagnostic of this rhythm.

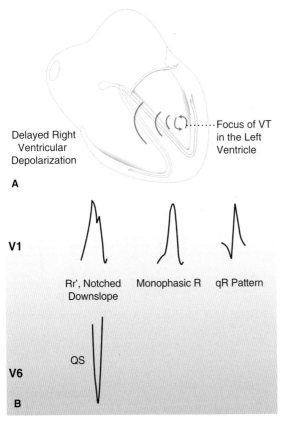

FIGURE 11.4 A. Diagram of left ventricular focus of VT.
B. QRS morphologies suggestive of VT with RBBB pattern.

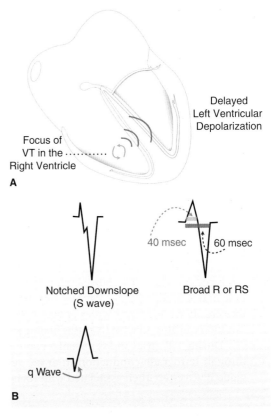

FIGURE 11.5 A. Diagram of right ventricular focus of VT.
B. QRS morphologies suggestive of VT with LBBB pattern.

The Rr' pattern in V1 is a specific, but insensitive morphology in VT with a RBBB pattern. It is also known as the "Marriott sign" or as the "Rabbit ear sign." The left ear is taller than the right.

Not all morphologic criteria for VT with RBBB morphology that have been described in the literature are illustrated.

The presence of any q/Q wave in lead V6 makes SVT with aberrancy secondary to LBBB unlikely. Recall that in LBBB, septal depolarization occurs from right to left, in the same direction as ventricular depolarization. The initial deflection of the QRS wave in the setting of LBBB is positive, and in the same direction as the rest of the QRS wave.

Polymorphic VT

As the name suggests, the QRS complexes in polymorphic VT change in width, shape, and axis. The rhythm is irregular. Polymorphic VT with a normal QTc is most often secondary to acute myocardial ischemia. Some complexes may appear pointing upward while others appear pointing downward.

Catecholaminergic Polymorphic VT

This type of VT is either bidirectional or polymorphic and is induced by exercise or emotional stress. Approximately half of these patients are found to have mutations in genes coding for the ryanodine receptor or the protein calsequestrin. Treatment includes beta-blocker therapy and placement of an ICD.

Torsades de Pointes

If polymorphic VT is associated with QTc prolongation, the rhythm is torsades de pointes. The QTc interval can be measured before the onset of or after the termination of the tachycardia. The waves of VT gradually increase and decrease in amplitude. The rate ranges from 180 to 250 bpm. This rhythm often self-terminates after seconds. It can degenerate into ventricular fibrillation.

Commonly the onset of torsades occurs after a long R-R cycle is followed by an early depolarization.

Ventricular Flutter

This is a regular monomorphic tachycardia resulting from a macroreentrant ventricular rhythm similar to the atrial reentrant circuit of atrial flutter. The ECG morphology may appear as a sine wave. This is a nonsustainable rhythm that deteriorates into ventricular fibrillation.

ECG changes secondary to motion artifact can look remarkably similar to ventricular flutter. Narrow QRS complexes will interrupt the large amplitude waves generated by motion artifact.

Ventricular Fibrillation

Ventricular fibrillation is a disorganized rhythm with rates exceeding 300 bpm. The shape and amplitude of each wave vary. VFib with very low-amplitude undulations may be mistaken for asystole.

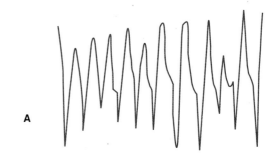

A

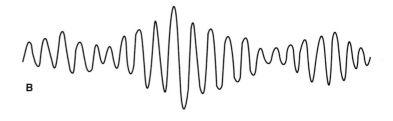

B

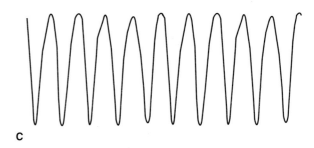

C

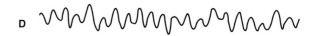

D

FIGURE 11.6 ECG appearance of **A.** polymorphic VT; **B.** Torsades de pointes; **C.** ventricular flutter; and **D.** ventricular fibrillation.

Supraventricular Causes of Wide-Complex Tachycardia

VT is far more common than supraventricular tachycardia with aberrancy. SVT with aberrancy should still be considered, however, in the differential of wide-complex tachycardias as treatment and outcomes differ.

Mechanisms

SVT can result in a wide-complex tachycardia if the AV node is bypassed by conduction down an accessory pathway or if a normal conduction pathway (bundle branch) distal to the AV node is blocked.

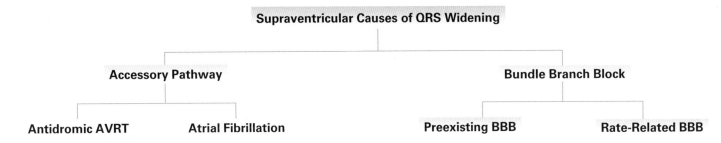

ECG Features

Preexcitation   A slurring of the initial inscription of the QRS wave may represent a delta wave. This results from ventricular preexcitation by an accessory pathway. A similar pattern of preexcitation seen on a patient's previous ECG makes the diagnosis of SVT more likely.

Preexistant BBB   SVT with aberrancy is the likely diagnosis if identical QRS morphology in the setting of normal sinus rhythm can be seen on a previous ECG.

Triphasic Waves   Triphasic morphology in leads V1 and V6 (Fig. 11.8) is an unlikely QRS morphology to result from an impulse generated by a single ventricular focus and is therefore suggestive of SVT.

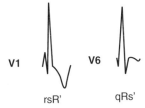

FIGURE 11.7 Triphasic appearance of QRS waves.

Antidromic Atrioventricular Reciprocating Tachycardia

This rhythm is also known as wide-complex atrioventricular reciprocating tachycardia (AVRT). In patients with Wolff–Parkinson–White Syndrome, narrow-complex AVRT due to orthodromic conduction is far more common than wide-complex AVRT due to antidromic conduction.

Mechanism

The reentrant circuit of AVRT is triggered by an ectopic impulse. In antidromic AVRT, the ectopic impulse encounters an AV node still in its refractory period and a bypass tract that is out of its refractory period and ready to conduct to the ventricles.

Activation of the ventricles occurs by antero-grade conduction down the bypass tract. Ventricular impulse spreads from myocardial cell to myocardial cell. Conduction then continues in a retrograde fashion from the ventricles to the atria through the AV node before reentering the reentrant circuit.

Rarely, retrograde conduction from the ventricles to the atria can occur through a second bypass tract.

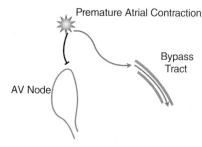

FIGURE 11.8 Initial event of reentrant tachycardia.

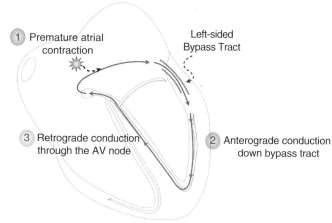

FIGURE 11.9 Antidromic AVRT with a left-sided bypass tract. Rhythm initiated by a premature atrial contraction (*blue star*).

ECG Features

QRS complexes are wide and regular. Because the ventricle is activated solely through the bypass tract, each QRS wave should show evidence of preexcitation (delta wave).

Location

Left-sided bypass tract: The left ventricle is the first to be activated. Spread of ventricular impulse occurs in a left-to-right direction. This results in positive QRS complexes in the right precordial lead V1. This is similar to the QRS morphology seen in RBBB.

Right-sided bypass tract: Ventricular activation spreads from the right ventricle to the left ventricle, away from the direction of V1. The QRS complex in V1 is therefore predominantly negative and similar to the morphology of a LBBB.

Mistaken for: Ventricular Tachycardia

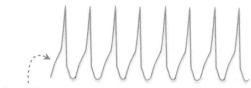

FIGURE 11.10 ECG appearance of lead V1 in antidromic AVRT with a left-sided bypass tract.

Atrial Fibrillation Down an Accessory Pathway

This is the most dangerous rhythm that can occur in a patient with a bypass tract capable of anterograde conduction.

Mechanism

Conduction from the disordered supraventricular rhythm of atrial fibrillation reaches the ventricles via both the AV Node/Purkinje system and the bypass tract (Fig. 11.12A).

The variability in QRS morphology (Fig. 11.12B) results from the variable contributions of the bypass tract and the normal conduction pathway to ventricular activation.

ECG Features

QRS morphology varies from one beat to the next. Each QRS complex is a fusion complex generated by simultaneous conduction coming from the normal and bypass pathways. QRS complexes show varying degrees of pre-excitation and delta wave morphology.

The ventricular rate is extremely rapid because the bypass tract is capable of conducting impulses much faster than the AV node.

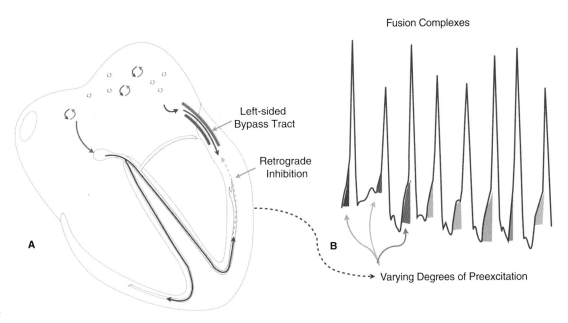

FIGURE 11.11 **A.** Diagram of atrioventricular conduction down both normal and accessory pathways. Atrial fibrillation. **B.** Appearance of QRS complexes. AFib in a patient with WPW.

Clinical Course

This rhythm can deteriorate into ventricular fibrillation or lead to hypotension and cardiac ischemia. Bypass tracts with a shorter refractory period are capable of conducting impulses to the ventricle at dangerously rapid rates.

Drugs to Avoid

The accessory pathway and pathway of normal ventricular conduction are not completely independent. Impulses carried through the His-Purkinje system can, in retrograde fashion, inhibit the bypass tract and thereby decrease the number of atrial impulses successfully conducted down the accessory pathway (dotted blue arrow, Fig. 11.12A). Any medication that inhibits the AV node can facilitate more rapid conduction down the accessory pathway and increase the risk of ventricular fibrillation. These medications include adenosine, beta blockers, calcium channel blockers, and digitalis. If the patient is stable, the preferred treatment is procainamide. Direct current cardioversion is indicated if the patient is unstable.

Aberrancy

Aberrancy refers to any disturbance in normal intraventricular conduction. In the context of discussing supraventricular arrhythmias with aberrancy, the term usually refers to conduction distorted by a bundle branch block (BBB).

Fixed/Preexisting Bundle Branch Block

Tachyarrhythmias occur in people with a preexisting BBB. Because the pattern of ventricular conduction does not change between normal sinus rhythm and a supraventricular tachycardia, the QRS morphology is the same. It is helpful to find an older ECG for QRS morphology comparison. If the morphologies are the same, the wide-complex tachycardia is supraventricular and the widening of the QRS can be attributed to the ventricular conduction delay caused by the preexisting BBB.

Rate-Related

Ectopic Atrial Impulse

This is also known as the Ashman phenomenon and occurs most often in the setting of atrial fibrillation. The refractory period of the cardiac period is directly related to the length of the preceding cycle (R-R interval). The slower the rate, the longer the cycle and the longer the refractory period following that cardiac cycle. Aberrancy is usually initiated by an ectopic atrial wave that arrives prematurely at the ventricular conduction system. This premature beat can encounter part of the ventricular conduction system (most often the right bundle branch) when it is in its refractory period. Conduction is essentially blocked in that part of the system. The QRS wave looks like that of a BBB.

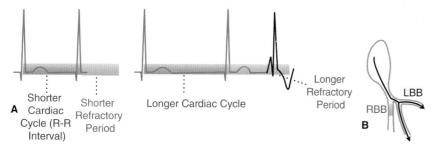

FIGURE 11.13 A. Relationship between lengths of cardiac cycle and refractory period. B. Diagram of right bundle branch block.

Critical Rate

The sinus node can accelerate to a cycle length that is shorter than the inherent refractory period of one of the bundle branches (most often that of the right bundle). The bundle branch is unable to recover in time for the rapid arrival of impulses from the atria.

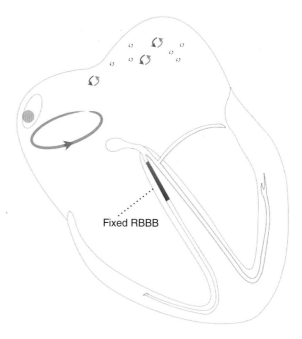

FIGURE 11.12 Fixed RBBB in the setting of sinus rhythm (*blue dot*), atrial flutter (*large red circle*) and atrial fibrillation (*smaller circles*).

Characteristics Suggestive of Aberrancy

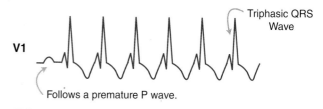

FIGURE 11.14 ECG appearance of a supraventricular taachyarrhythmia with aberrancy.

Different Causes of Wide-Complex Tachycardia

The differential diagnosis of wide-complex tachycardia is not limited to ventricular tachycardia and SVT with aberrancy. Sinus tachycardia with widened QRS complexes can mimic VT or SVT with aberrancy. The diagnosis of sinus tachycardia with QRS widening is especially important because underlying causes are both fatal and treatable.

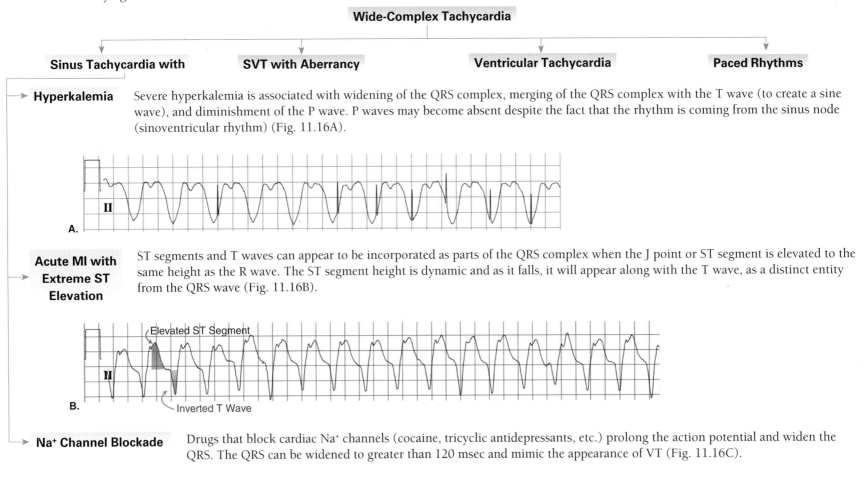

Wide-Complex Tachycardia

Sinus Tachycardia with | **SVT with Aberrancy** | **Ventricular Tachycardia** | **Paced Rhythms**

Hyperkalemia — Severe hyperkalemia is associated with widening of the QRS complex, merging of the QRS complex with the T wave (to create a sine wave), and diminishment of the P wave. P waves may become absent despite the fact that the rhythm is coming from the sinus node (sinoventricular rhythm) (Fig. 11.16A).

Acute MI with Extreme ST Elevation — ST segments and T waves can appear to be incorporated as parts of the QRS complex when the J point or ST segment is elevated to the same height as the R wave. The ST segment height is dynamic and as it falls, it will appear along with the T wave, as a distinct entity from the QRS wave (Fig. 11.16B).

Na⁺ Channel Blockade — Drugs that block cardiac Na⁺ channels (cocaine, tricyclic antidepressants, etc.) prolong the action potential and widen the QRS. The QRS can be widened to greater than 120 msec and mimic the appearance of VT (Fig. 11.16C).

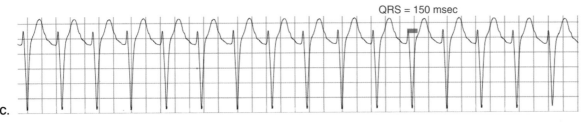

FIGURE 11.15 Wide-complex tachycardia secondary to A. hyperkalemia, B. myocardial infarction, and C. tricyclic antidepressant toxicity.

ECG 11.1a A 46-year-old male complains of his heart racing for 2 hours.

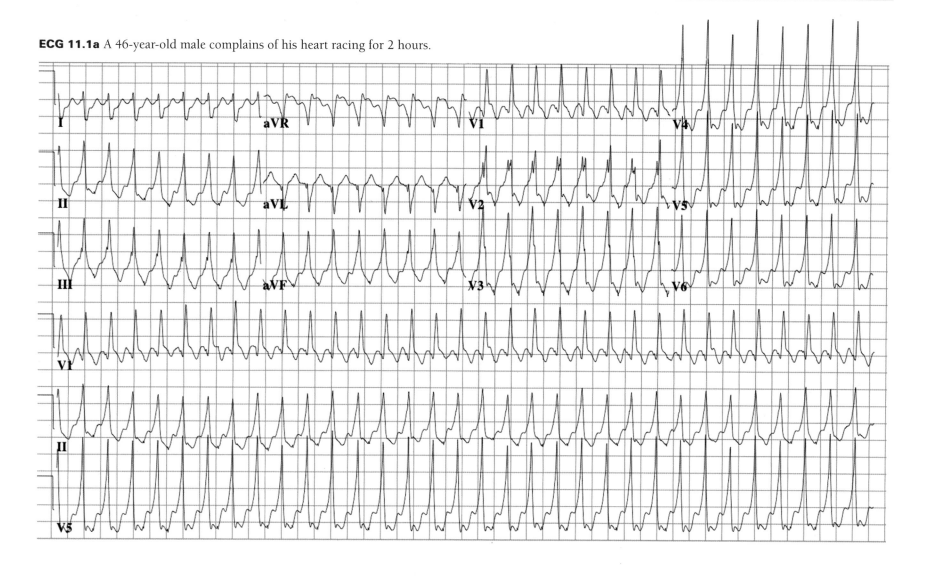

ECG 11.1b A 46-year-old male complains of his heart racing for 2 hours.

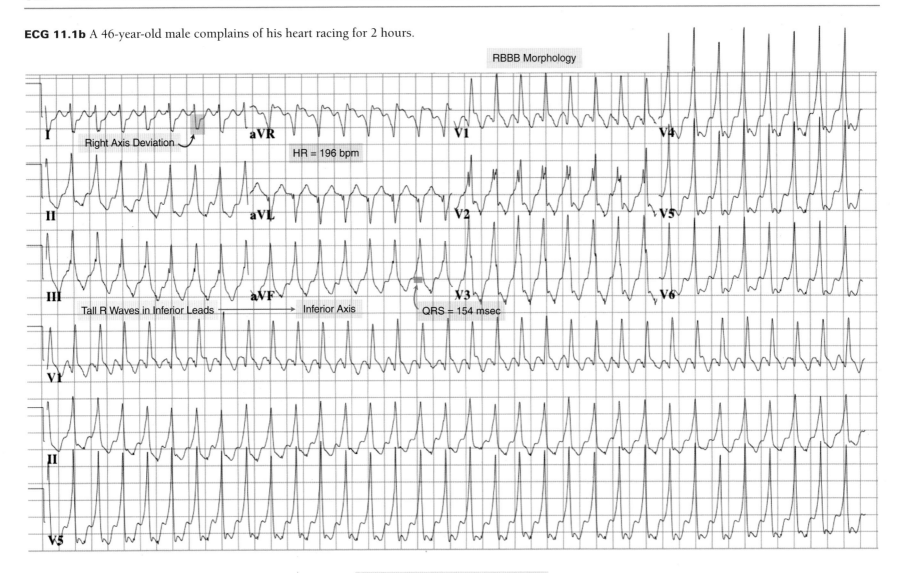

RBBB Morphology

Right Axis Deviation

aVR

HR = 196 bpm

V1

V4

aVL

V2

V5

aVF

Tall R Waves in Inferior Leads

Inferior Axis

QRS = 154 msec

V3

V6

VI

II

V5

Ventricular Tachycardia—LVOT

This patient converted to normal sinus rhythm after cardioversion with 150 Joules. He had a recurrent episode during his hospital course and underwent direct current cardioversion again with return to sinus rhythm. He underwent placement of an automated implantable cardioverter-defibrillator (AICD), which has fired several times in response to recurrent episodes of VT while on mexilitine and sotalol. He underwent successful radiofrequency ablation of a VT focus in the left ventricular outflow tract (LVOT). The combination of RBBB morphology and an inferior axis is typical for LVOT VT. A feature of this ECG suggestive of VT is a QRS width >140 msec with RBBB morphology.

ECG 11.2a

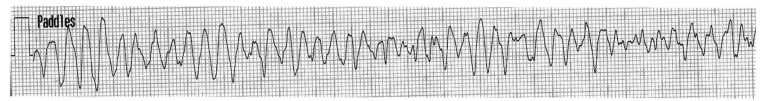

ECG 11.3a A 67-year-old male became unresponsive immediately after an exercise stress test.

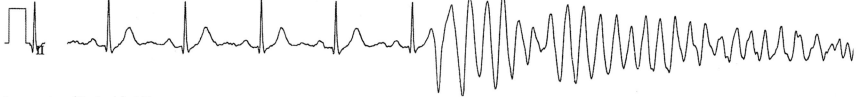

Image courtesy of Ben Sandefur, MD.

ECG 11.4a An 85-year-old female on coumadin is found to have bilateral subdural hemorrhages. This rhythm occurs while fresh frozen plasma is infusing.

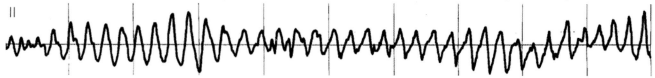

ECG 11.2b

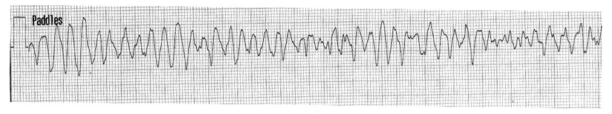

The rhythm is irregular. The morphology and amplitude of each wave are different. There are no discernible QRS or T waves.

Ventricular Fibrillation

ECG 11.3b A 67-year-old male became unresponsive immediately after an exercise stress test.

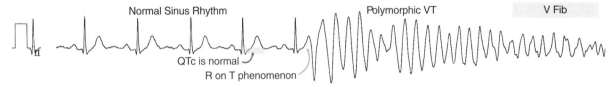

Polymorphic VT Degenerating into V Fib

This patient was shocked with 300 J within 1 minute of the onset of the abnormal rhythm and returned to normal sinus rhythm. VT in this rhythm begins with an R wave occurring near the apex of the preceding T wave (R on T phenomenon). This represents ventricular depolarization from an ectopic beat occurring during the relative refractory period of the previous beat while myocardial cells were still repolarizing. While QTc prolongation predisposes to R on T phenomenon, the QTc in this patient was normal. The rhythm, therefore cannot be defined as torsades de pointes. Myocardial ischemia from the stress test may have been the underlying cause of this patient's dysrhythmia.

ECG 11.4b An 85-year-old female on coumadin is found to have bilateral subdural hemorrhages. This rhythm occurs while fresh frozen plasma is infusing.

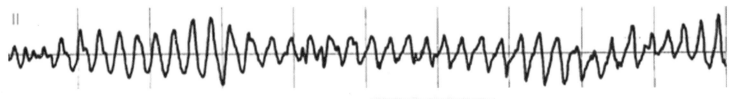

Torsades de Pointes

ECG 11.4c This patient's ECG 1 hour later:

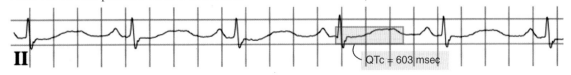

QTc Prolongation

Recall that intracranial injuries are associated with QTc prolongation and subsequent Torsades de Pointes.

ECG 11.5a

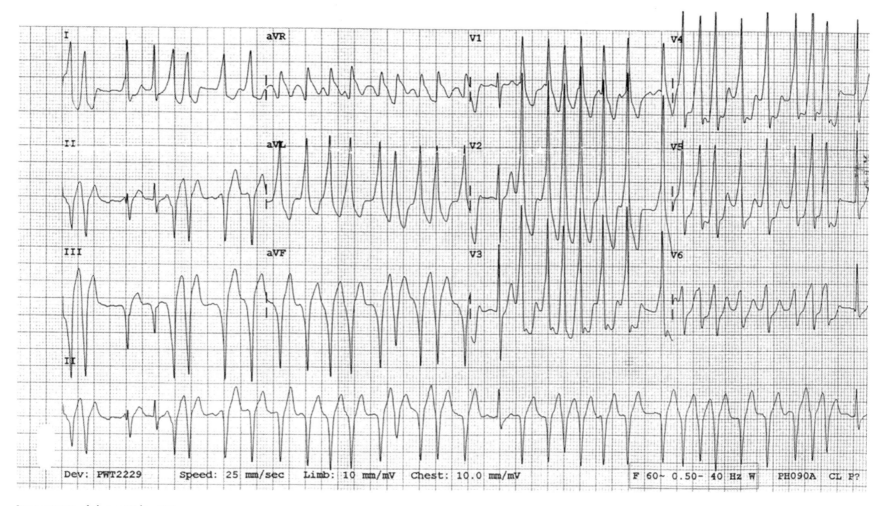

Dev: PWT2229   Speed: 25 mm/sec   Limb: 10 mm/mV   Chest: 10.0 mm/mV   F 60~ 0.50- 40 Hz W   PH090A   CL P?

Image courtesy of Thomas Nielan, MD.

ECG 11.5b

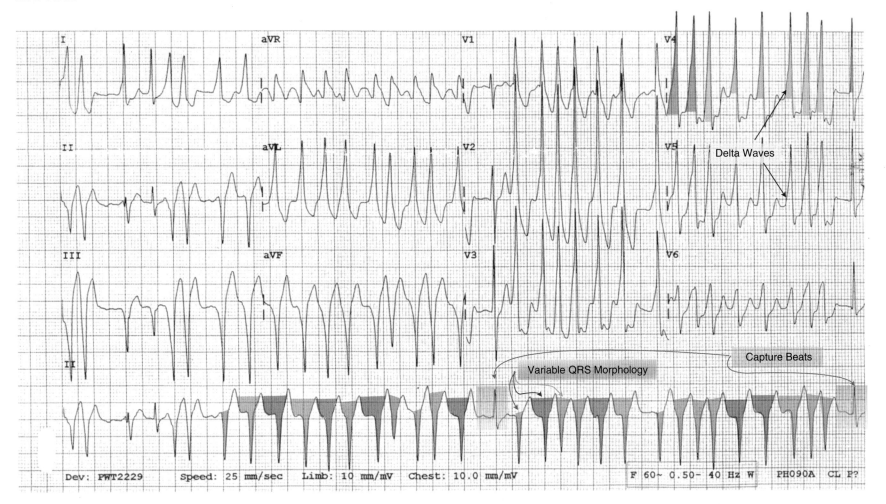

Atrial Fibrillation with Aberrancy (WPW)

The most striking feature of this ECG is the beat-to-beat variation in QRS morphology. This results from variable contributions of the accessory and normal conduction pathways to each ventricular impulse. Variable QRS morphology in an irregular, wide-complex tachycardia indicates atrial fibrillation down an accessory pathway. Administration of a nodal blocking agent in this setting could facilitate conduction down the accessory pathway at an even faster rate.

Note the occasional normal-appearing QRS complexes (highlighted in red boxes). These represent ventricular activation occurring from the normal conduction pathway without contribution from the accessory pathway.

ECG 11.6a An 81-year-old male with a history of myocardial infarction develops acute dyspnea while exercising on a treadmill.

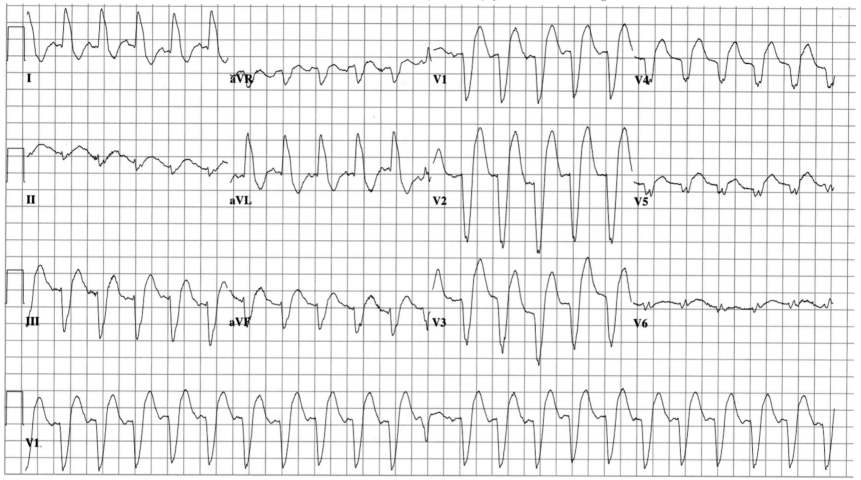

ECG 11.6b An 81-year-old male with a history of myocardial infarction develops acute dyspnea while exercising on a treadmill.

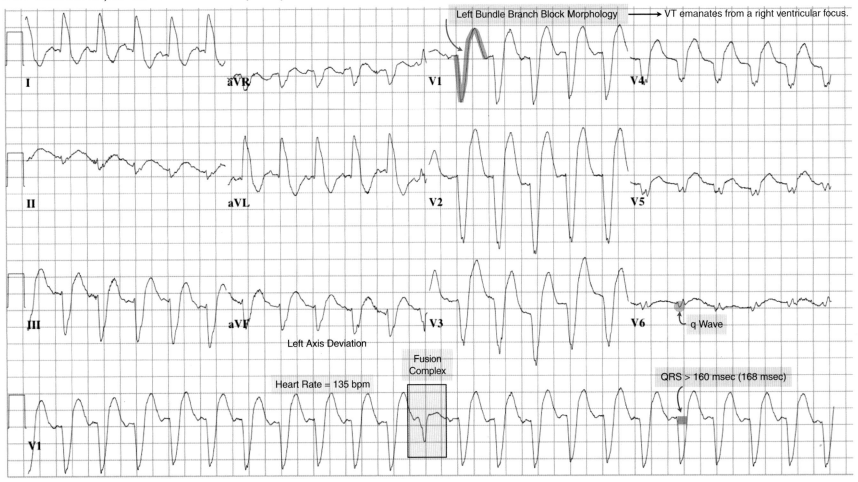

Ventricular Tachycardia

The most important clue to the ECG diagnosis of VT is this patient's age and clinical history of coronary artery disease. An ECG diagnosis can be made absent of any history in this case because there is a fusion complex. A fusion complex signifies that the origin of at least one of two separate impulses is ventricular. Other ECG findings suggesting VT in this ECG are marked QRS prolongation (beyond 160 msec), left axis deviation, and a q wave in lead V6.

ECG 11.7a A 63-year-old homeless male with daily cocaine use; He develops chest pain and this rhythm 3 minutes after a treadmill stress test.

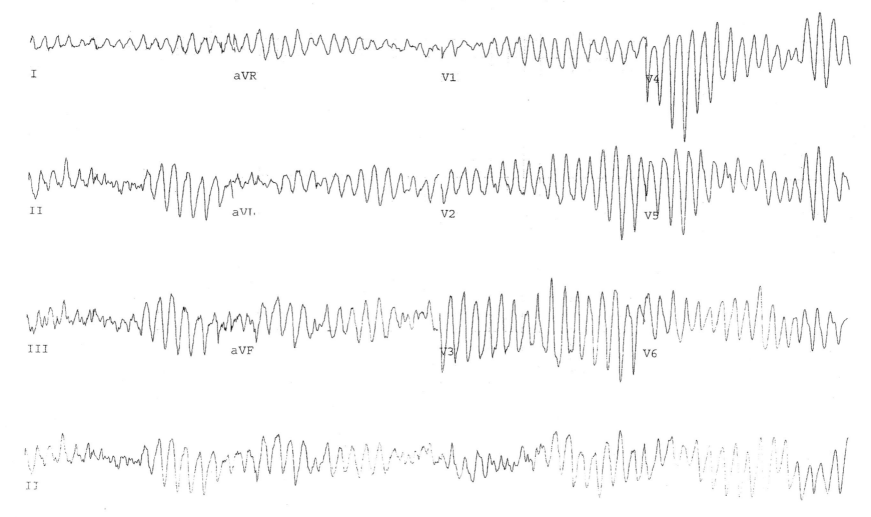

Image courtesy of Maya Yiadom, MD.

ECG 11.7b A 63-year-old homeless male with daily cocaine use; He develops chest pain and this rhythm 3 minutes after a treadmill stress test.

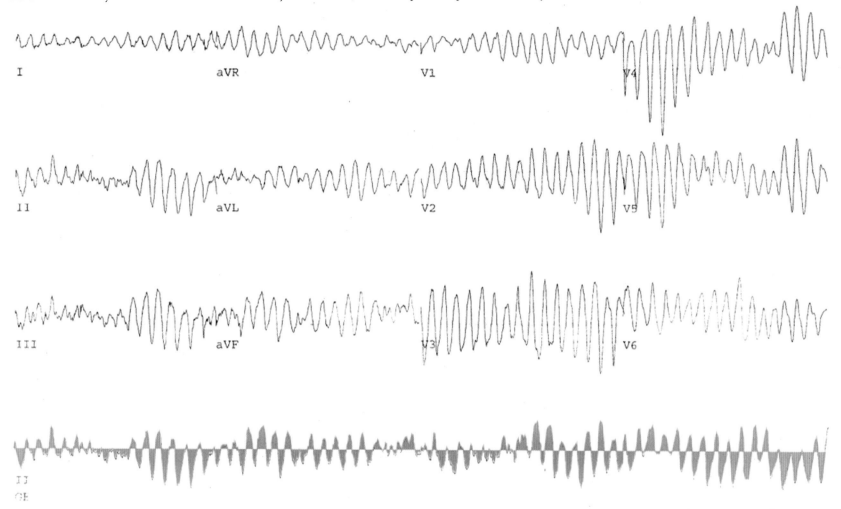

Torsades de Pointes

Recall that cocaine can cause QTc prolongation by inhibiting potassium channels involved in repolarization.

ECG 11.8a A 50-year-old female presents with recurrent episodes of palpitations.

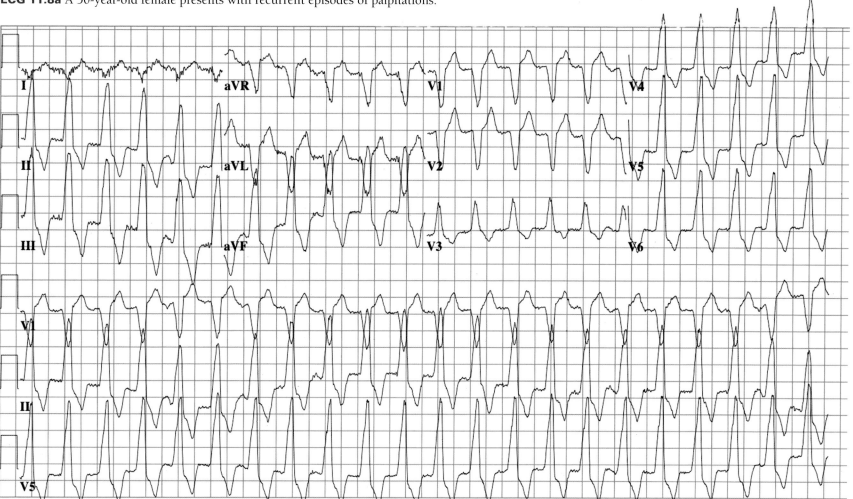

ECG 11.8b A 50-year-old female presents with recurrent episodes of palpitations.

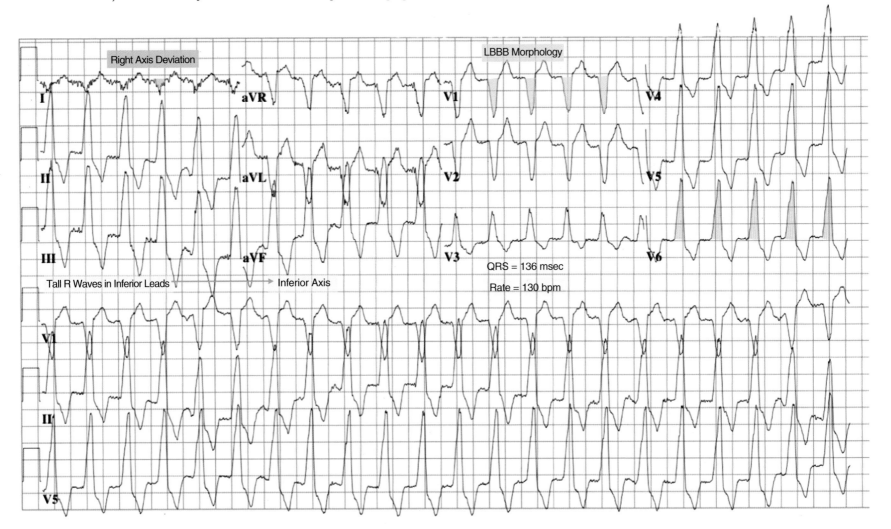

Right Axis Deviation

LBBB Morphology

I aVR V1 V4

II aVL V2 V5

III aVF V3 V6

Tall R Waves in Inferior Leads

Inferior Axis

QRS = 136 msec

Rate = 130 bpm

V1

II

V5

Right Ventricular Outflow Tract Tachycardia

Resist the temptation to call this SVT with aberrancy. This patient was found to have RVOT ventricular tachycardia. Electrophysiologic mapping revealed an area on the septal aspect of the RVOT to be the source of her ventricular tachycardia. She underwent successful radiofrequency ablation of this area. The combination of LBBB morphology and inferior axis (either normal axis or RAD) is typical of RVOT.

ECG 11.9a A 29-year male with several episodes of chest pain with associated diaphoresis and light-headedness while watching television.

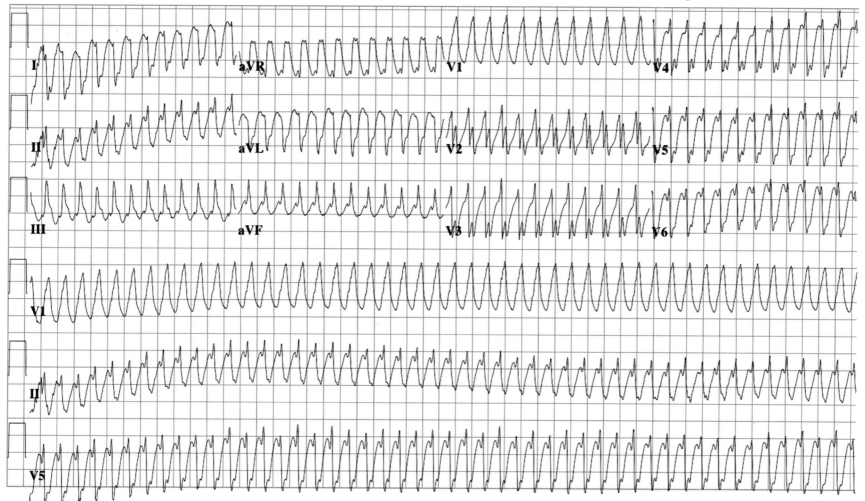

ECG 11.9b A 29-year-old male with several episodes of chest pain with associated diaphoresis and light-headedness while watching television.

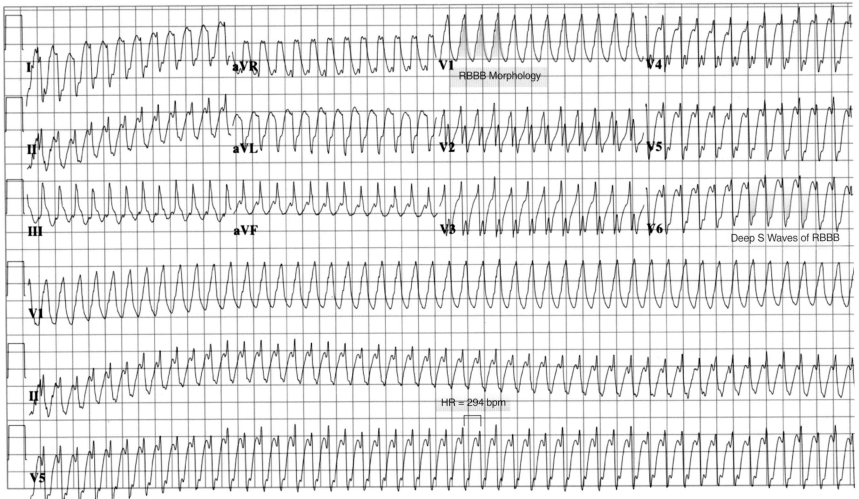

Atrial Flutter with Aberrancy

This is atrial flutter with 1:1 conduction. Ventricular rates that exceed 260 bpm are likely secondary to atrial flutter. In the electrophysiology lab, this patient was noted to have aberrant ventricular conduction matching the QRS morphology in this rhythm while he underwent rapid atrial pacing at a rate of 220 beats per minute. He underwent successful ablation of atrial flutter at the cavotricuspid isthmus. Aberrancy in this patient was rate-related.

ECG 11.10a A 52-year-old male with sarcoidosis senses his heart racing.

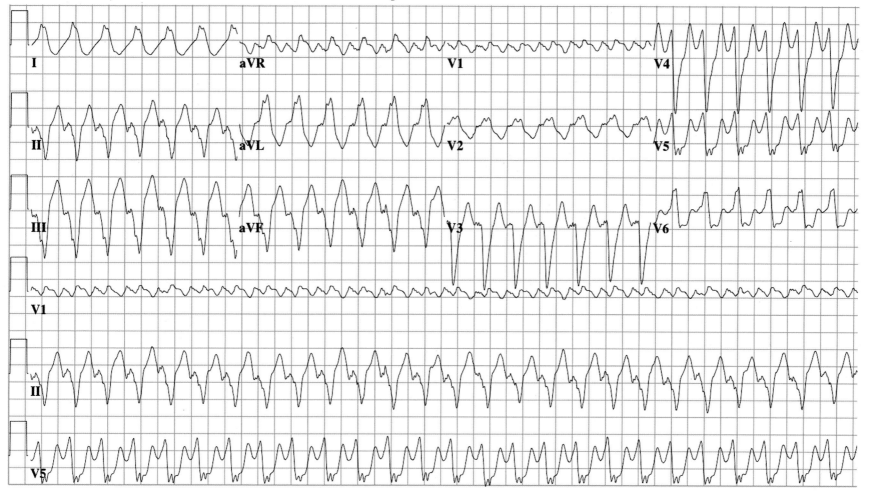

ECG 11.10b A 52-year-old male with sarcoidosis senses his heart racing.

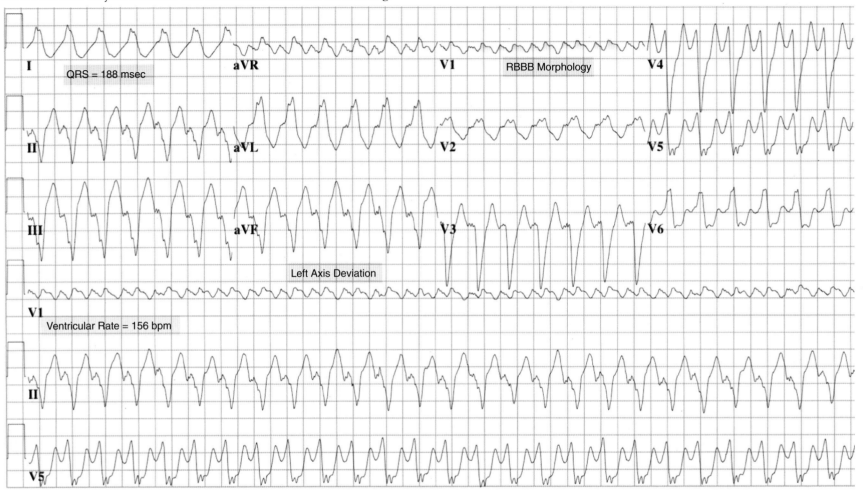

QRS = 188 msec

RBBB Morphology

Left Axis Deviation

Ventricular Rate = 156 bpm

Ventricular Tachycardia

This patient had a history of cardiac sarcoidosis complicated by severe cardiomyopathy and recurrent VT. This patient had a functioning ICD in place at the time of this ECG which was programmed to shock for any ventricular rate above 170 bpm. The patient became hypotensive in the ED and was transcutaneously shocked with return of sinus rhythm.

After this episode, his ICD was reprogrammed to shock for ventricular rates above 145 bpm.

ECG 11.11a A 52-year-old male with complains of progressive dyspnea at rest (while watching television) for the past day.

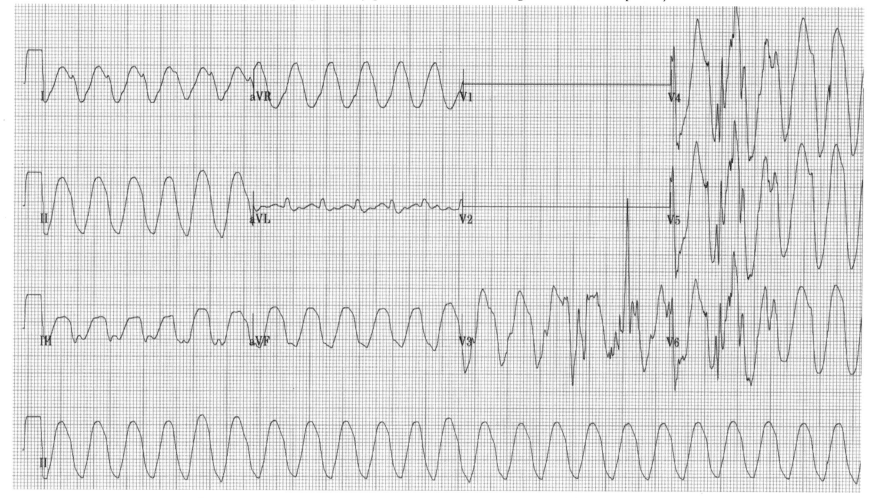

Image Courtesy of Gerard Beltran, DO.

ECG 11.11b A 52-year-old male with complains of progressive dyspnea at rest (while watching television) for the past day.

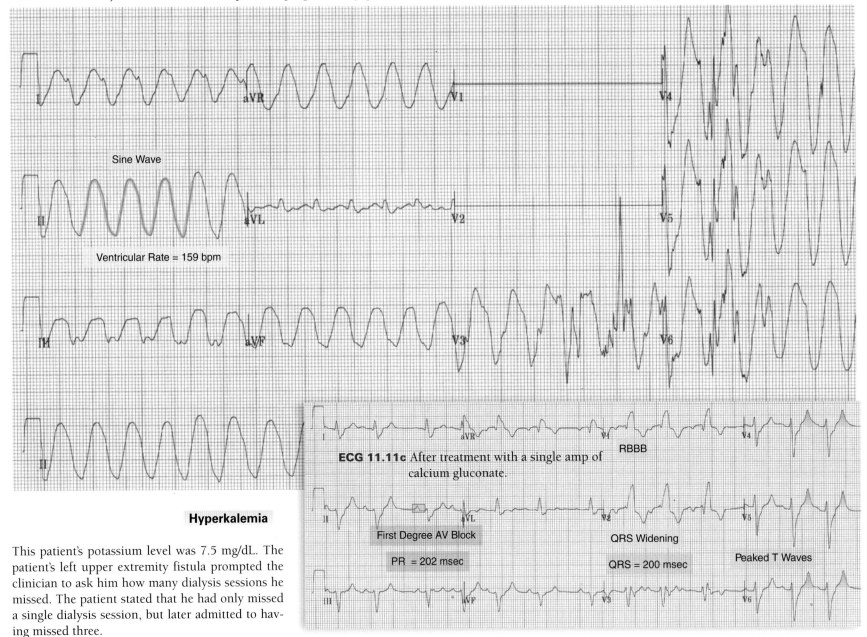

Sine Wave

Ventricular Rate = 159 bpm

Hyperkalemia

This patient's potassium level was 7.5 mg/dL. The patient's left upper extremity fistula prompted the clinician to ask him how many dialysis sessions he missed. The patient stated that he had only missed a single dialysis session, but later admitted to having missed three.

ECG 11.11c After treatment with a single amp of calcium gluconate.

RBBB

First Degree AV Block

PR = 202 msec

QRS Widening

QRS = 200 msec

Peaked T Waves

ECG 11.12a A 17-year-old male feels light-headed during wrestling practice and drives himself to the nearest emergency department.

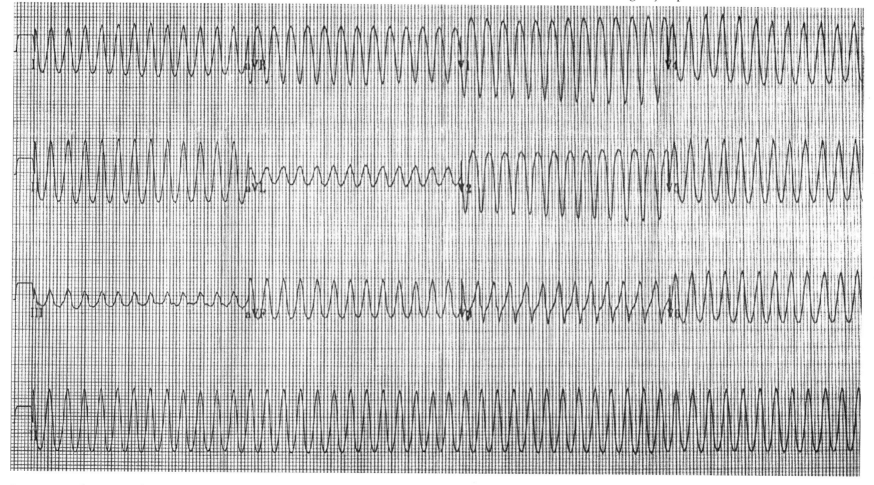

Image courtesy of Pierre Borczuk, MD.

ECG 11.12b A 17-year-old male feels light-headed during wrestling practice and drives himself to the nearest emergency department.

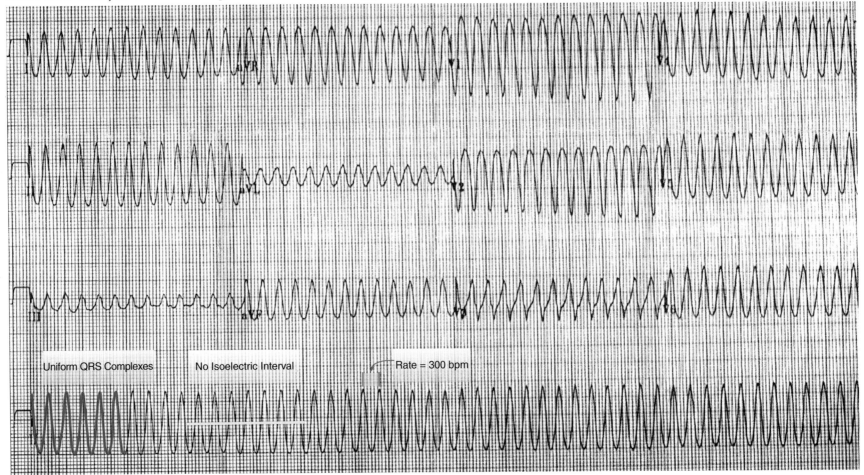

Ventricular Flutter

The patient became hypotensive and was shocked once with return of sinus rhythm. In the electrophysiology lab, he was found to have inducible ventricular fibrillation. He underwent AICD placement and had 20 episodes of VT/VFib in the next several months. Cardiac MRI and left ventricular biopsy findings were suggestive of myocarditis as an underlying cause of his ventricular arrhythmias.

ECG 11.13a

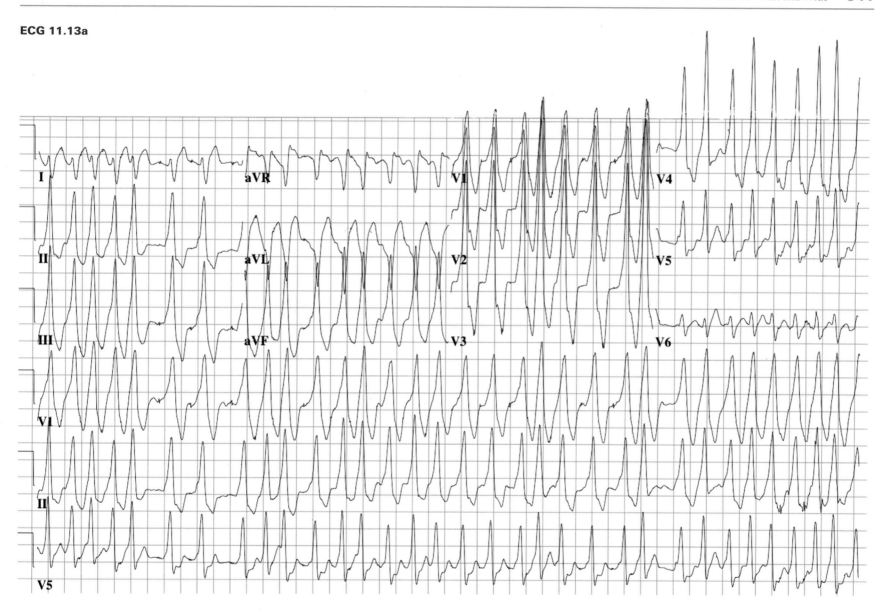

ECG 11.13b

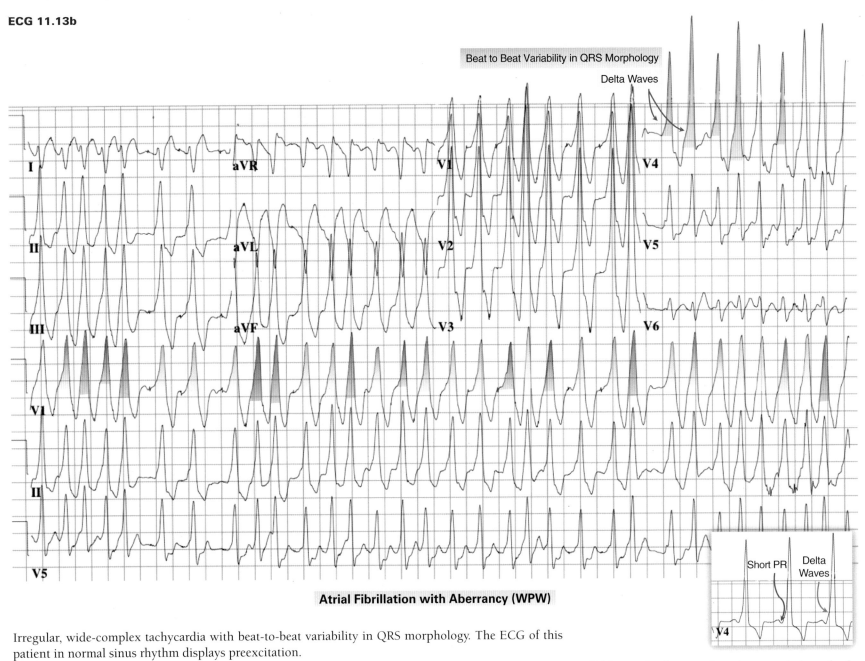

Beat to Beat Variability in QRS Morphology

Delta Waves

I   aVR   V1   V4

II   aVL   V2   V5

III   aVF   V3   V6

V1

II

V5

Atrial Fibrillation with Aberrancy (WPW)

Short PR   Delta Waves

V4

Irregular, wide-complex tachycardia with beat-to-beat variability in QRS morphology. The ECG of this patient in normal sinus rhythm displays preexcitation.

ECG 11.13c Same patient, in normal sinus rhythm.

ECG 11.14a

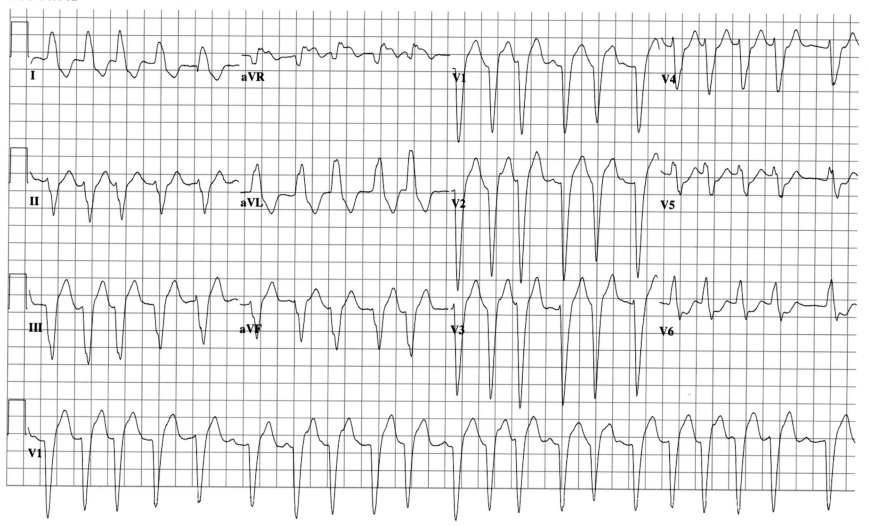

ECG 11.14b

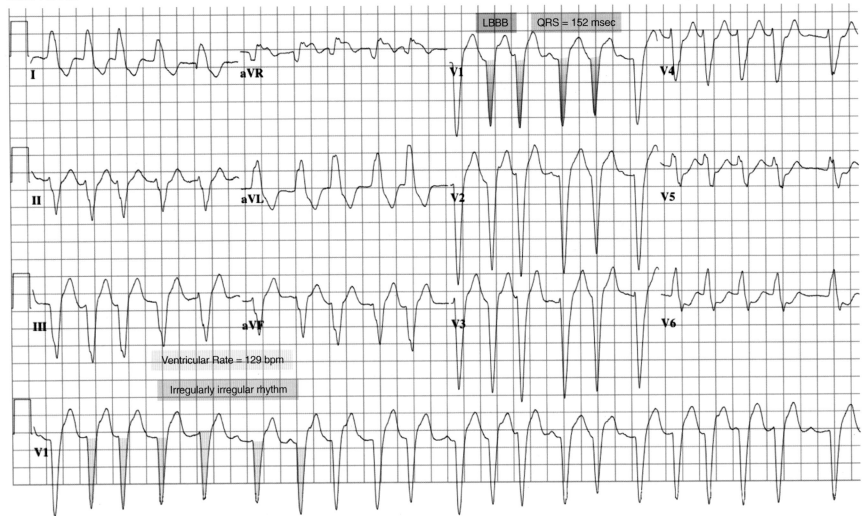

LBBB   QRS = 152 msec

I   aVR   V1   V4

II   aVL   V2   V5

III   aVF   V3   V6

Ventricular Rate = 129 bpm

Irregularly irregular rhythm

V1

Atrial Fibrillation with Left Bundle Branch Block

ECG 11.15a

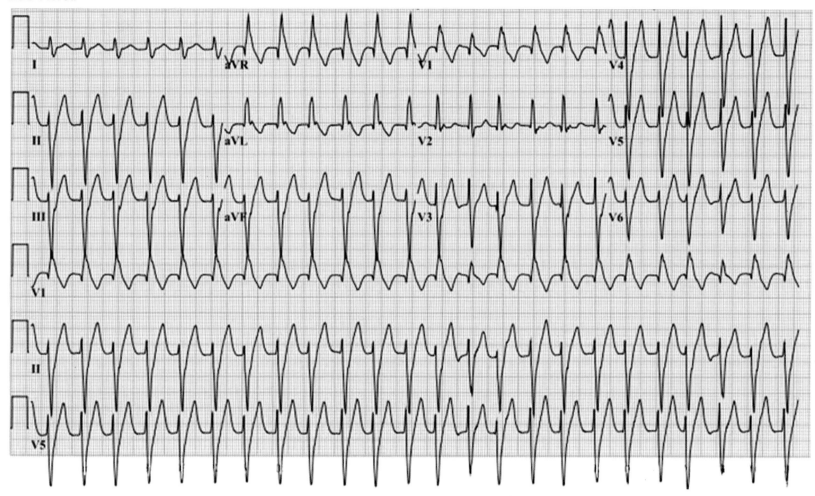

Image courtesy of Takashi Shiga, MD.

ECG 11.15b

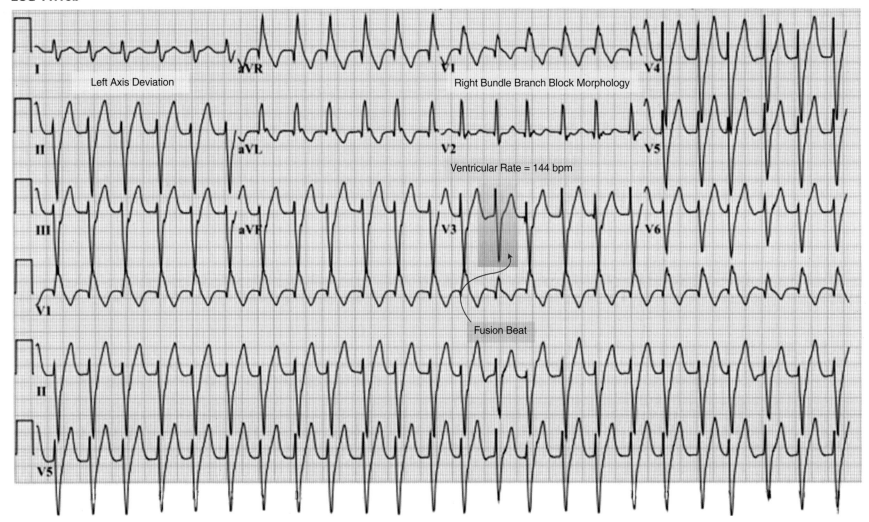

Left Axis Deviation

Right Bundle Branch Block Morphology

Ventricular Rate = 144 bpm

Fusion Beat

Fascicular Ventricular Tachycardia

This patient was diagnosed with fascicular VT. The combination of a RBBB morphology and left axis deviation suggests that the posterior fascicle is the origin of this arrhythmia. QRS complexes in fascicular VT are typically closer to 120 msec wide. This tachycardia responds well to verapamil and adenosine.

ECG 11.16a A 75-year-old female with symptomatic paroxysmal atrial fibrillation and coronary artery disease developed sudden onset chest pressure and light-headedness while carrying heavy bags through the airport.

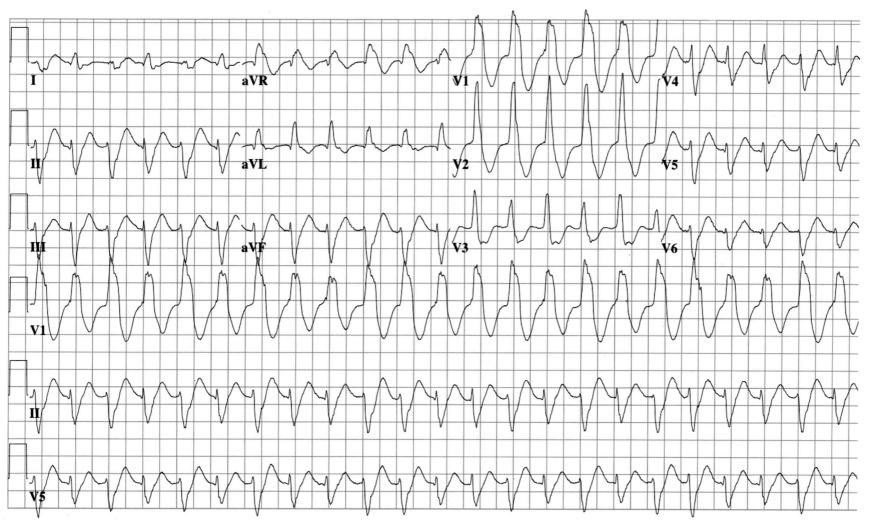

ECG 11.16b A 75-year-old female with symptomatic paroxysmal atrial fibrillation and coronary artery disease developed sudden onset chest pressure and light-headedness while carrying heavy bags through the airport.

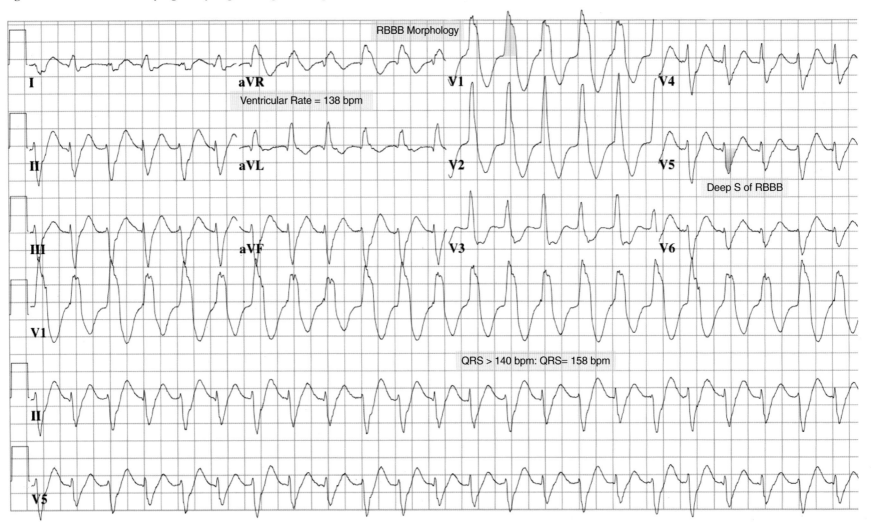

Ventricular Tachycardia

This patient was found in the electrophysiology lab to have two separate foci in the left ventricle and one focus in the right ventricle where sustained VT could be induced. She underwent radiofrequency ablation of these sites.

ECG 11.17a

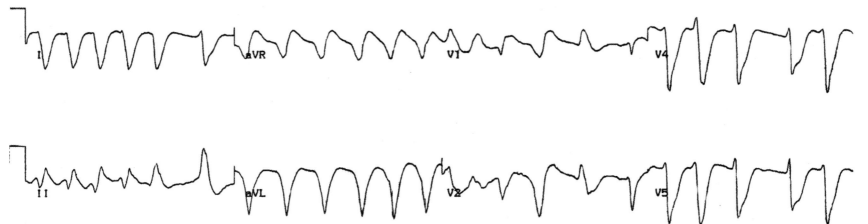
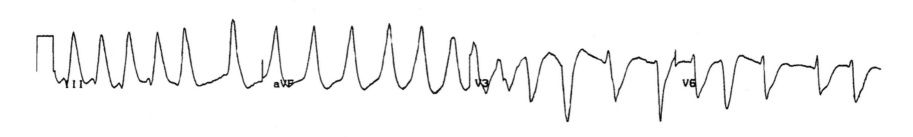
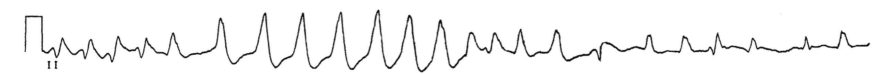

Image courtesy of Keith Marill, MD.

ECG 11.17b

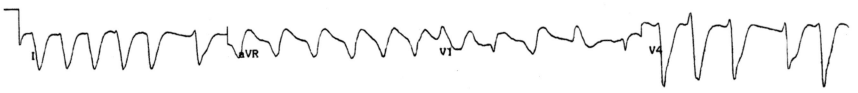

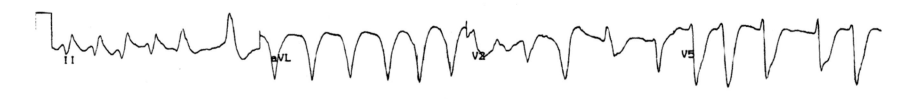

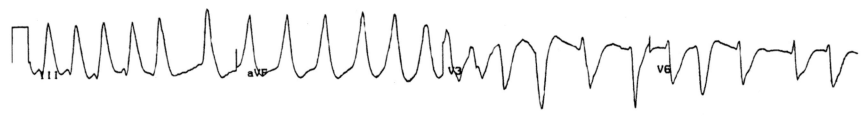

Highly Variable QRS Morphology

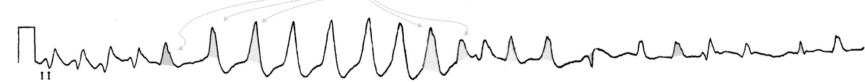

Polymorphic Ventricular Tachycardia

ECG 11.18a A 52-year-old woman with a history of myocardial infarction and congestive heart failure presents with shortness of breath.

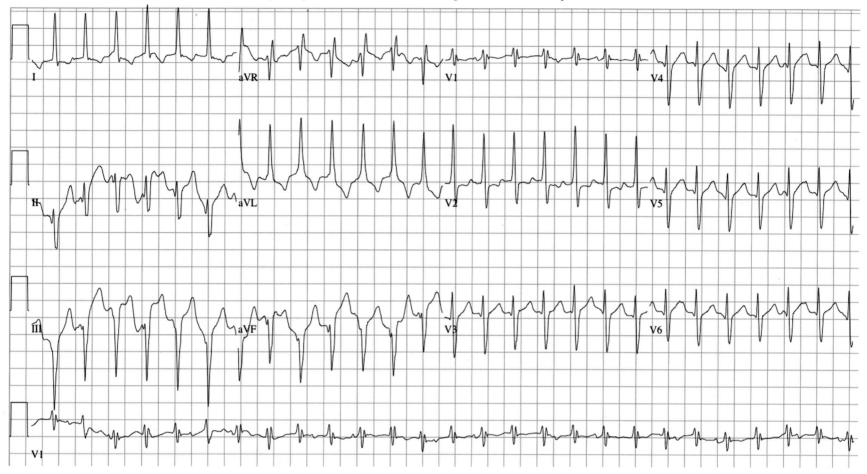

Image courtesy of Keith Marill, MD.

ECG 11.18b A 52-year-old woman with a history of myocardial infarction and congestive heart failure presents with shortness of breath.

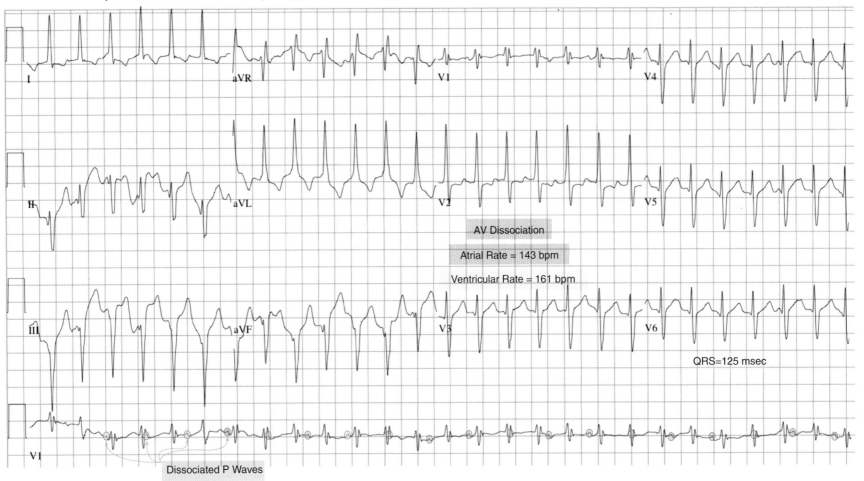

AV Dissociation

Atrial Rate = 143 bpm

Ventricular Rate = 161 bpm

QRS=125 msec

Dissociated P Waves

Ventricular Tachycardia

This ECG was initially misread as supraventricular tachycardia, given the narrow appearance of the QRS. Close inspection of lead V1, however, reveals AV dissociation.

ECG 11.19a A 65-years-old male with diabetes is brought into the emergency department in cardiac arrest.

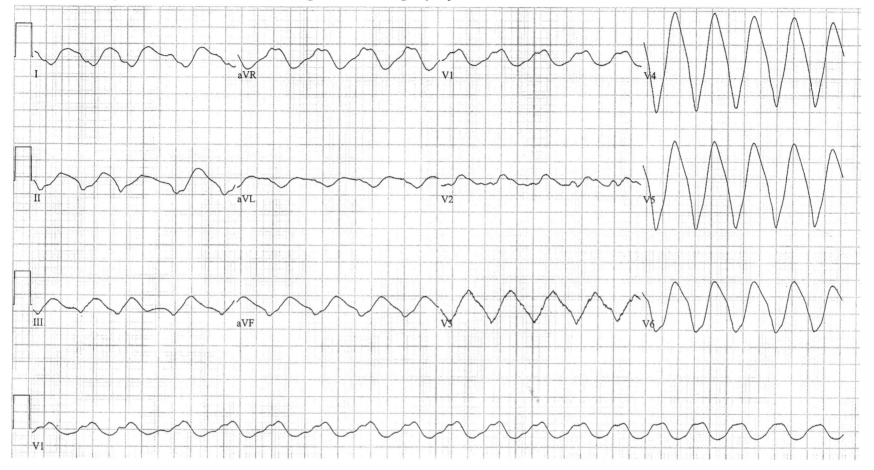

ECG 11.19b A 52-year-old woman with a history of myocardial infarction and congestive heart failure presents with shortness of breath.

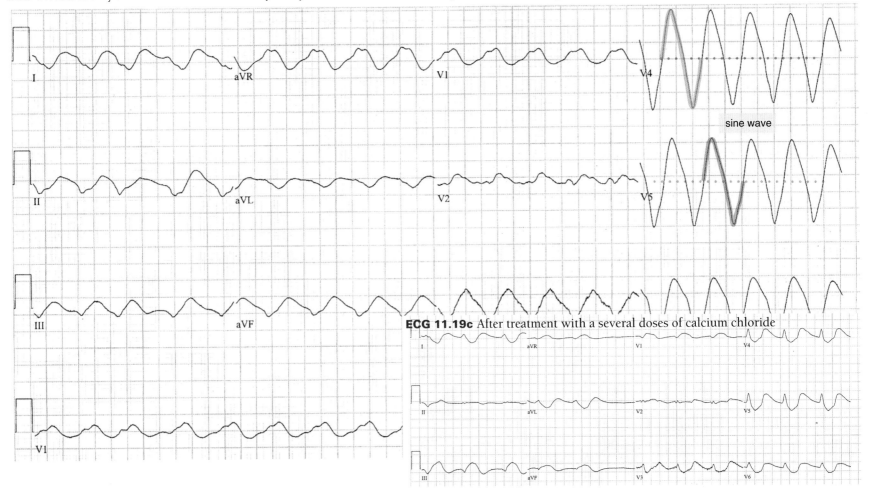

Severe Hyperkalemia

This patient's potassium level was 9.7 mg/dL. He was found to have new acute renal failure. After several doses of calcium chloride, the sine wave would transition to wide, but discernible QRS complexes (ECG 11.19c).

References

1. Pellegrini CN, Scheinman MM. Clinical management of ventricular tachycardia. *Curr Probl Cardiol* 2010;35:453–504.
2. Morady F, Baerman JM, DiCarlo LA Jr, et al. A prevalent misconception regarding wide-complex tachycardias. JAMA 1985;254:2790–2792.
3. Wellens HJ, Bar FW, Lie KI. The value of the electrocardiogram in the differential diagnosis of a tachycardia with a widened QRS complex. *Am J Med* 1978;64:27–33.
4. Brugada P, Brugada J, Mont L, et al. A new approach to the differential diagnosis of a regular tachycardia with a wide QRS complex. *Circulation* 1991;83:1649–1659.
5. Akhtar M, Shenasa M, Jazayeri M, et al. Wide QRS complex tachycardia. Reappraisal of a common clinical problem. *Ann Intern Med* 1988;109:905–912.

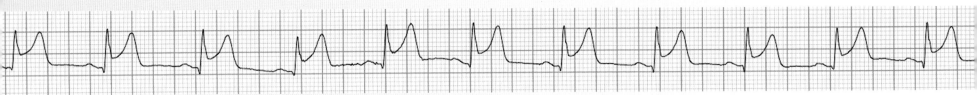

Coronary Anatomy

The right and left main coronary arteries arise from the right and left aortic sinuses located at the aortic root. The left main coronary artery branches into the left anterior descending and left circumflex artery.

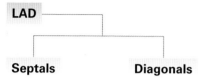

The left anterior descending artery travels down the interventricular groove toward the apex. It may wrap around the apex to supply blood to the posterior-apical wall. The left anterior descending supplies blood to the anteroseptal, anterior, and anterolateral walls of the left ventricle. The LAD divides into diagonal branches that supply the base of the left ventricle and septal branches that are oriented perpendicular to the LAD to supply blood to the interventricular septum.

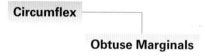

The circumflex artery wraps around the left atrioventricular groove and supplies blood to both anterior and posterior aspects of the lateral wall.

The major branches of the circumflex are the obtuse marginal (OM) arteries. They supply blood to the lateral free wall of the left ventricle.

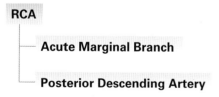

The right coronary artery (RCA) runs along the right atrioventricular groove and supplies blood to the right ventricle through its acute marginal branch. It wraps around to the posterior wall of the right ventricle before branching into the posterior descending artery (PDA). The PDA descends toward the apex along the posterior interventricular groove and supplies blood to the inferior septum and wall, the right bundle branch, and the posteromedial papillary muscle of the mitral valve.

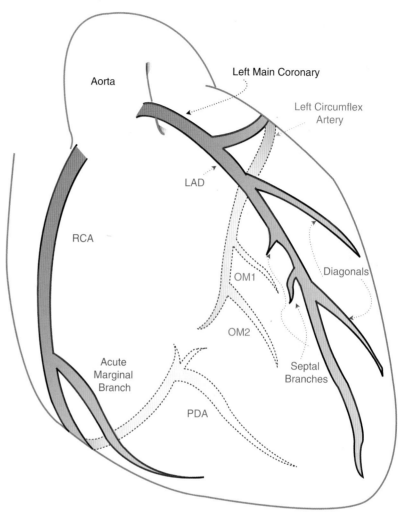

FIGURE 12.1 Simplified diagram of the coronary arteries and their branches depicted from an anterior view of a heart with right-dominant circulation.

Right Coronary Dominance In 85% of patients, the RCA is considered dominant, giving rise to the PDA and a posterolateral branch that supplies blood to the left ventricle. In 15% of patients, the PDA branches off the left circumflex artery.[1]

Subendocardial Ischemia

Pathophysiology

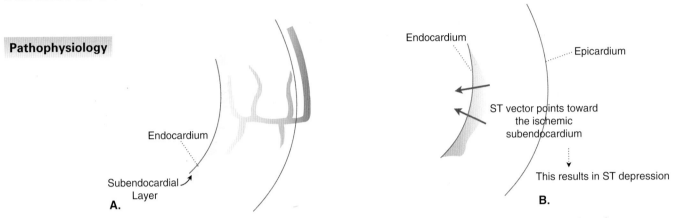

FIGURE 12.2 A. Relationship of coronary artery to layers of the ventricular wall. B. Vectors resulting from subendocardial ischemia.

The coronary arteries supply blood to the cardiac muscle by piercing the epicardium along which it runs, and branching into the epicardial, myocardial, and subendocardial vessels. Subendocardial tissue receives the most distal branches and thus the most distal coronary blood supply, making it the layer most susceptible to coronary ischemia.

ECG Features

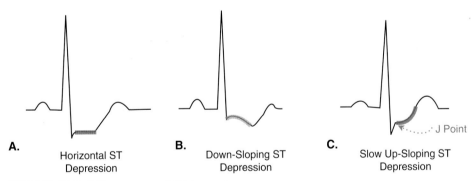

FIGURE 12.3 Different types of ST depression.

ST depression is a nonspecific finding for subendocardial ischemia. The pattern of ST depression (≥1 mm) is typically horizontal or down-sloping. ST depression can also have an up-sloping pattern when the J point is depressed.

The T waves of subendocardial ischemia often remain upright but with decreased amplitude. This differs from LVH with strain pattern in which the T waves are inverted.

The leads that demonstrate ST depression *do not* anatomically correspond to the region of the left ventricle which is affected by myocardial ischemia.[2] Cardiac markers may be elevated with ST depression if there is associated myocardial necrosis.

ST Elevation MI

Pathophysiology

ST elevation MI (STEMI) results from complete thrombotic occlusion or persistent vasospasm of an epicardial coronary artery. Insufficient perfusion results in epicardial or transmural injury.

Prinzmetal angina: Coronary vasospasm occludes distal blood flow. When it persists for more than 20 minutes, transmural infarction can result.

Current of Injury   Acute ischemia alters the action potential of the myocardial cell in several ways. Voltage differences in the action potential between normal and ischemic cells set up a current, the vector of which results in ST elevation.

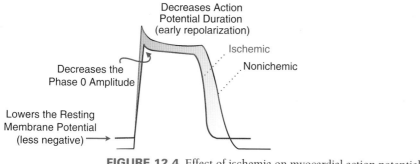

FIGURE 12.4 Effect of ischemia on myocardial action potential.

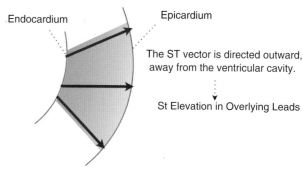

FIGURE 12.5 Vector resulting from MI.

ECG Evolution

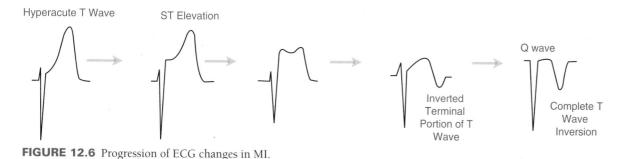

FIGURE 12.6 Progression of ECG changes in MI.

Signs of Reperfusion

Resolution of ST Elevation   Resolution of ST elevations by more than 70% is associated with reperfusion. The degree of ST segment resolution has been shown to be related to infarct size, left ventricular function, and clinical outcome.[3,4]

Early T Wave Inversion   The appearance of early T wave inversion has been associated with reperfusion and decreased mortality.[5]

ST Elevation

ST elevation in myocardial infarction (MI) can have different morphologies. It is important to recognize them all.

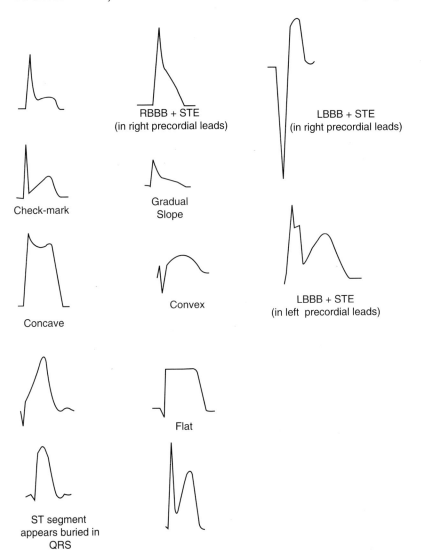

FIGURE 12.7 Different morphologies of ST segments in acute MI.

Localizing the Infarct

Different patterns of ST elevation on an ECG correlate with different sites of coronary artery occlusion. The territory and extent of MI can be inferred from the pattern of lead involvement. The diagram below is a color-coded representation of different ST elevation patterns as they correlate to the coronary anatomy of someone with right-coronary dominance.

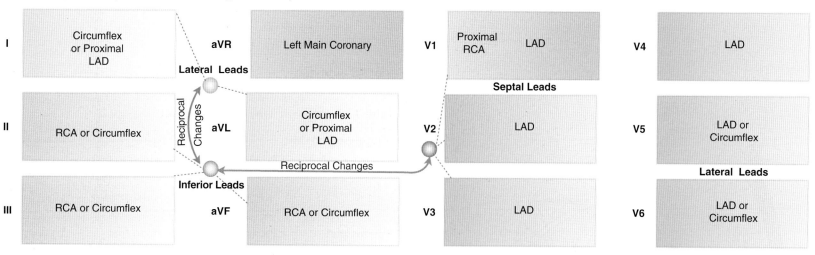

Anterior MI

When the occlusion is located at the mid or distal aspects of the LAD, ST segments will be elevated in V1-V3. Reciprocal depressions can be seen in II, III, and aVF.

Anterolateral MI

Occlusion of the proximal LAD or left main coronary can result in an extensive anterolateral MI.

The ST segment in aVR can be elevated to a greater extent than in V1 in left main coronary artery occlusion.[6]

Right Ventricular MI

ST elevation in V1, especially in the setting of ST elevations in the inferior leads, can represent infarction of the right ventricle. This results from occlusion of the proximal RCA. Placing right-sided leads (V3R-V5R) can help increase the sensitivity of ECG for the diagnosis of right ventricular MI.

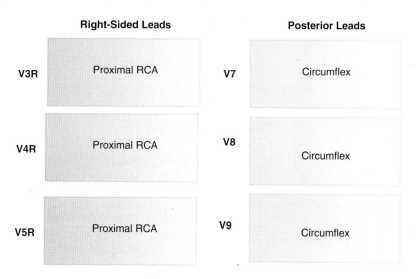

FIGURE 12.8 A map of ECG leads and their associated coronary artery anatomy. Colored circles represent groupings of ECG leads.

Inferior MI

Inferior MI can result from occlusion of either the left circumflex or RCA. ST segments are elevated in II, III, and aVF.

Reciprocal ST depressions occur in leads I and aVL and leads V1-V3.

Posterior MI

Lead V1 can be considered as a mirror image of posterior leads. ST depressions in V1 can be reflections of ST elevations in posterior leads (V7-V9). Occlusion of the left circumflex artery can cause this type of MI.

Anterior MI

The LAD supplies a significant area of the left ventricular wall. Complete occlusion of the LAD can result in extensive myocardial necrosis and severely compromised cardiac output. Septal and diagonal branches arise from the LAD. The pattern of infarction varies based on whether the occlusion occurs proximal or distal to these branches.

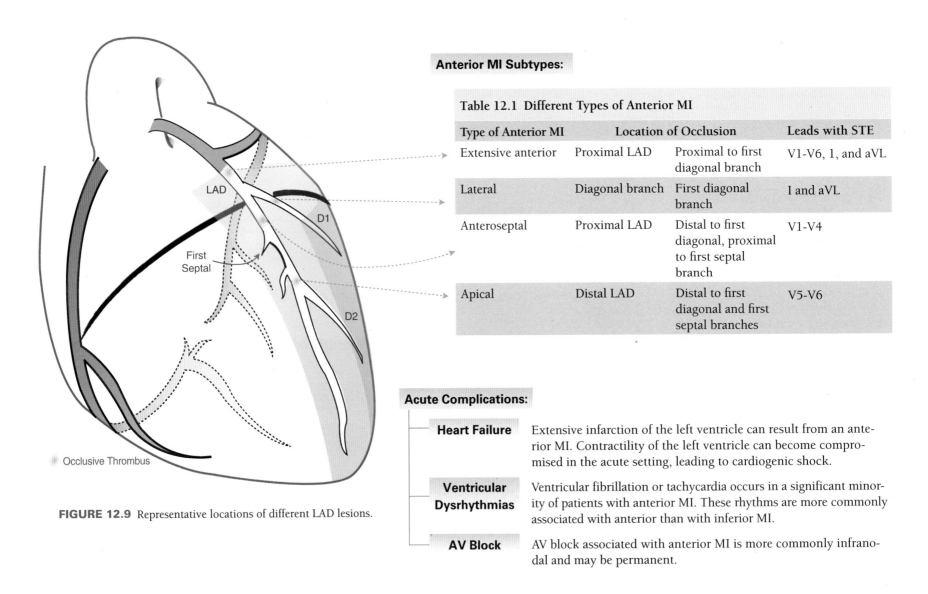

Anterior MI Subtypes:

Table 12.1 Different Types of Anterior MI

Type of Anterior MI	Location of Occlusion		Leads with STE
Extensive anterior	Proximal LAD	Proximal to first diagonal branch	V1-V6, 1, and aVL
Lateral	Diagonal branch	First diagonal branch	I and aVL
Anteroseptal	Proximal LAD	Distal to first diagonal, proximal to first septal branch	V1-V4
Apical	Distal LAD	Distal to first diagonal and first septal branches	V5-V6

LAD

D1

First Septal

D2

Occlusive Thrombus

FIGURE 12.9 Representative locations of different LAD lesions.

Acute Complications:

Heart Failure Extensive infarction of the left ventricle can result from an anterior MI. Contractility of the left ventricle can become compromised in the acute setting, leading to cardiogenic shock.

Ventricular Dysrhythmias Ventricular fibrillation or tachycardia occurs in a significant minority of patients with anterior MI. These rhythms are more commonly associated with anterior than with inferior MI.

AV Block AV block associated with anterior MI is more commonly infranodal and may be permanent.

Inferior MI

An inferior MI results in ST elevations in leads II, III, and aVF. Reciprocal ST depressions appear in leads I and aVL.

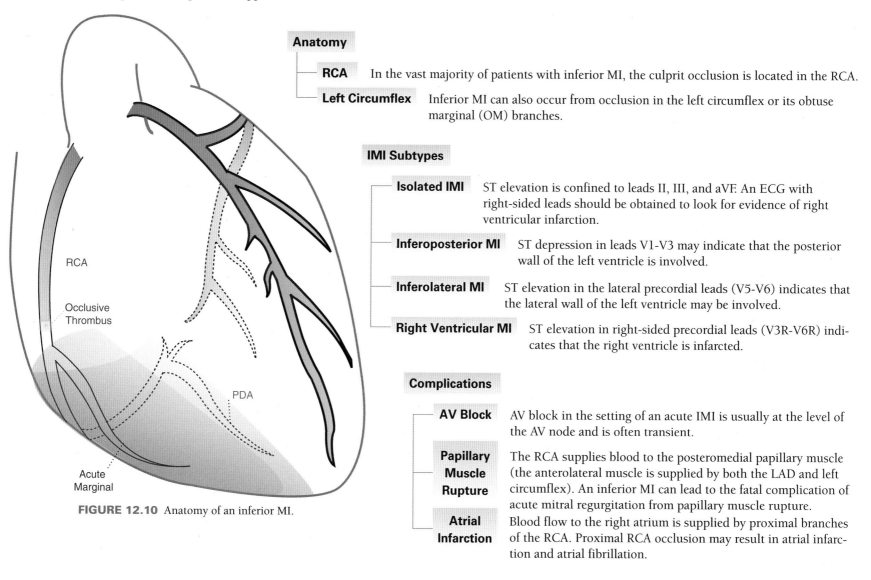

Anatomy

RCA In the vast majority of patients with inferior MI, the culprit occlusion is located in the RCA.

Left Circumflex Inferior MI can also occur from occlusion in the left circumflex or its obtuse marginal (OM) branches.

IMI Subtypes

Isolated IMI ST elevation is confined to leads II, III, and aVF. An ECG with right-sided leads should be obtained to look for evidence of right ventricular infarction.

Inferoposterior MI ST depression in leads V1-V3 may indicate that the posterior wall of the left ventricle is involved.

Inferolateral MI ST elevation in the lateral precordial leads (V5-V6) indicates that the lateral wall of the left ventricle may be involved.

Right Ventricular MI ST elevation in right-sided precordial leads (V3R-V6R) indicates that the right ventricle is infarcted.

Complications

AV Block AV block in the setting of an acute IMI is usually at the level of the AV node and is often transient.

Papillary Muscle Rupture The RCA supplies blood to the posteromedial papillary muscle (the anterolateral muscle is supplied by both the LAD and left circumflex). An inferior MI can lead to the fatal complication of acute mitral regurgitation from papillary muscle rupture.

Atrial Infarction Blood flow to the right atrium is supplied by proximal branches of the RCA. Proximal RCA occlusion may result in atrial infarction and atrial fibrillation.

FIGURE 12.10 Anatomy of an inferior MI.

Posterior Myocardial Infarction

Posterior MIs occur in isolation in a significant minority (3%–7%) of STEMIs.[7,8] Because no leads in the standard 12-lead ECG directly face the posterior wall of the left ventricle, the 12-lead ECG is an insensitive tool for diagnosing this type of infarction. Diagnosis of a posterior MI is often missed or delayed. Patients with a posterior MI benefit from early PCI and thrombolysis.

Anatomy

Posterior MIs usually result from occlusion of the left circumflex artery (or its first OM branch). The left circumflex artery supplies blood to the lateral and posterior walls of the left ventricle. Posterior MIs are commonly associated with lateral and inferior infarctions.

ECG Features

ST Depression V1-V3

These leads can be a mirrored representation of the posterior left ventricular (PLV) wall. ST depression in V1-V3, therefore, may actually represent posterior ST elevation.

Prominent R Waves V1

A tall R wave in V1 is abnormal. A tall R wave in V1 could represent the mirror image of a deep Q wave coming from the posterior wall. This, however, can be a marker of an old posterior MI.

ST Elevation in Posterior Leads

Posterior MI can only be confirmed on EKG by demonstrating ST elevation in posterior leads V7-V9. These leads are placed in the same horizontal plane as leads V4-V6. V7 is placed at the left posterior axillary line, V8 at the scapular tip, and V9 to the left of the spinal column.

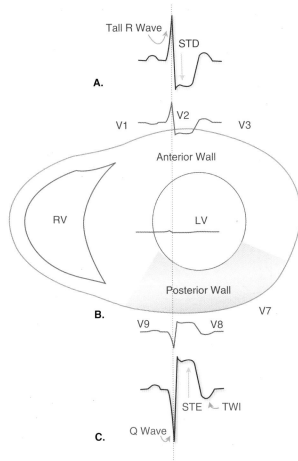

FIGURE 12.11 **A.** ECG appearance in anterior precordial leads. **B.** Axial view of a heart with posterior wall infarction. **C.** ECG appearance in posterior leads.

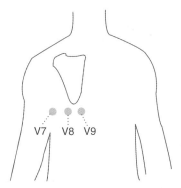

FIGURE 12.12 Positioning of posterior leads.

Table 12.2 Differential Diagnosis of ST Depression in V1
Posterior STEMI
Reciprocal changes to an inferior MI
Anterior subendocardial ischemia

Right Ventricular MI

Infarction of the right ventricle occurs in approximately 50% of inferior MIs.[9] Right ventricular MIs may also rarely occur in isolation. Life-threatening complications from a right ventricular infarction can occur early in the acute presentation.

Anatomy

Infarction of the right ventricle results from occlusion of the RCA proximal to the first acute marginal branch. The marginal branch is critical in supplying blood to the free wall of the right ventricle.

ECG Features

STE in V1

ST elevation in lead V1 is a relatively specific finding, but sensitivity is very poor. ST elevation is most prominent in V1 with declining degrees of elevation in V2 and V3. ST elevation in leads V1-V3 may lead to the incorrect diagnosis of an anteroseptal MI. The degree of ST elevation should increase in V2 and V3 in an anteroseptal MI.

STE in III > STE in II

ST segments in an RV MI are elevated in II, III, and aVF. Because lead III is a right-sided limb lead, ST elevation is greater in lead III than in lead II (a left-sided limb lead) in an RV MI. This may be a more sensitive finding than ST elevation in V4R.[9]

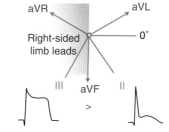

FIGURE 12.14 ST elevation in II and III as they relate to their leftward and rightward lead positions.

STE in V4R-V6R

Right-sided precordial leads should be recorded in all patients with an inferior MI. ST elevation ≥1mm in V4R-V6R is diagnostic of an RV MI. V4R is the most sensitive lead. This is a transient finding and may be absent for 24–48 hours after symptom onset.[9]

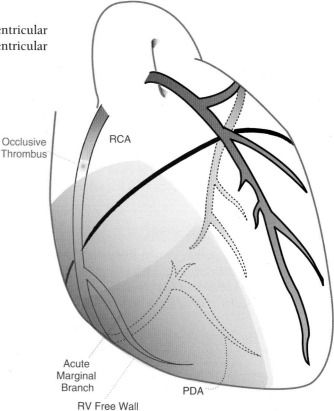

FIGURE 12.13 Proximal RCA occlusion resulting in infarction of the right ventricular lateral and posterior walls (*areas shaded in blue*).

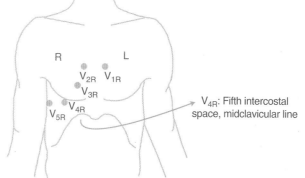

FIGURE 12.15 Positioning of right-sided precordial leads.

Complications of a Right Ventricular MI

Lower oxygen demand, collateral blood supply from the LAD, and a thinner myocardium are factors that limit the morbidity and mortality in right ventricular MI relative to those associated with a left ventricular MI. However, extension of an inferior MI to involve the right ventricle is associated with increased morbidity and mortality compared to inferior MIs that occur in isolation. Right ventricular MIs are also associated with their own hemodynamic complications.

Hypotension

In a minority of patients with right ventricular MI, right ventricular failure (both systolic and diastolic dysfunction of the right ventricle) results in altered hemodynamics.[10] The presence of hypotension should raise concern for a right ventricular MI. Hypotension, jugular venous distention, and clear lungs are described as a clinical triad associated with RV MI.[11] The classic hemodynamic finding on right-heart catheterization is a disproportionate elevation in right-sided filling pressures. Right ventricular dysfunction often resolves in several weeks, suggesting that the myocardium of the right ventricle is stunned in the acute setting and not necrotic.[12] Early identification of an RV MI is critical in preventing iatrogenic hypotension by the administration of preload-reducing agents (nitroglycerin).

Systolic Dysfunction

Decreased cardiac output from the right ventricle results in decreased preload delivered to the left side of the heart. Left ventricular output suffers and results in hypotension. Treatment is aimed at increasing right ventricular preload by delivering intravenous crystalloid.

Diastolic Dysfunction

Decreased compliance of the right ventricle leads to increased diastolic filling pressures of both the right ventricle and atrium. This can result in the bowing of the interventricular septum into the left ventricular space during diastole. The amount of left ventricular diastolic filling becomes limited.

Hypoxemia

R-to-L Shunt

Patients with a patent foramen ovale in the setting of elevated RV and RA pressures can develop a right-to-left shunt leading to hypoxemia.

Pulmonary Emboli

Embolization of a right ventricular thrombus from the cavity of an infarcted right ventricle to the pulmonary circulation is another important cause of hypoxemia to consider.

Bradycardia

Vagal Stimulation

Reflex stimulation of afferent vagal fibers that run along the RCA may result in sinus bradycardia.

AV Block

In most patients, the blood supply to the AV node is from the AV nodal branch of the RCA. Persistent AV block may indicate AV nodal dysfunction in an ischemic AV node. However, in many cases, AV block in the acute setting of an RV MI is from vagal stimulation.

Atrial Fibrillation

Occlusion of the proximal RCA can lead to right atrial infarction. This can increase the risk of supraventricular tachyarrhythmias including atrial fibrillation.

Acute Pulmonary Edema

The RCA is the single blood supply to the posteromedial papillary muscle of the mitral valve. Proximal RCA occlusion can result in papillary muscle rupture and subsequent life-threatening mitral regurgitation.

Pericarditis

Pericarditis accounts for approximately 5% of the causes of non-ischemic chest pain in the emergency department.[13] In the vast majority of cases, this cause is unknown or secondary to viral infection. Less common causes include malignancy, uremia, chest wall irradiation, chest trauma, autoimmune disease, medications, recent myocardial infarction, and bacterial infections.

Clinical Characteristics

The chest pain of acute pericarditis often has a sudden onset. It is described as retrosternal (or left sided), pleuritic, and positional (relieved by sitting forward, worse supine). The pain can radiate to the trapezius ridge or down the left arm. Symptoms typically last less than 2 weeks.

ECG Features

Diffuse ST elevation is the classic finding in acute pericarditis. ST segments are elevated in all leads except aVR and often V1. Elevated ST segments are typically concave. The ECG characteristics of acute pericarditis evolve through four stages.[14]

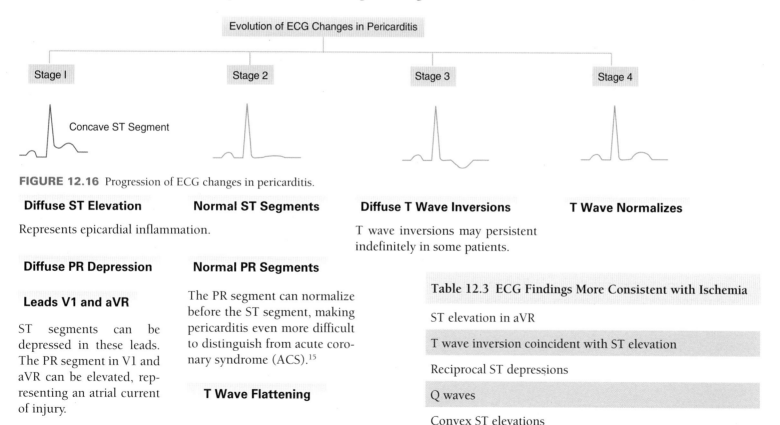

FIGURE 12.16 Progression of ECG changes in pericarditis.

Diffuse ST Elevation

Represents epicardial inflammation.

Diffuse PR Depression

Leads V1 and aVR

ST segments can be depressed in these leads. The PR segment in V1 and aVR can be elevated, representing an atrial current of injury.

Normal ST Segments

Normal PR Segments

The PR segment can normalize before the ST segment, making pericarditis even more difficult to distinguish from acute coronary syndrome (ACS).[15]

T Wave Flattening

Diffuse T Wave Inversions

T wave inversions may persistent indefinitely in some patients.

T Wave Normalizes

Table 12.3 ECG Findings More Consistent with Ischemia
ST elevation in aVR
T wave inversion coincident with ST elevation
Reciprocal ST depressions
Q waves
Convex ST elevations

Left Ventricular Aneurysm

Left ventricular aneurysms are dyskinetic segments of the left ventricular wall that bulge out during both systole and diastole. LV aneurysm develops in less than 5% of all patients with STEMI.[16]

Anatomy	LV aneurysms most commonly complicate large anterior MIs and occur in the anterior or anterolateral wall of the left ventricle.
	Less often, aneurysms can occur in the inferior or posterior walls after infarction involving these areas.
Pathology	The aneurysmal wall is thin and consists of fibrous and necrotic myocardial tissue. Rupture, however, is rare.

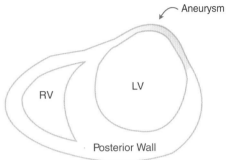

FIGURE 12.17 Anterior LV aneurysm.

ECG Features

Q Waves	Deep Q waves commonly accompany the elevated ST segments resulting from an LV aneurysm.
STE	ST elevation occurs most often in the anterior precordial leads. The ST segment is often concave. Elevation of the ST segments is thought to be secondary to traction on the normal myocardium by the scarred tissue forming the aneurysm.
Absent Reciprocal Depression	Reciprocal ST depression is notably *absent*.
Absence of Dynamic Changes	The morphology of the QRS waves is unchanged over time. ST elevation appears fixed and unrelated to the patient's complaint or resolution of chest pain.

Persistent ST elevation after MI does not always indicate left ventricular aneurysm. ST elevation may indicate regional wall motion abnormality in an infarcted area. Imaging studies can help differentiate wall motion abnormality from a true aneurysm.

Clinical Course	Larger aneurysms may both decrease left ventricular stroke volume and increase oxygen demand of surrounding viable myocardium. Patients may subsequently develop heart failure or angina.

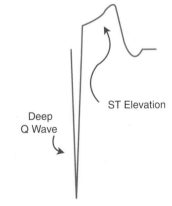

FIGURE 12.18 ECG appearance of an anterior LV aneurysm.

Benign Early Repolarization

Benign early repolarization (BER) is a pattern of ST elevation occurring in approximately 1–2% of the population, more commonly in young adults and in men.[17] It is important to recognize this pattern and be able to distinguish it from acute MI and pericarditis.

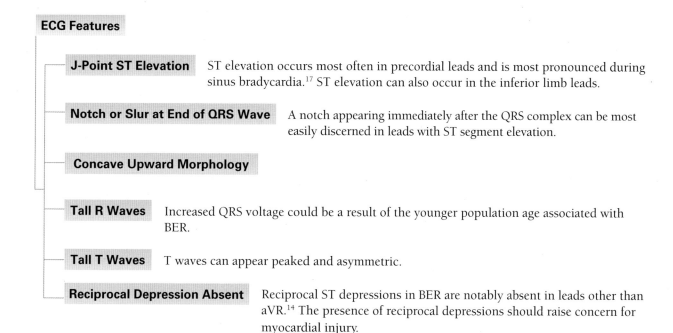

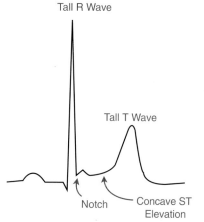

ECG Features

J-Point ST Elevation ST elevation occurs most often in precordial leads and is most pronounced during sinus bradycardia.[17] ST elevation can also occur in the inferior limb leads.

Notch or Slur at End of QRS Wave A notch appearing immediately after the QRS complex can be most easily discerned in leads with ST segment elevation.

Concave Upward Morphology

Tall R Waves Increased QRS voltage could be a result of the younger population age associated with BER.

Tall T Waves T waves can appear peaked and asymmetric.

Reciprocal Depression Absent Reciprocal ST depressions in BER are notably absent in leads other than aVR.[14] The presence of reciprocal depressions should raise concern for myocardial injury.

FIGURE 12.19 ECG appearance of BER.

Differential Unlike pericarditis and MI, the ECG abnormalities associated with BER are relatively constant.

Pericarditis PR segment depression may not reliably distinguish between BER and pericarditis.[18] Notching and slurring at the end of the QRS complex, however, is present in BER but is not a feature in pericarditis.[19]

Myocardial Infarction Convexity of the ST segment, reciprocal changes, presence of Q waves, and lower R wave amplitudes are findings more suggestive of MI than BER.

Takotsubo Cardiomyopathy

Takotsubo cardiomyopathy is a nonischemic cardiomyopathy in which the ventricular myocardium becomes acutely weakened and dysfunctional.

Other names for this syndrome include apical ballooning syndrome, stress-induced cardiomyopathy, broken heart syndrome, and neurogenic stunning syndrome.

The base of the left ventricle is hyperkinetic, and the apex instead of contracting along with the base, balloons outward during systole.

The area of the left ventricle affected does not correspond to a particular vascular territory.

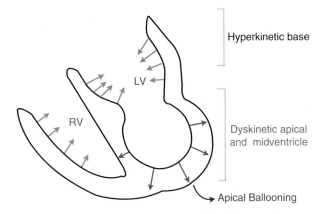

FIGURE 12.20 Apical ballooning of the left ventricle in systole. Arrows indicate direction of contraction forces.

Angiographic Appearance	The shape that the LV acquires during this ballooning phase has been described as reminiscent of the trap (takot-subo) used in Japan for catching an octopus.
ECG Appearance	ST segments in the precordial leads are elevated and mimic the appearance of an anterior STEMI. The ST segment normalizes over a short period of time (hours), and T waves become inverted. There is no reliable way to distinguish Takotsubo cardiomyopathy from STEMI on ECG. The diagnosis is made by coronary angiography.
Clinical Presentation	Acute chest pain or heart failure in a postmenopausal woman. The onset of this syndrome often follows an acute emotional or stressful event. Cardiac markers can become elevated. Coronary angiography reveals the absence of an occlusive thrombus.
Prognosis	Left ventricular dysfunction most often resolves completely within days to weeks after symptom onset. Complications include left heart failure, and, rarely, death.

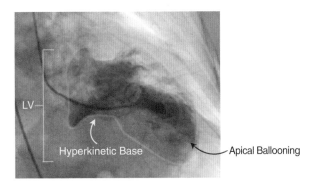

FIGURE 12.21 Image obtained from a left ventricular angiography in a patient with Takotsubo cardiomyopathy.

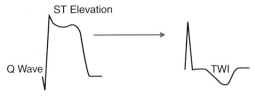

FIGURE 12.22 Evolution of ECG appearance in Takotsubo cardiomyopathy.

Left Bundle Branch Block and ST Segment Deviation

ST segments deviate in ECGs with left bundle branch block (LBBB). They deviate in a predictably discordant pattern. Discordance is a term used to describe segments on opposite sides of an isoelectric line (shown as a faint blue line below). In leads with negative QRS waves (right-sided precordial leads, V1-V2), one can expect to see elevated ST segments and positive T waves. In left-sided leads (V5-V6) with positive QRS waves, one can expect to see ST depression and T wave inversion. This pattern is referred to as "appropriate discordance."

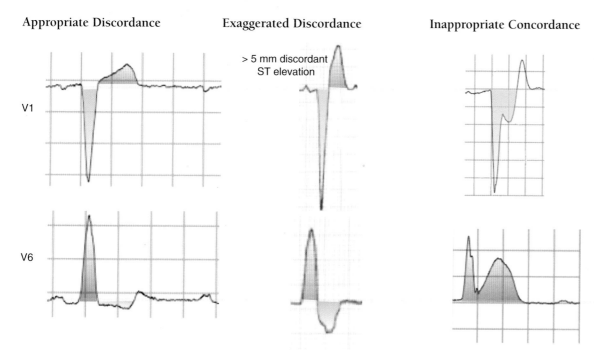

FIGURE 12.23 Comparison of abnormal findings in LBBB to the normal appearance of LBBB in leads V1 and V6.

Discordance associated with LBBB can mask ischemic changes. However, ST segments may deviate in ways that suggest MI. Both inappropriate concordance and exaggerated discordance are concerning ECG findings.

Sgarbossa *et al* derived and validated a scoring system for diagnosing MI in the presence of LBBB.[20] A score greater than or equal to 3 is highly specific for and positively predictive of acute MI.[21] However, it is important to remember that the sensitivity and negative predictive value of these criteria were low in their studied populations.

Inappropriate Concordance	**Concordant STE**	Concordant ST elevation ≥1 mm in any lead	5 Points
	Concordant STD	Concordant ST depression ≥1 mm in leads V1-V3	3 Points
Exaggerated Discordance	**Discordant STE**	Discordant STE ≥5 mm in any lead	2 Points

Mimics of ST Elevation MI

An awareness of conditions that can masquerade as STEMI is critical in limiting the attendant adverse effects of thrombolysis or percutaneous coronary intervention and minimizing delay of appropriate treatment for conditions other than ACS.

Takotsubo Cardiomyopathy	This clinical entity is often indistinguishable from an acute anterior MI. The diagnosis is made by coronary angiography.
Pericarditis	ST elevations are concave up and are diffuse (sparing lead aVR). Reciprocal ST depressions are notably absent except in lead aVR, and T waves remain upright until the ST segments are normalized. Diffuse PR segment depression (except in lead aVR) helps to distinguish pericarditis. In cases of focal pericarditis, ST elevations may be more localized to a group of leads.
Myocarditis	ST elevations are diffuse and can resemble those of acute MI or pericarditis.
Pulmonary Embolism	ST elevation is an uncommon ECG finding in pulmonary embolism but can mimic anteroseptal or inferior MI.[22–24]
LV Aneurysm	ST elevation that persists for several weeks after an acute MI could be secondary to the formation of a left ventricular aneurysm. Large Q waves accompany the elevated ST segments. Reciprocal ST depressions are notably absent.
Brugada Pattern	ST segments in the right precordial leads, V1 and V2, are by definition elevated in all three Brugada patterns. The ST segment is either coved or saddle-back shaped. Reciprocal changes are notably absent.
Hypothermia	A J wave (Osborn wave) can be of high amplitude and mistaken for the kind of ST elevation seen in acute MI.
LBBB	Repolarization abnormalities accompany the depolarization abnormalities in LBBB. In segments with predominantly negative QRS complexes, the ST segments will be elevated in a discordant fashion. Exaggerated discordance (ST elevation > 5 mm) and inappropriate concordance raise concern for MI.
LVH	Repolarization abnormalities in a hypertrophied myocardium generate the same type of discordance as seen in LBBB. In the precordial leads with negative QRS complexes, the ST segments may be elevated.
Hyperkalemia	ST elevation is an uncommon finding in hyperkalemia. When present, the degree of ST elevation can be dramatic and the elevation can localize in an anatomic distribution to precordial or limb leads. The ST elevation corrects with normalization of potassium levels.[25] Look for other ECG abnormalities suggestive of hyperkalemia.
Hypercalcemia	Severe hypercalcemia has been described in case reports to cause ECG changes that mimic acute ST elevation MI.[26–28] These changes resolve with lowering serum calcium levels.
Benign Early Repolarization	Concave ST elevation in the precordial leads may be a normal finding, particularly in young men. Additional findings that support the diagnosis of BER include the presence of a notch at the end of the QRS complex, absence of reciprocal depression, tall R waves, and peaked T waves. These findings tend to be more pronounced during sinus bradycardia.
Cardioversion	ST segments can become transiently (lasting minutes) depressed or elevated immediately following electrical direct current cardioversion.[29] This may be less common with biphasic defibrillation.[30]

ECG 12.1a A 47-year-old male with a history of prior MI presents with shortness of breath, substernal chest pain, hypotension, and diaphoresis.

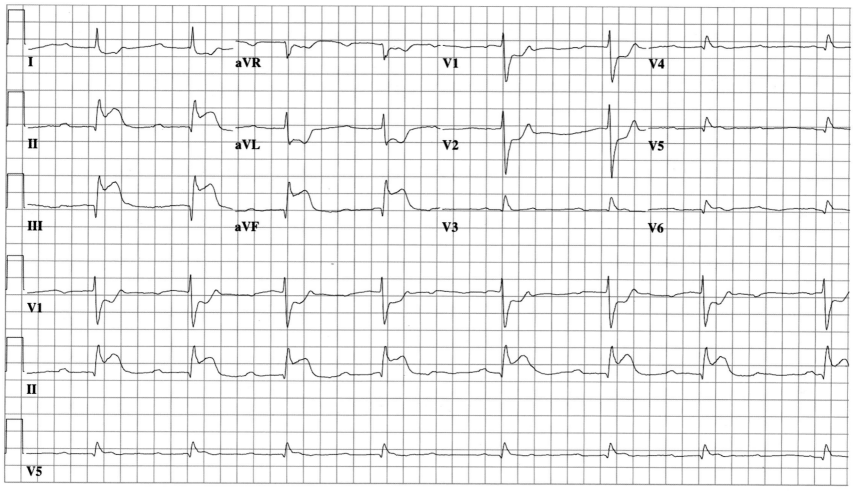

ECG 12.1b A 47-year-old male with a history of prior MI presents with shortness of breath, substernal chest pain, hypotension, and diaphoresis.

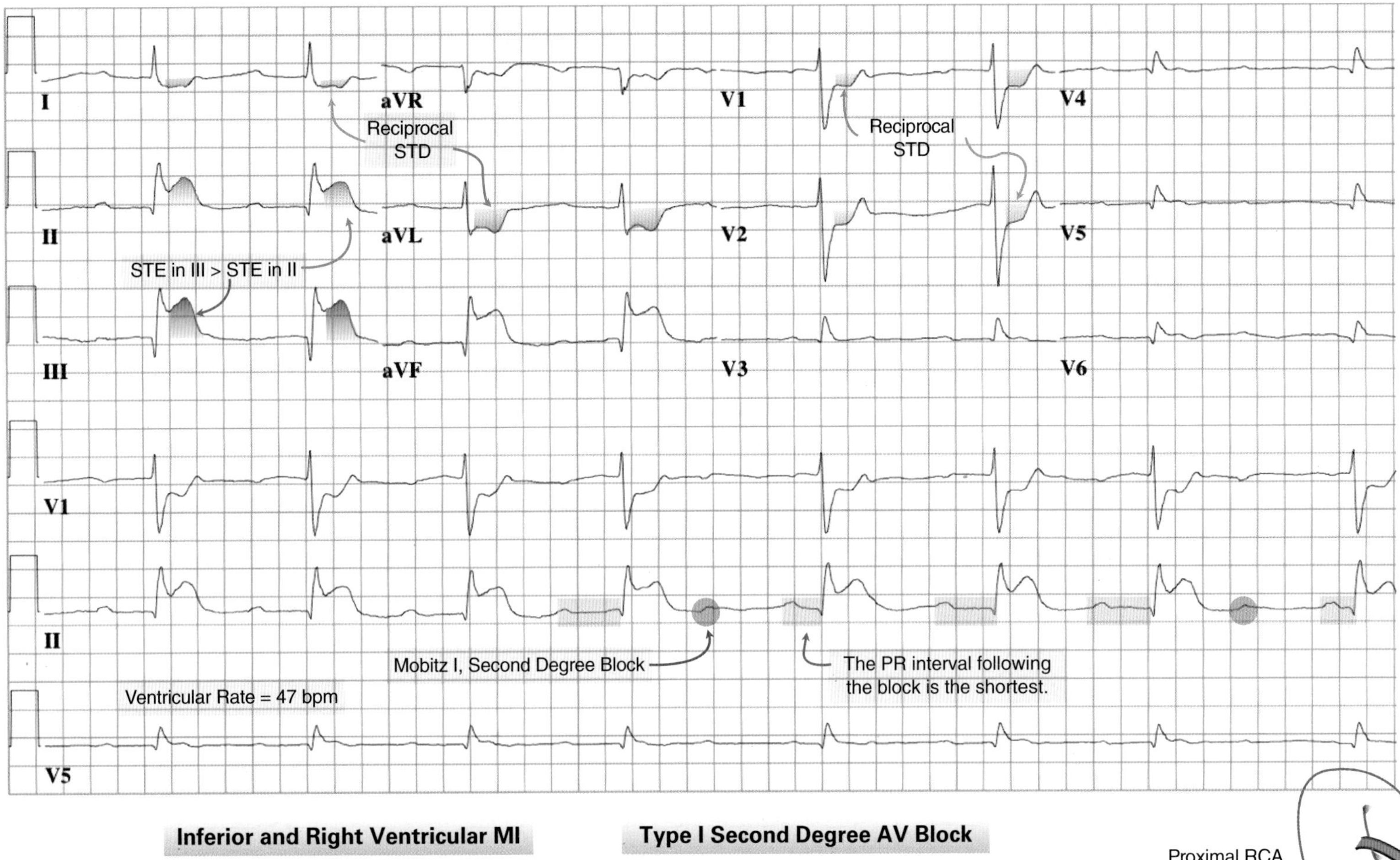

I

aVR
Reciprocal
STD

V1

V4

II

aVL

V2

Reciprocal
STD

V5

STE in III > STE in II

III

aVF

V3

V6

V1

II

Mobitz I, Second Degree Block

The PR interval following
the block is the shortest.

Ventricular Rate = 47 bpm

V5

Inferior and Right Ventricular MI   **Type I Second Degree AV Block**

This patient arrived with a blood pressure of 80/40. His heart rate was intermittently between 30 and 40 bpm en route to the ED. Cardiac catheterization revealed total occlusion of the proximal RCA.

The clue in this ECG that the infarction involved the right ventricle was the greater degree of ST elevation in lead III than in lead II. Lead III reflects the right side of the heart more than lead II. An ECG that includes right-sided leads was not recorded in this patient.

The ST segment in V1 may fail to show ST elevation (or as in this ECG, may show ST depression) because it may more strongly reflect reciprocal changes to the ST elevations in the inferior leads. When injury to the inferior wall is less extensive, right-sided precordial leads demonstrate ST elevations.[31]

This patient's hypotension was likely the result of a right ventricular dysfunction and preload dependence. Right atrial pressures during right-heart catheterization were elevated (16 mm Hg), reflecting right heart failure.

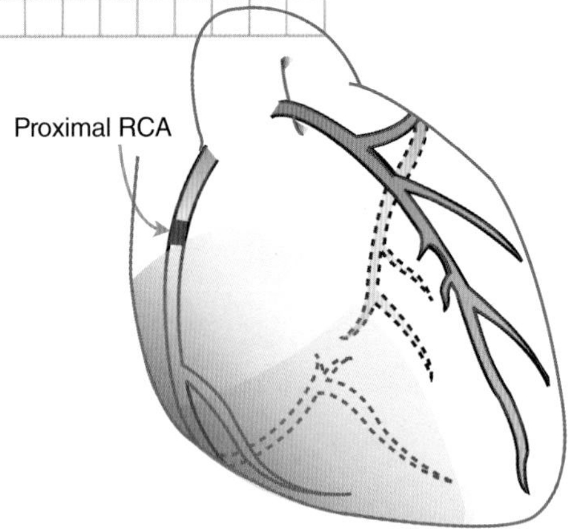

Proximal RCA

FIGURE 12.24 Territory infarcted by proximal RCA occlusion.

ECG 12.2a A 67-year-old male with a history of prior MI presents with shortness of breath, substernal chest pain, hypotension, and diaphoresis.

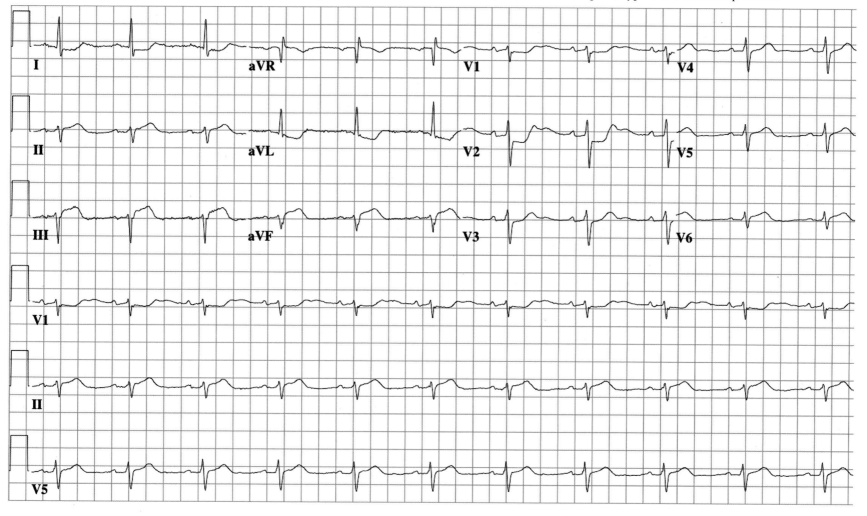

ECG 12.2b A 67-year-old male with a history of prior MI presents with shortness of breath, substernal chest pain, hypotension, and diaphoresis.

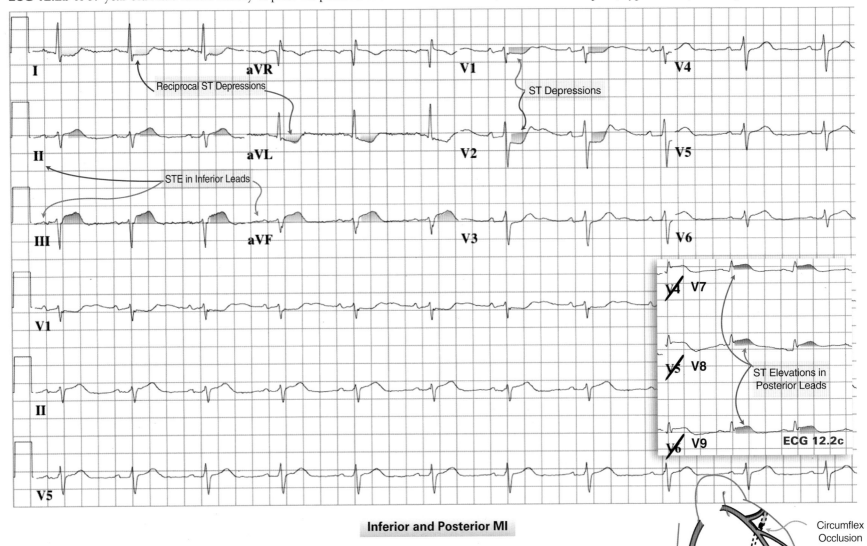

Inferior and Posterior MI

ST elevations in the inferior leads with reciprocal ST depressions in the lateral limb leads (I and aVL) indicate that this patient is having an inferior MI. The differential for ST depressions in leads V1 and V2 includes reciprocal changes to inferior injury and posterior MI. ST depressions in leads V1 and V2 led the clinicians to suspect that the posterior wall was involved in this infarction. Posterior leads applied to this patient (ECG 12.2c) demonstrated ST elevation.

This patient was found during cardiac catheterization to have complete occlusion of the mid circumflex artery.

FIGURE 12.25 Territory infarcted by a left circumflex occlusion.

ECG 12.3a A 36-year-old male complains of light-headedness for 4 months following a motor vehicle collision.

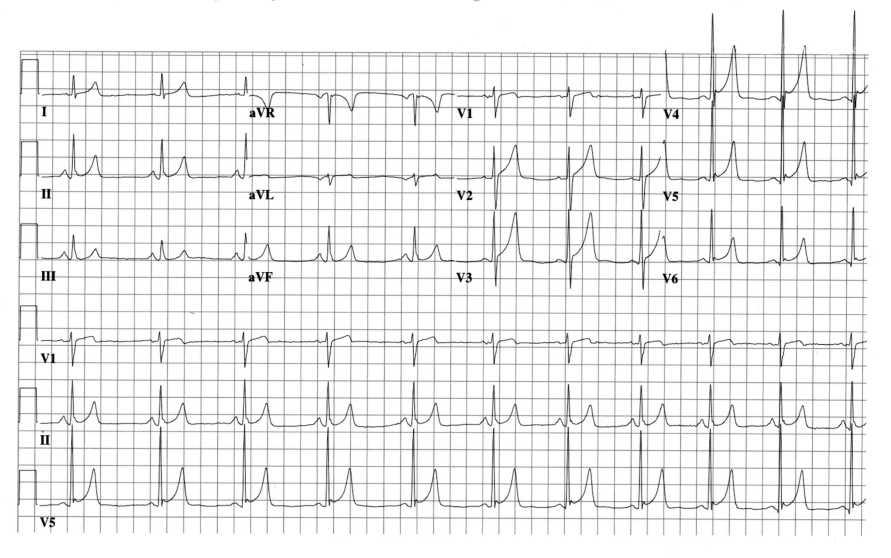

ECG 12.3b A 36-year-old male complains of light-headedness for 4 months following a motor vehicle collision.

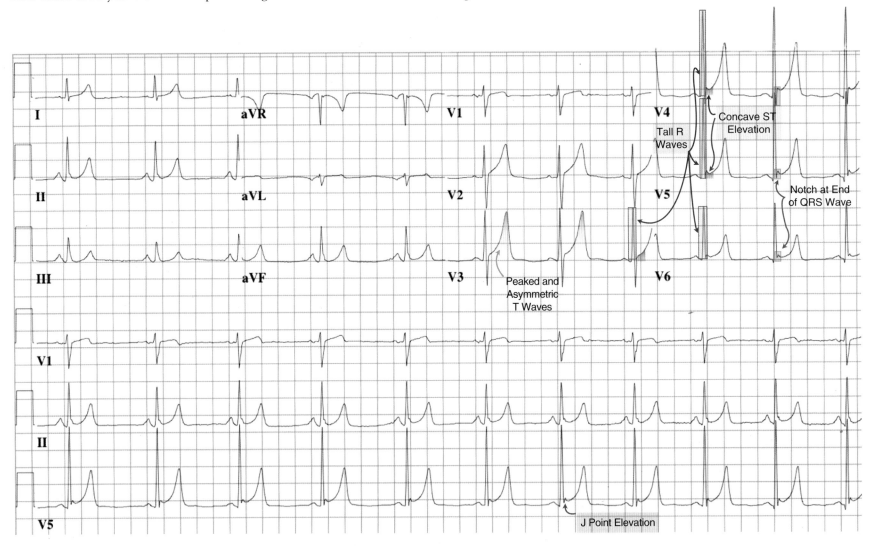

Benign Early Repolarization

There are several characteristics of this ECG, which favor the diagnosis of BER. The ST segments are concave upward and elevated at the J point. The terminal portion of the QRS is notched in leads V3-V6. R and T waves are tall.

Note the absence of reciprocal ST depression.

ECG 12.4a A 60-year-old male presents to the emergency department with intermittent crushing substernal chest pain for 2 days.

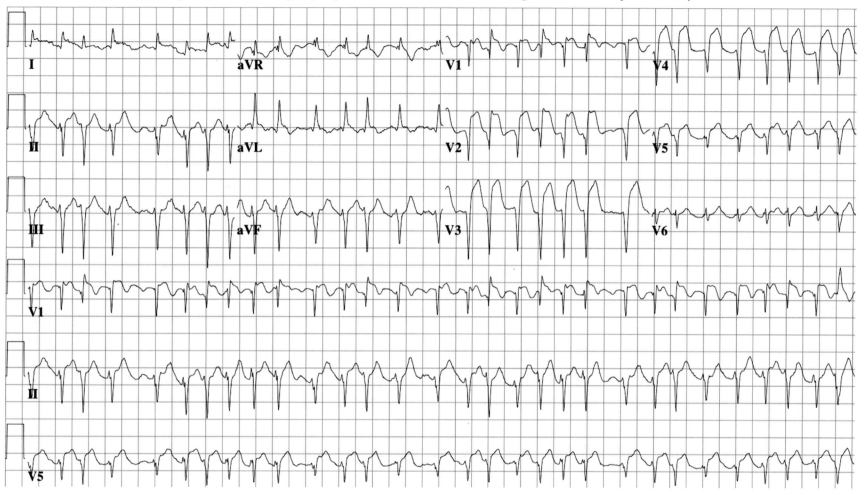

ECG 12.4b A 60-year-old male presents to the emergency department with intermittent crushing substernal chest pain for 2 days.

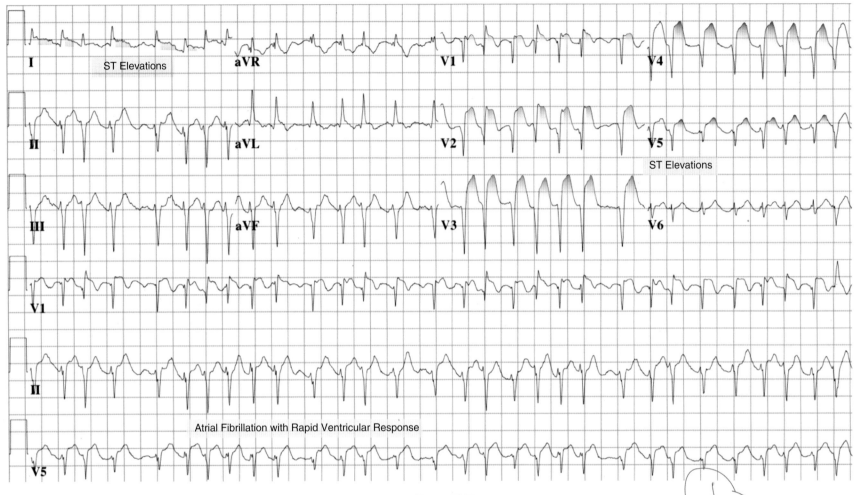

Anterior STEMI

This ECG demonstrates impressive ST elevations in V1-V5 and in lead I. This patient had total occlusion of the mid-LAD just distal to the first diagonal branch. Note the rhythm is atrial fibrillation with rapid ventricular response. A systematic approach to interpreting this ECG might help prevent overlooking the ST segment elevations and being distracted by the rate and rhythm disturbances.

FIGURE 12.26 Territory infarcted by a mid-LAD lesion distal to the first diagonal branch.

ECG 12.5a A 47-year-old male complained of 2 hours of severe chest pain. He appeared pale and diaphoretic.

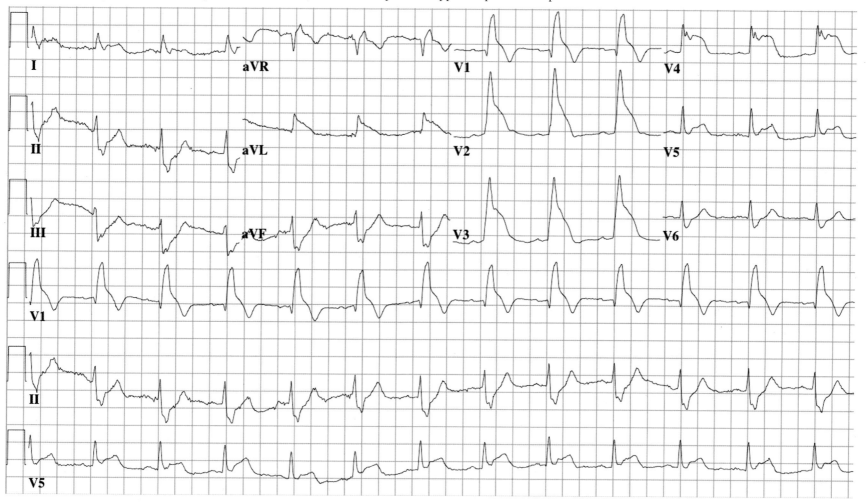

ECG 12.5b A 47-year-old male complained of 2 hours of severe chest pain. He appeared pale and diaphoretic.

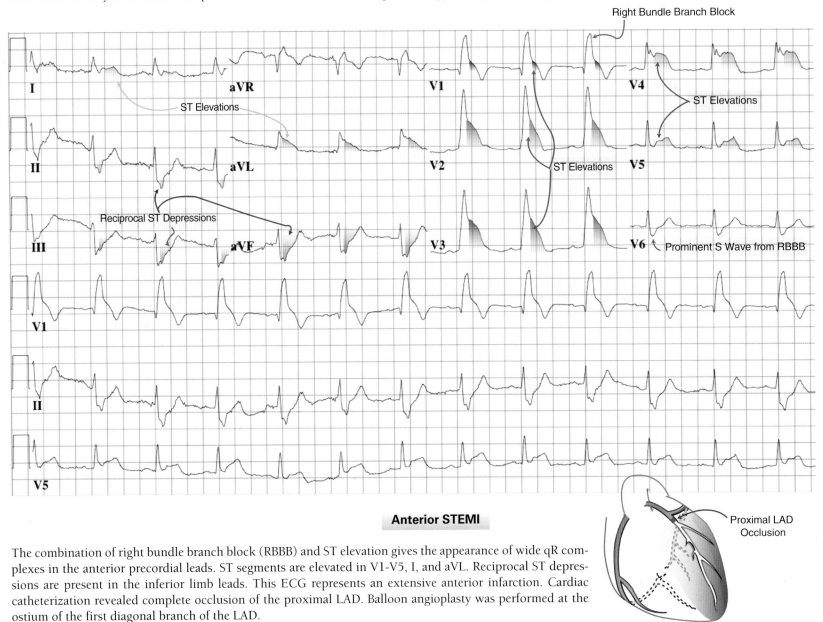

Anterior STEMI

The combination of right bundle branch block (RBBB) and ST elevation gives the appearance of wide qR complexes in the anterior precordial leads. ST segments are elevated in V1-V5, I, and aVL. Reciprocal ST depressions are present in the inferior limb leads. This ECG represents an extensive anterior infarction. Cardiac catheterization revealed complete occlusion of the proximal LAD. Balloon angioplasty was performed at the ostium of the first diagonal branch of the LAD.

FIGURE 12.27 Territory infarcted by an LAD lesion, proximal to the first diagonal branch.

ECG 12.6a A 61-year-old male wakes with chest pain and diaphoresis.

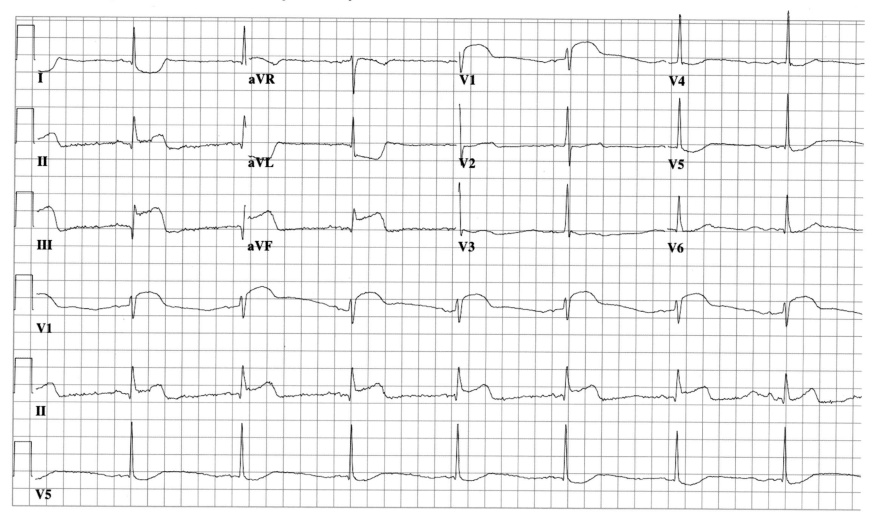

ECG 12.6b A 61-year-old male wakes with chest pain and diaphoresis.

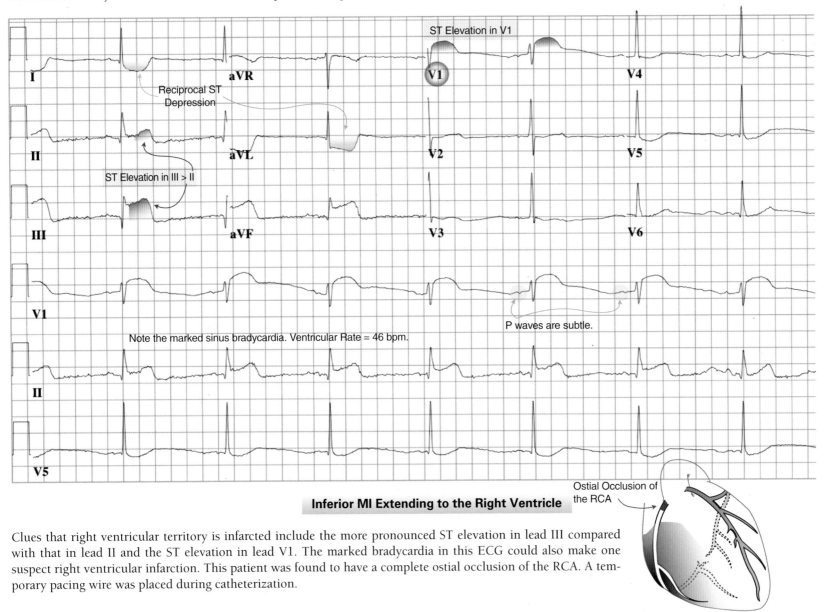

Inferior MI Extending to the Right Ventricle

Clues that right ventricular territory is infarcted include the more pronounced ST elevation in lead III compared with that in lead II and the ST elevation in lead V1. The marked bradycardia in this ECG could also make one suspect right ventricular infarction. This patient was found to have a complete ostial occlusion of the RCA. A temporary pacing wire was placed during catheterization.

FIGURE 12.28 Territory infarcted by a proximal RCA lesion.

ECG 12.7a A 60-year-old woman with mesothelioma complains of dyspnea 1 day after thoracotomy.

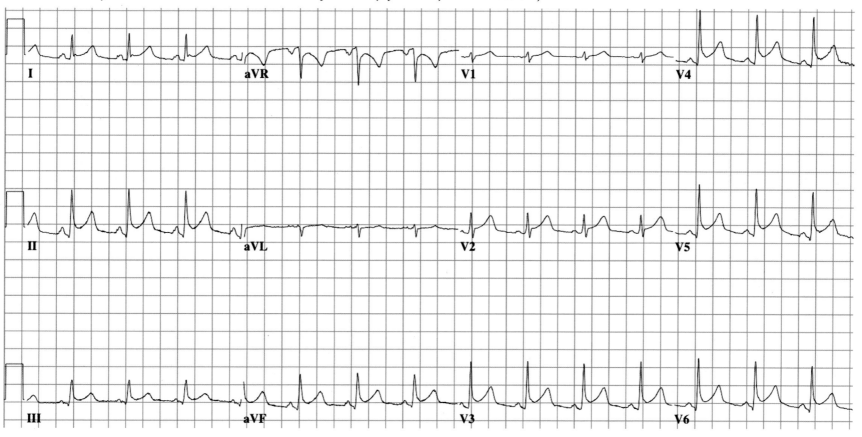

ECG 12.7b A 60-year-old woman with mesothelioma complains of dyspnea 1 day after thoracotomy.

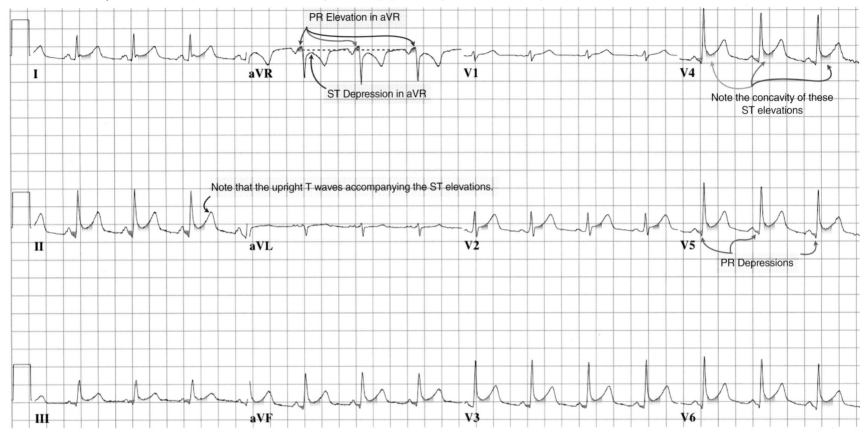

Pericarditis

ECG 12.8a A 53-year-old male presents to an urgent care center with chest pain that started after running on a treadmill.

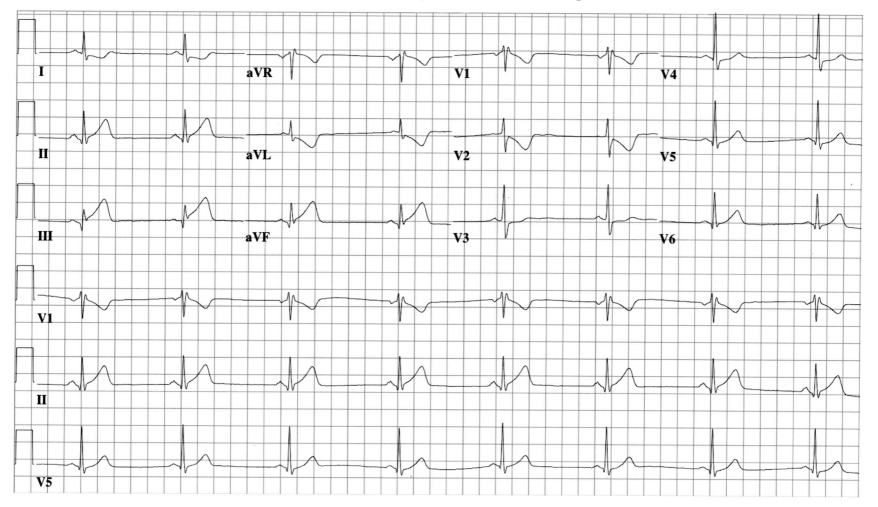

ECG 12.8b A 53-year-old male presents to an urgent care center with chest pain that started after running on a treadmill.

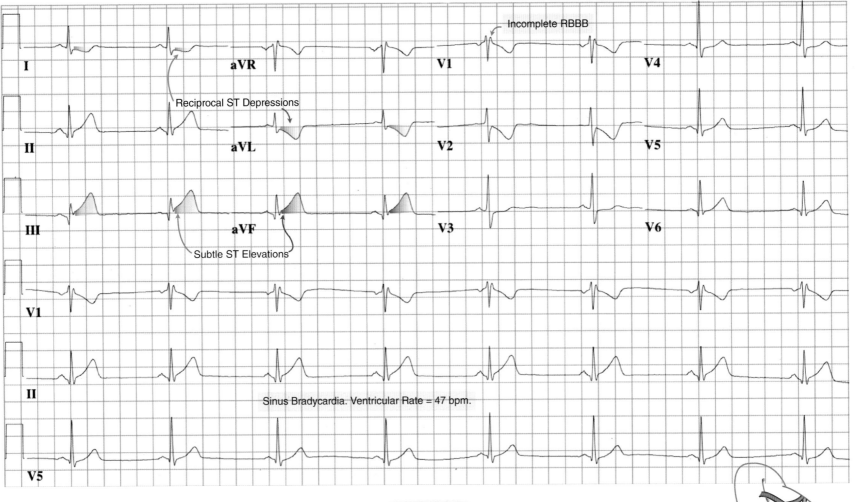

Inferior MI

This patient was found to have thrombotic occlusion of the mid-RCA with mild hypokinesis of the inferior wall.

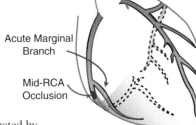

FIGURE 12.29 Territory infarcted by mid-RCA occlusion.

ECG 12.9a

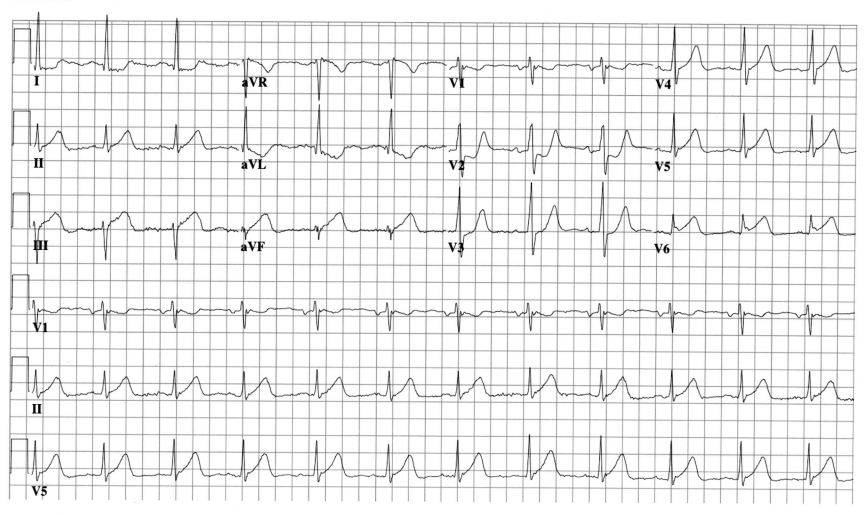

Image courtesy of Roberta Capp, MD.

ECG 12.9b

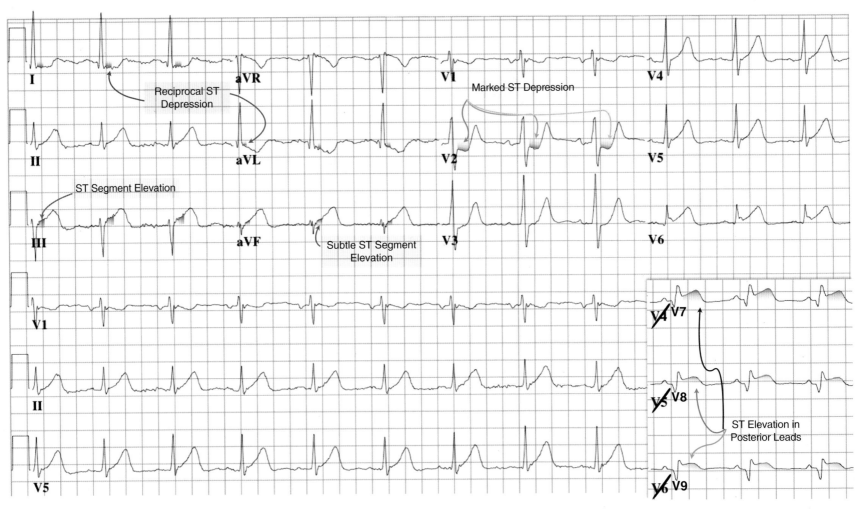

Inferior and Posterior MI

The ST elevations in the inferior leads are not obvious at first glance. ST elevation in these leads is associated with reciprocal depression in leads I and aVL. The tall R wave and marked ST depression in lead V2 led the clinicians caring for this patient to suspect posterior MI. Posterior leads demonstrated ST elevation.

ECG 12.10a A 75-year-old woman complains of 2 days of dyspnea, 6 months after being hospitalized for a MI.

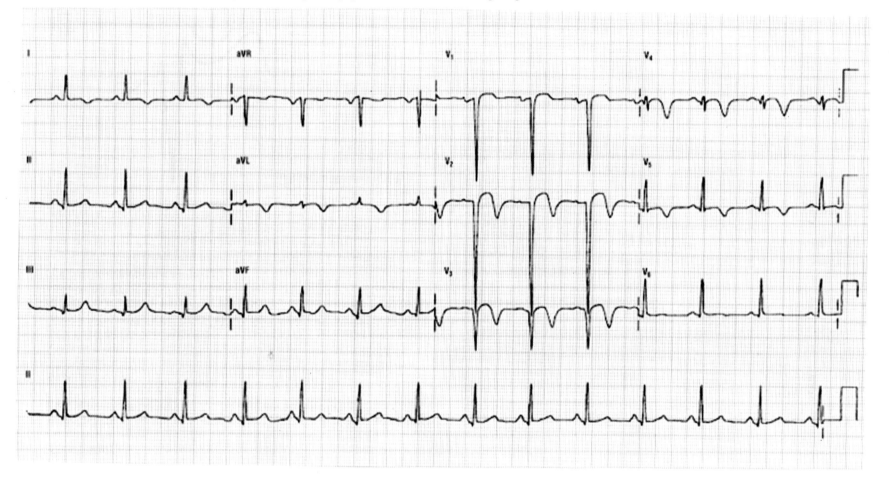

Image courtesy of Josh Kosowsky, MD.

ECG 12.10b A 75-year-old woman complains of 2 days of dyspnea, 6 months after being hospitalized for a MI.

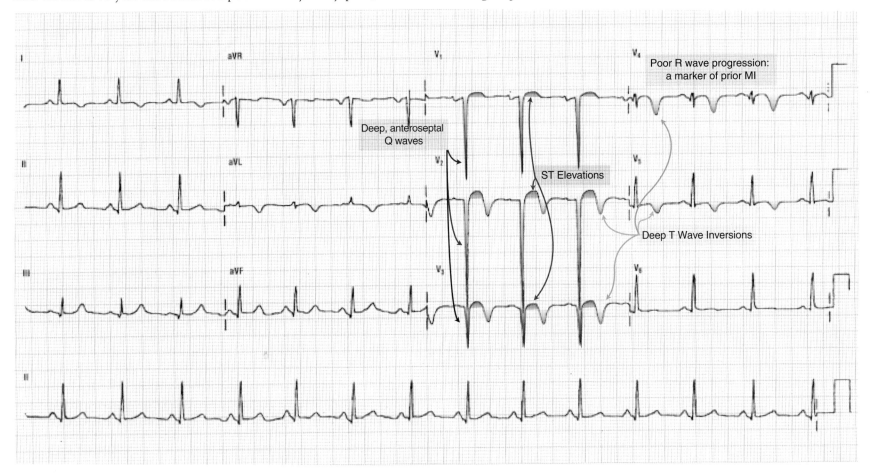

Left Ventricular Aneurysm

The deep anteroseptal Q waves and inverted T waves that accompany these ST elevations suggest LV aneurysm. Note the absence of reciprocal ST depressions.

ECG 12.11a A 62-year-old male with a history of an anterior MI treated with a stent to the LAD 3 years prior presents with chest pain and shortness of breath.

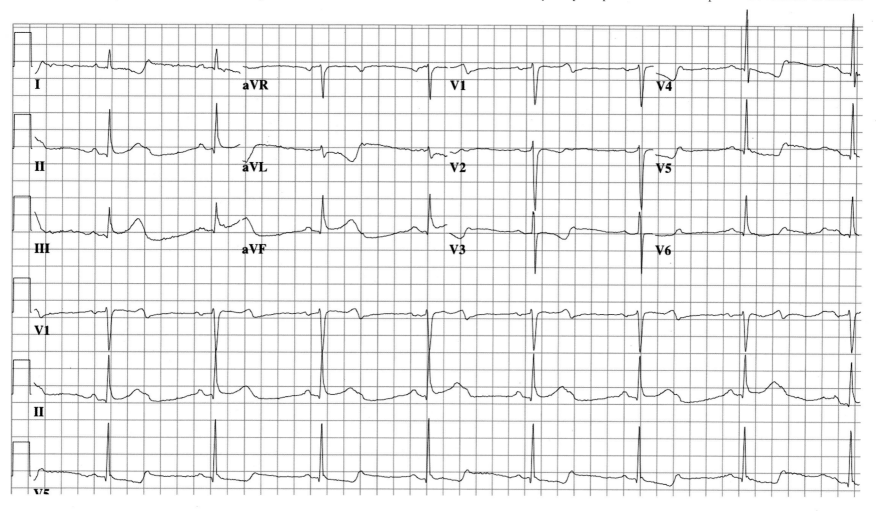

ECG 12.11b A 62-year-old male with a history of an anterior MI treated with a stent to the LAD 3 years prior presents with chest pain and shortness of breath.

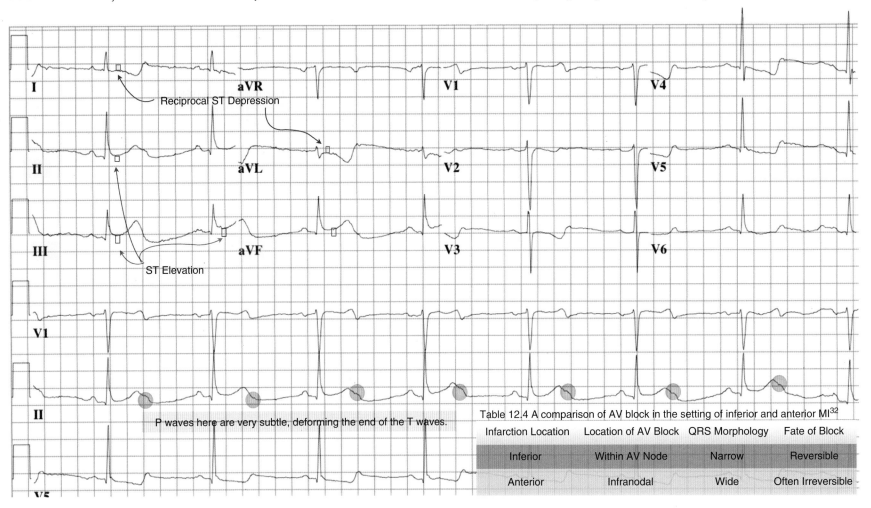

Table 12.4 A comparison of AV block in the setting of inferior and anterior MI[32]

Infarction Location	Location of AV Block	QRS Morphology	Fate of Block
Inferior	Within AV Node	Narrow	Reversible
Anterior	Infranodal	Wide	Often Irreversible

Inferior MI with Second Degree 2:1 AV block

Do not forget to look for rhythm disturbances in ECGs demonstrating acute ischemia.

This patient was found to have complete occlusion of the proximal RCA. ECGs following cardiac catheterization demonstrated normal sinus rhythm.

ECG 12.11c Taken from lead V1 of an ECG performed on this patient 12 minutes later.

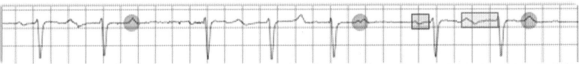

Second Degree AV Block Mobitz I

ECG 12.12a A 59-year-old presents with stuttering chest pain.

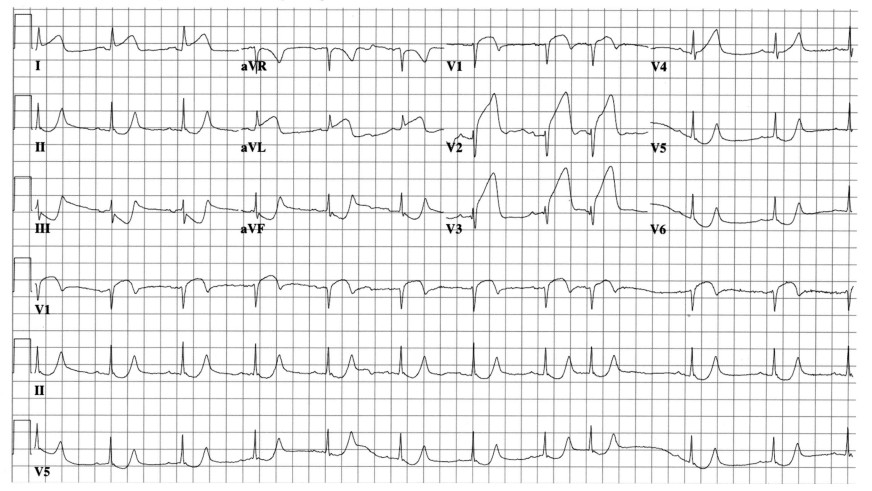

ECG 12.12b A 59-year-old presents with stuttering chest pain.

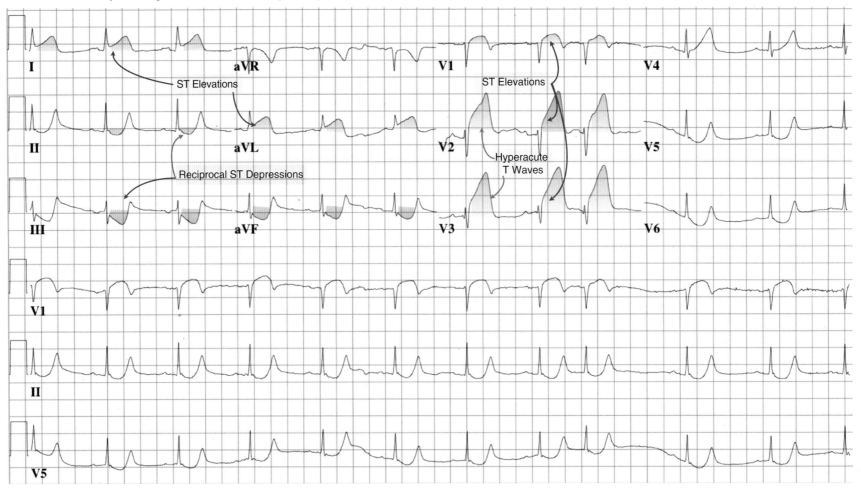

Anterior STEMI

This patient suffered a v-fib arrest on his way to the cardiac catheterization lab and had return of spontaneous circulation. He was found to have complete occlusion of the proximal LAD involving the first diagonal branch without collateral flow and cardiogenic shock, requiring placement of an intra-aortic balloon pump and administration of vasopressors.

ECG 12.13a A 79-year-old woman awakes with epigastric burning and presents to an urgent care clinic.

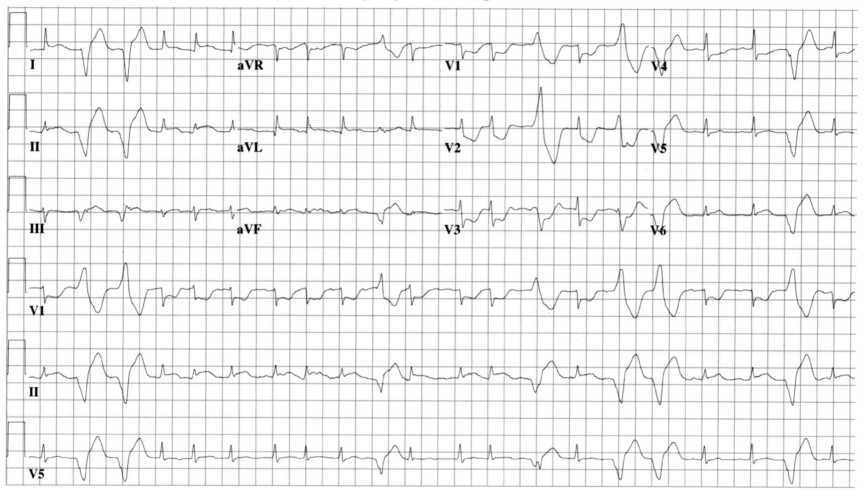

ECG 12.13b A 79-year-old woman awakes with epigastric burning and presents to an urgent care clinic.

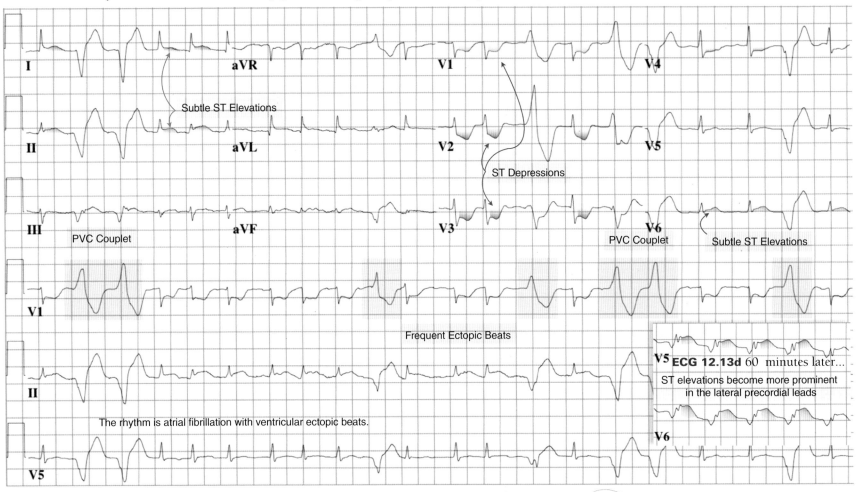

I   aVR   V1   V4

Subtle ST Elevations

II   aVL   V2   V5

ST Depressions

III   aVF   V3   V6

PVC Couplet   PVC Couplet   Subtle ST Elevations

V1

Frequent Ectopic Beats

II

The rhythm is atrial fibrillation with ventricular ectopic beats.

V5

Posterior MI

V5 **ECG 12.13d** 60 minutes later...
ST elevations become more prominent
in the lateral precordial leads

V6

ECG 12.13c This patient's rhythm deteriorated.

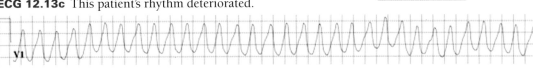

V1

Ventricular Tachycardia

This patient was found to have complete thrombotic occlusion of the left circumflex artery. She had three episodes of ventricular tachycardia and developed cardiogenic shock.

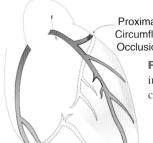

Proximal
Circumflex
Occlusion

FIGURE 12.30 Territory
infracted by a proximal
circumflex occlusion.

ECG 12.14a A 37-year-old female developed aching in her left arm followed by chest pain and shortness of breath while driving.

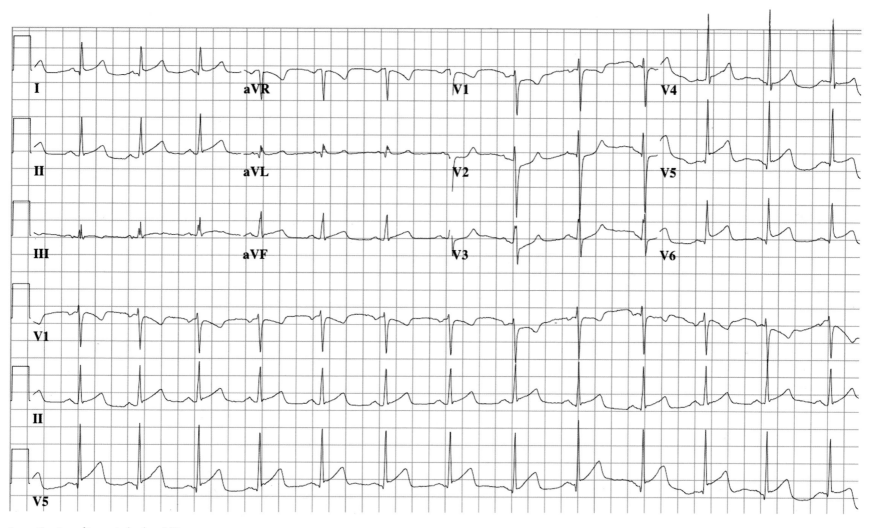

Image Courtesy of James Andruchow, MD.

ECG 12.14b A 37-year-old female developed aching in her left arm followed by chest pain and shortness of breath while driving.

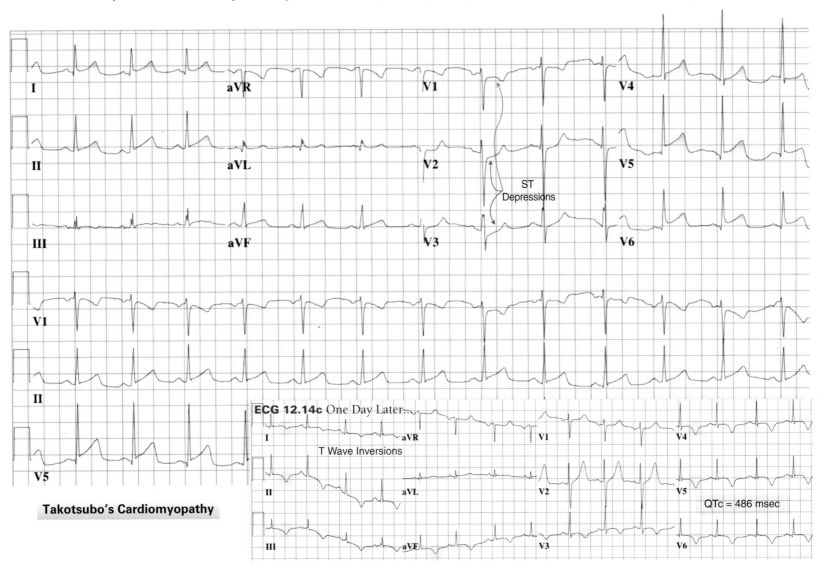

ECG 12.14c One Day Later...

T Wave Inversions

QTc = 486 msec

Takotsubo's Cardiomyopathy

These ST elevations (leads II, aVF, V3-V6, and I) raised concern for inferolateral ischemia. The patient was taken urgently to the catheterization lab. The initial troponin T level was 1.44 ng/mL (normal <0.03 ng/mL). Her coronary arteries were found to be patent. Apical ballooning of the left ventricle was observed consistent with Takotsubo's cardiomyopathy. Further history revealed that the patient was distressed by her ongoing divorce.
The following day her ECG was notable for widespread T wave inversions and QTc prolongation, consistent with the electrocardiographic progression of this disease. This patient was markedly younger than the population typically observed to have Takotsubo's cardiomyopathy.

ECG 12.15a A 83-year-old female with hypertension complained of general body aches and intermittent diaphoresis for 2 days.

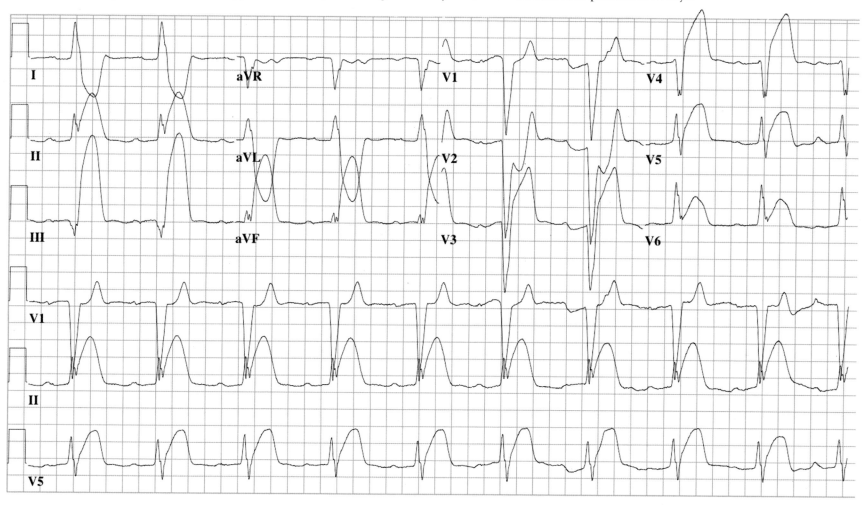

ECG 12.15b A 83-year-old female with hypertension complained of general body aches and intermittent diaphoresis for 2 days.

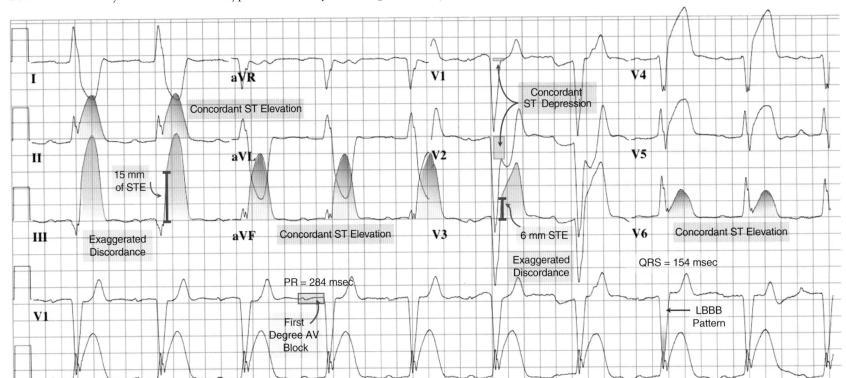

Inferoposterior MI and LBBB

The ST elevations and hyperacute T waves on this ECG are dramatic. The LBBB was a new ECG finding for this patient. In the setting of LBBB, findings in this ECG suggestive of STEMI include the following:

1. Concordant ST elevation in leads II, aVF, V5 and V6
2. Concordant ST depression in leads V1 and V2
3. Exaggerated discordant ST elevation in leads III, V3, and V4.

This patient was found to have 99% proximal occlusion of a large, dominant RCA. Intermittent AV block and atrial fibrillation occurred for several days after initial presentation.

ECG 12.16a A 53-year-old male has a cardiac arrest while driving. He developed ventricular fibrillation in the field and was shocked twice with return of spontaneous circulation. He arrived intubated with a pulse.

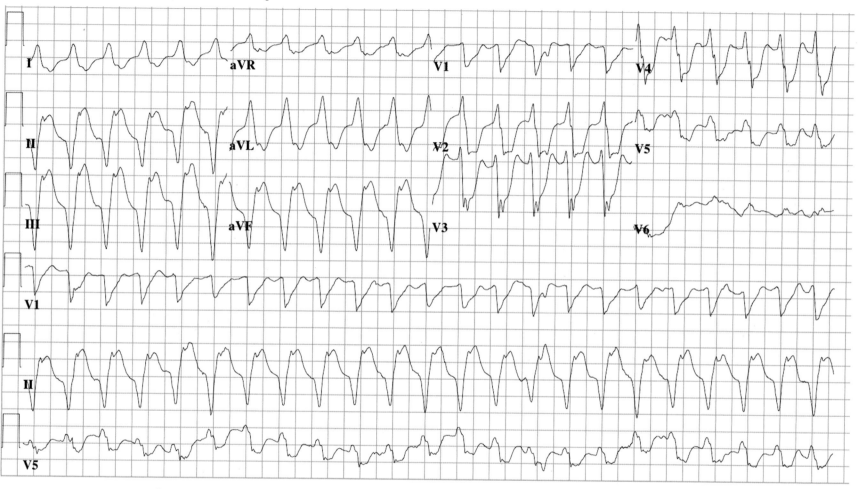

ECG 12.16b A 53-year-old male has a cardiac arrest while driving. He developed ventricular fibrillation in the field and was shocked twice with return of spontaneous circulation. He arrived intubated with a pulse.

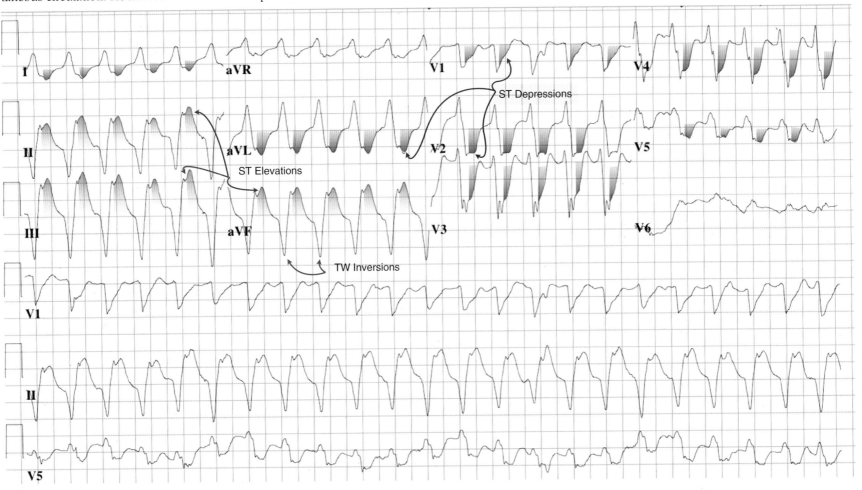

Inferoposterior MI

Initially, this rhythm was misinterpreted as ventricular tachycardia. The elevation of the ST segments to an amplitude higher than that of the peak of the QRS wave gives the illusion of a widened QRS (ECG 12.16c).

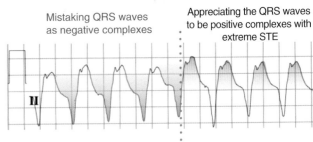

ECG 12.16c

ECG 12.17a Same patient, 25 minutes later.

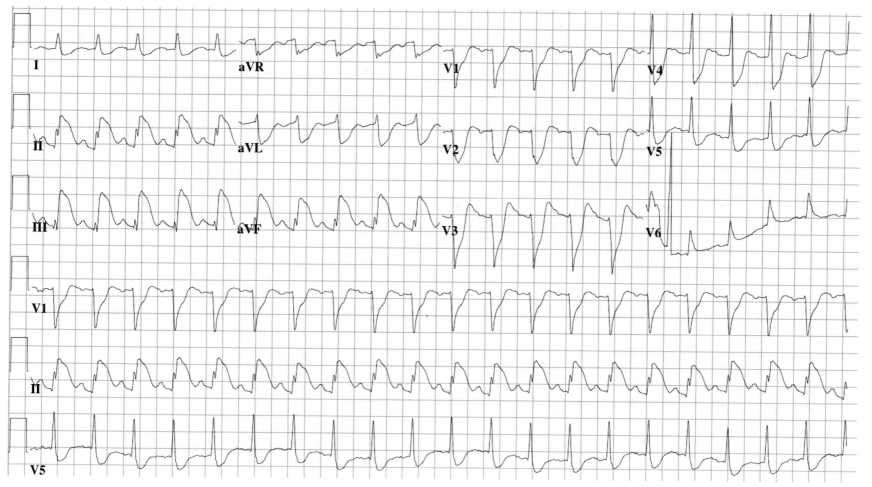

ECG 12.17b Same patient, 25 minutes later.

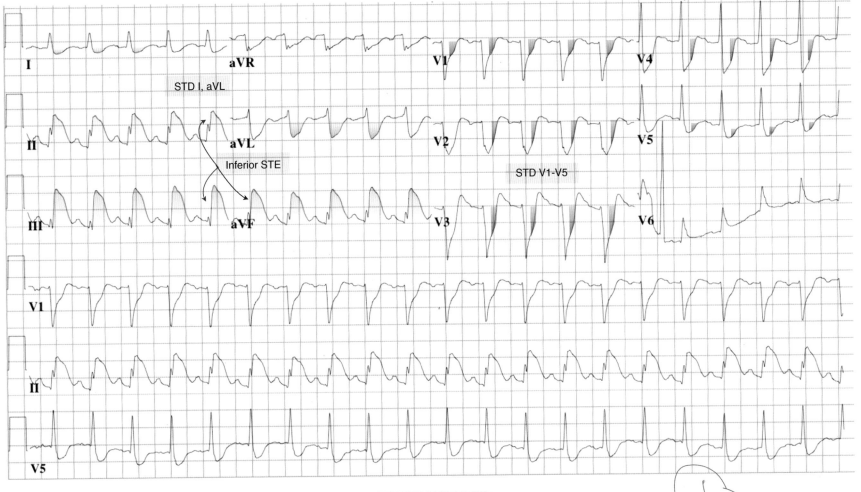

STD I, aVL

Inferior STE

STD V1-V5

Evolving Inferior MI

The ST elevations in the inferior leads are more distinct in this ECG. This patient was taken to the cardiac catheterization lab and found to have complete occlusion of the distal third of a right-dominant RCA.

FIGURE 12.31 Territory infarcted by a distal RCA occlusion.

ECG 12.18a A 25-year-old male awoke with pleuritic chest pain.

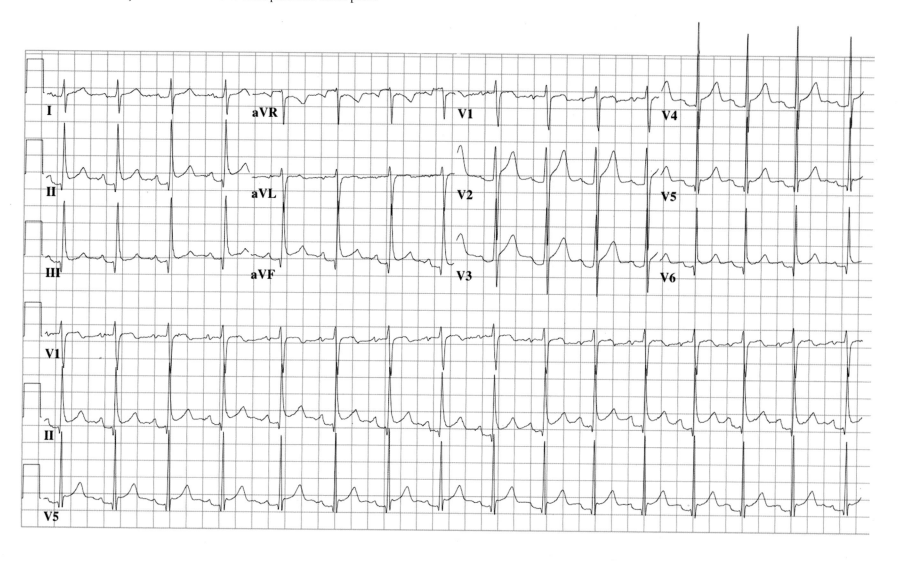

ECG 12.18b A 25-year-old male awoke with pleuritic chest pain.

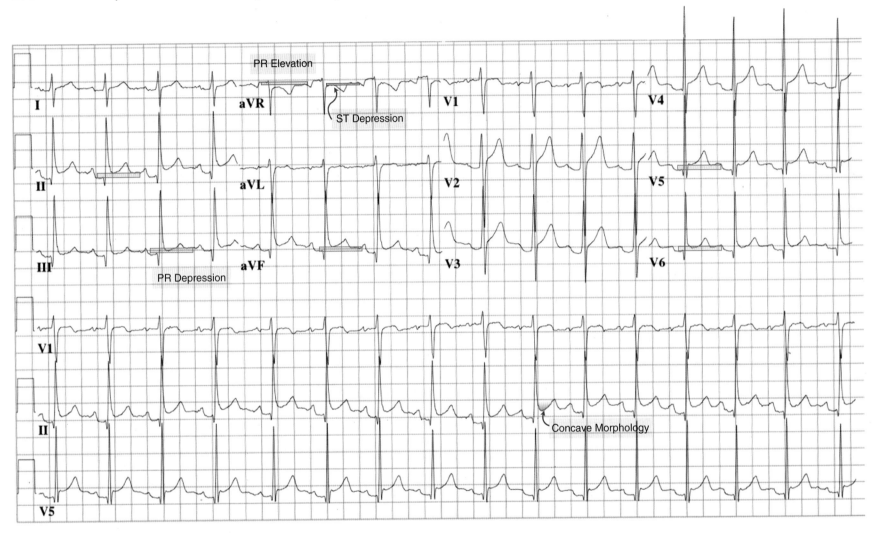

Pericarditis

ECG 12.19a A 47-year-old man has witnessed a collapse at home. He is defibrillated twice.

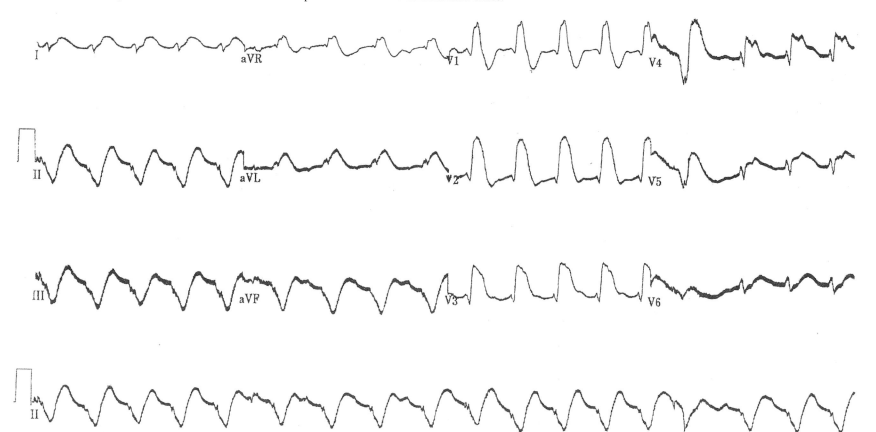

ECG 12.19b A 47-year-old man has witnessed a collapse at home. He is defibrillated twice.

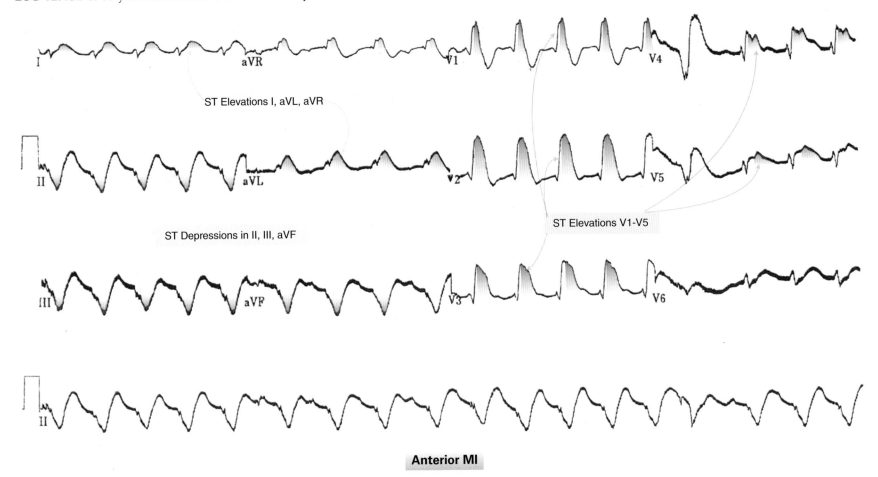

ST Elevations I, aVL, aVR

ST Depressions in II, III, aVF

ST Elevations V1-V5

Anterior MI

This ECG was initially interpreted as ventricular tachycardia. The patient was taken to the catheterization lab where he was found to have complete occlusion of the proximal LAD without collateral blood supply.

ECG 12.20a A 70-year-old female with congestive heart failure presents with substernal heaviness.

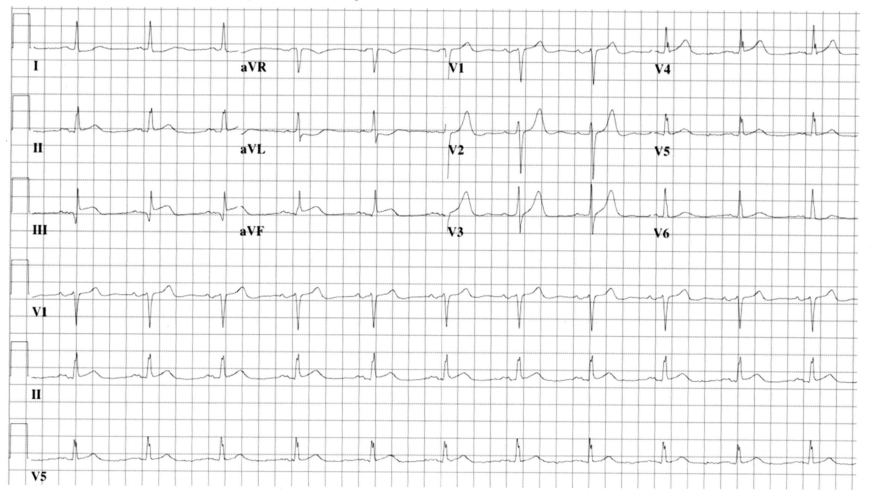

ECG 12.20b A 70-year-old female with congestive heart failure presents with substernal heaviness.

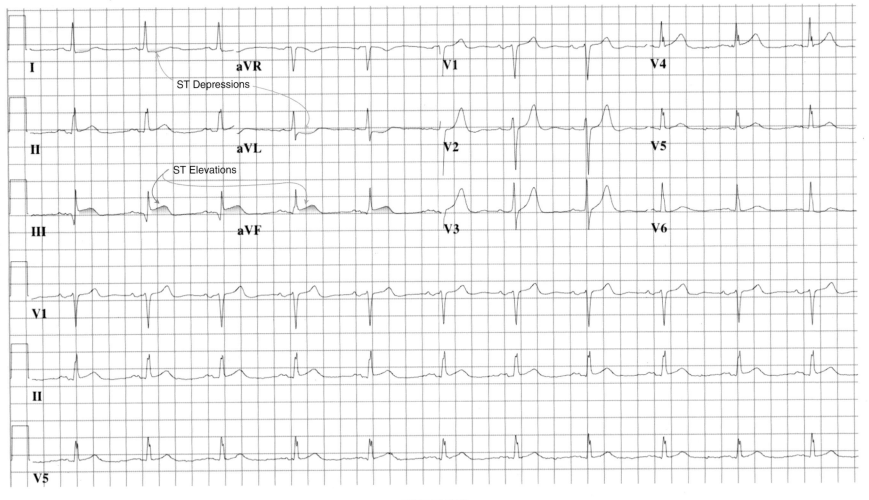

Inferior MI

ST elevations can be subtle. This patient was found to have occlusion of the PDA with extension into the posterior left ventricular (PLV) branch.

ECG 12.21a A 42-year-old female with known coronary artery disease and stents in the left circumflex artery presents with jaw pain and chest discomfort.

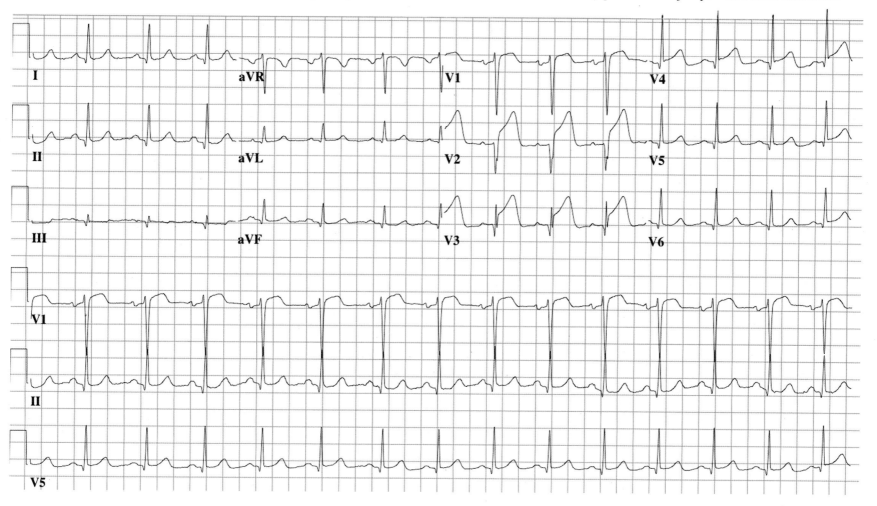

ECG 12.21b A 42-year-old female with known coronary artery disease and stents in the left circumflex artery presents with jaw pain and chest discomfort.

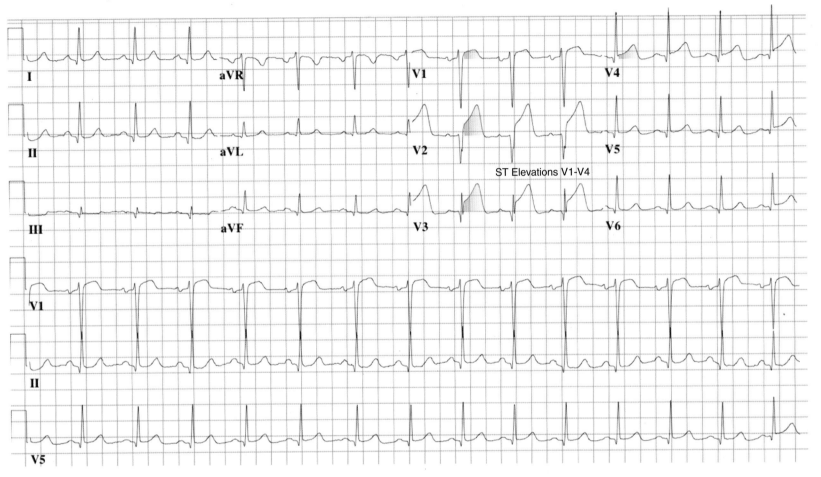

Anterior MI

This patient was found to have 99% occlusion of the mid-LAD.

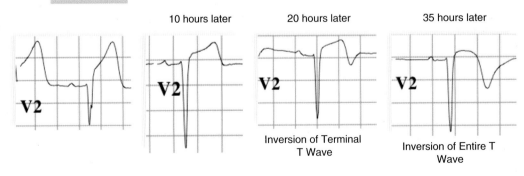

ECG 12.22a A 19-year-old male 2 days after a pericardial window and penetrating trauma to the heart.

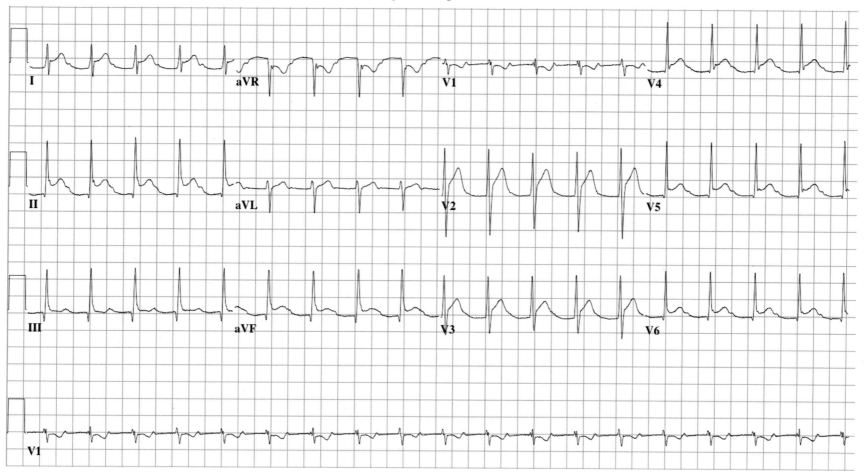

Image courtesy of Jonathan Elmer, MD.

ECG 12.22b A 19-year-old male two days after a pericardial window and penetrating trauma to the heart.

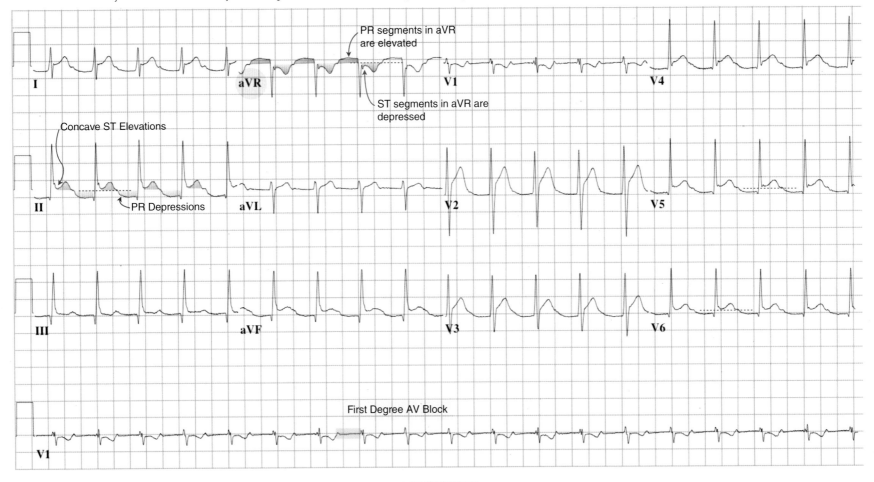

Pericarditis

The rhythm of this ECG is sinus tachycardia with first degree AV block. ST segments are diffusely elevated (except in leads aVR and V1).

ECG 12.23a A 68-year-old male is found slumped in his chair after completing a 4-mile run.

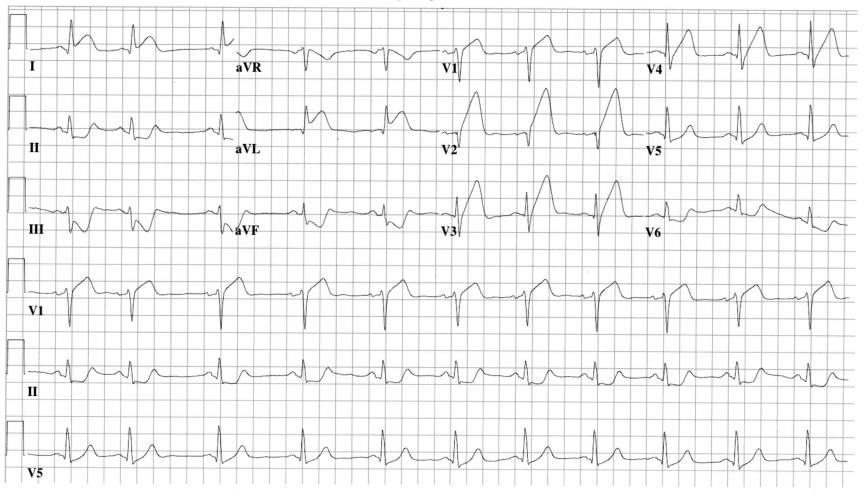

ECG 12.23b A 68-year-old male is found slumped in his chair after completing a 4-mile run.

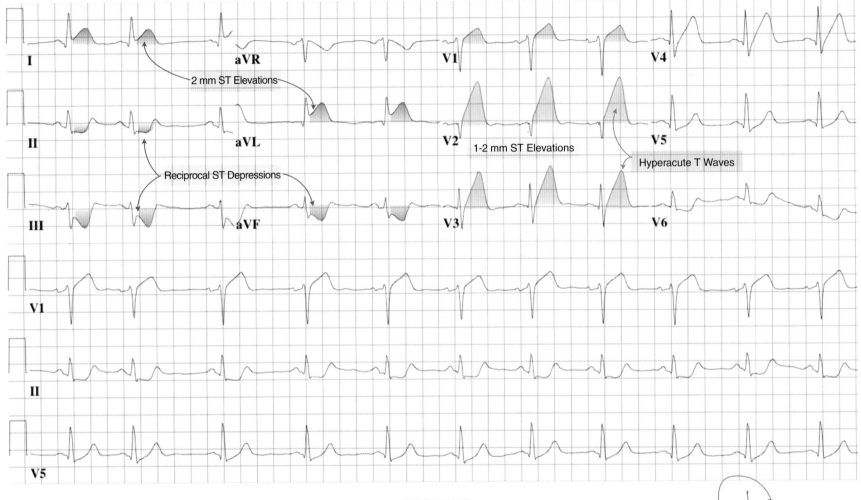

Anterior MI

This ECG demonstrates ST elevations in leads I and aVL in addition to elevations in the precordial leads. This provides a clue that the culprit lesion for this STEMI is in the proximal aspect of the left anterior descending artery (proximal to the first diagonal branch). This patient was found to have complete thrombotic occlusion in the proximal LAD.

FIGURE 12.32 Territory infarcted by a proximal LAD lesion.

ECG 12.24a A 19-year-old male diagnosed with influenza 4 days prior to presentation develops nonpleuritic chest pain.

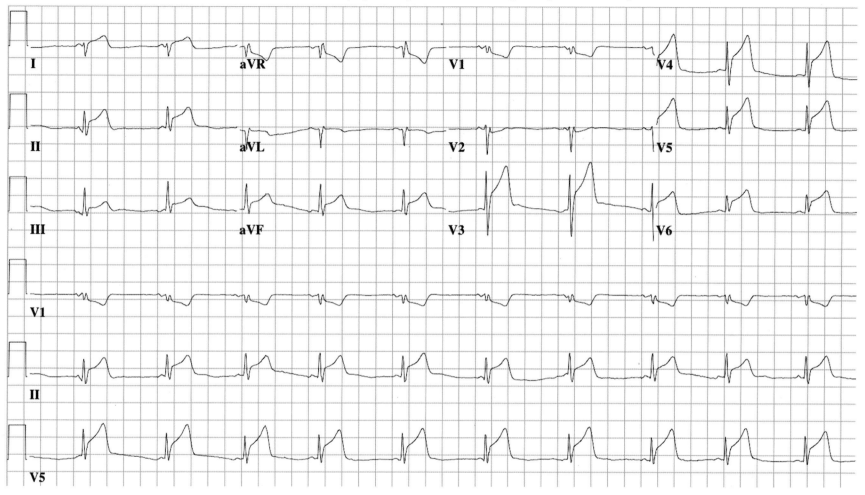

ECG 12.24b A 19-year-old male diagnosed with influenza 4 days prior to presentation develops nonpleuritic chest pain.

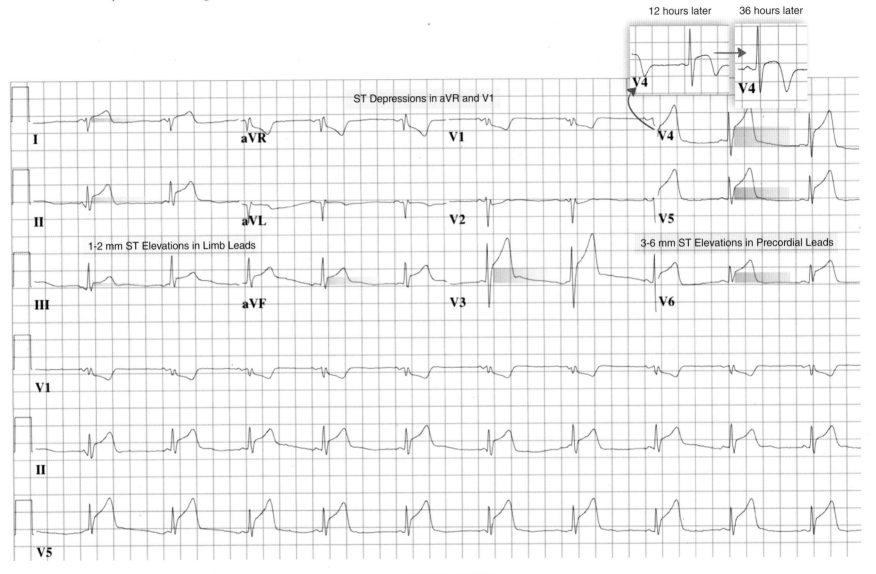

Acute Myocarditis

This ECG demonstrates diffuse ST elevations in multiple vascular territories. PR depression is absent. Subsequent ECG showed terminal T wave inversion and complete T wave inversion in the presence of persistently elevated ST segments. This patient's troponin was markedly elevated. Cardiac MRI findings were consistent with the diagnosis of myocarditis.

ECG 12.25a A 68-year-old female with hypertension came to the emergency department after several hours of substernal chest pain.

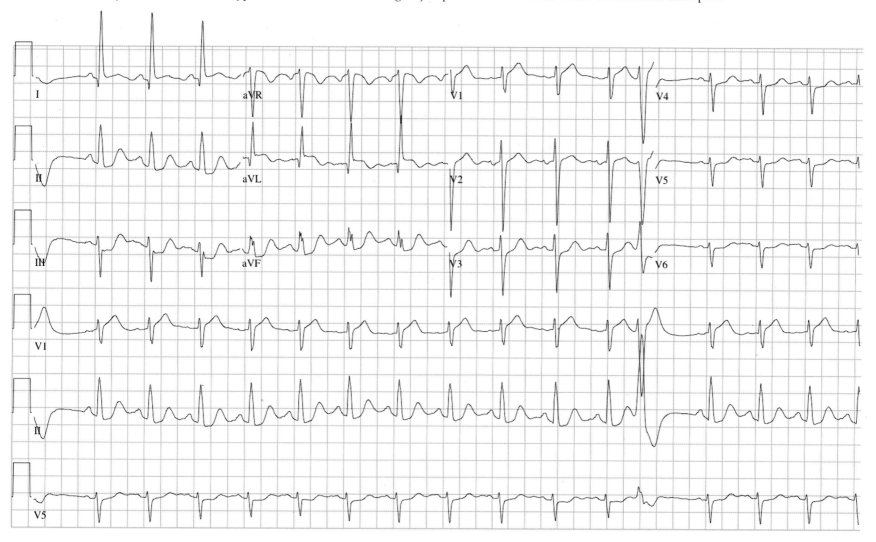

ECG 12.25b A 68-year-old female with hypertension came to the emergency department after several hours of substernal chest pain.

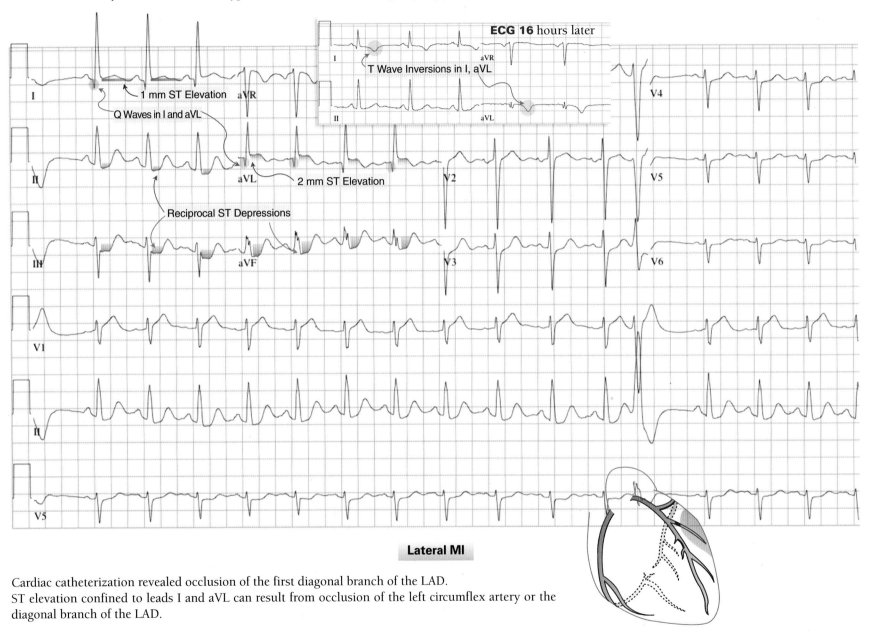

Lateral MI

Cardiac catheterization revealed occlusion of the first diagonal branch of the LAD.
ST elevation confined to leads I and aVL can result from occlusion of the left circumflex artery or the diagonal branch of the LAD.

FIGURE 12.33 Territory infarcted by occlusion of the first diagonal branch.

ECG 12.26a A 79-year-old female with hypertension presents with intermittent chest pain for the past 2 days. She is hypotensive.

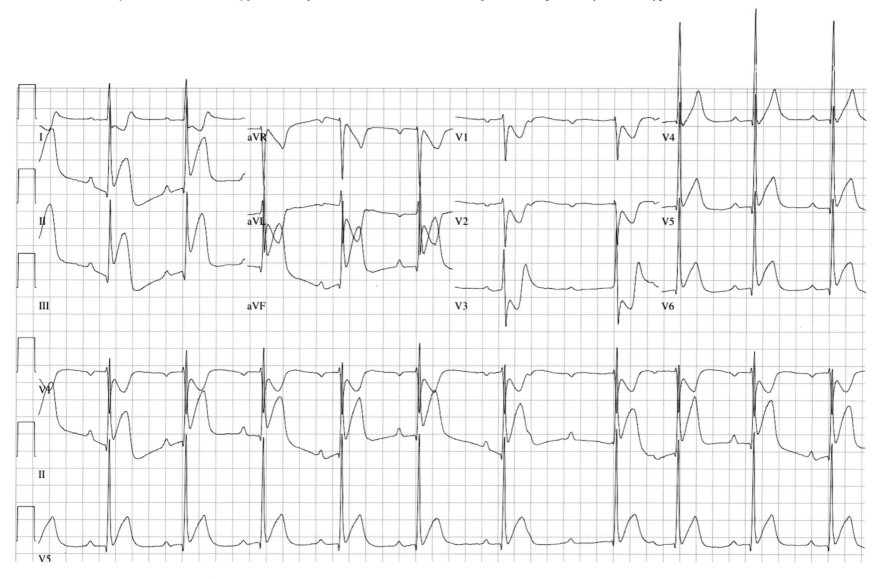

ECG 12.26b A 79-year-old female with hypertension presents with intermittent chest pain for the past 2 days. She is hypotensive.

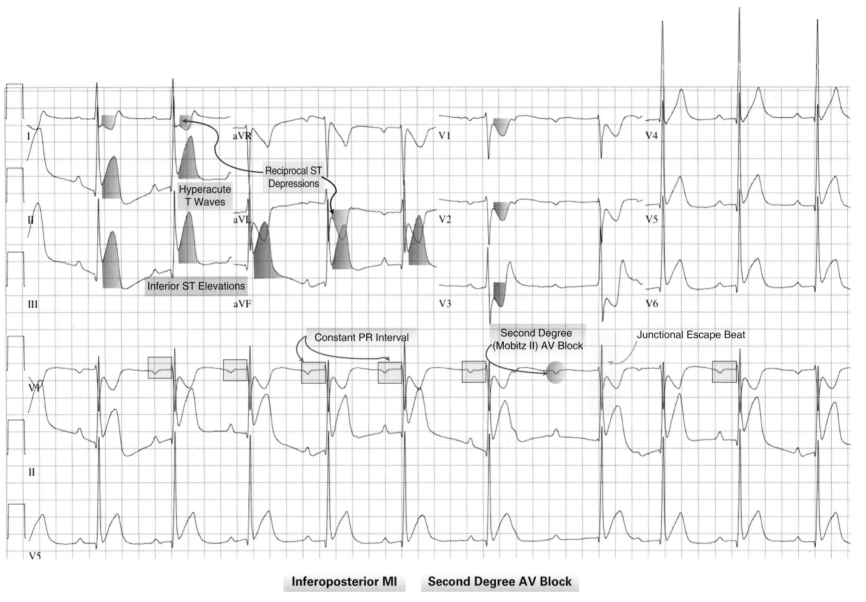

Inferoposterior MI   **Second Degree AV Block**

This patient was found to have occlusion of the RCA proximal to the PDA. Immediately prior to cardiac catheterization, she developed complete heart block and underwent placement of a temporary pacing wire. She had two episodes of ventricular fibrillation with immediate return of spontaneous circulation after defibrillation.

ECG 12.27a An 89-year-old woman with a history of an inferior MI presents with chest pain radiating to the axilla and hypotension.

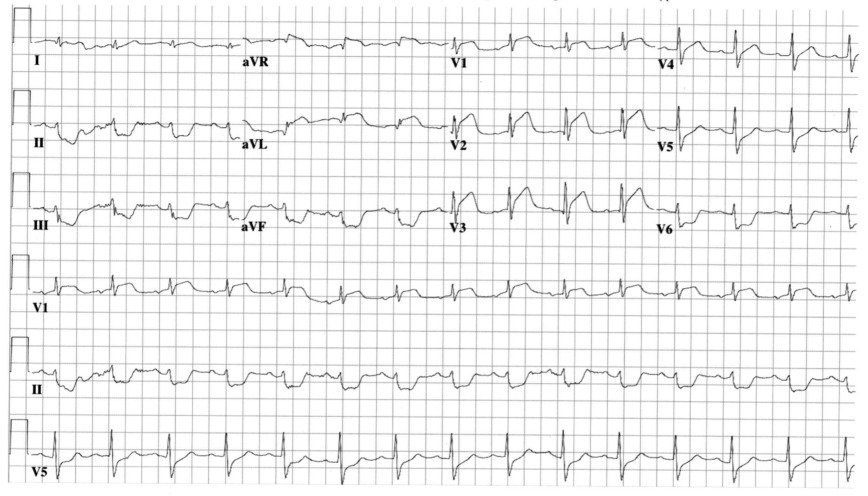

ECG 12.27b An 89-year-old woman with a history of an inferior MI presents with chest pain radiating to the axilla and hypotension.

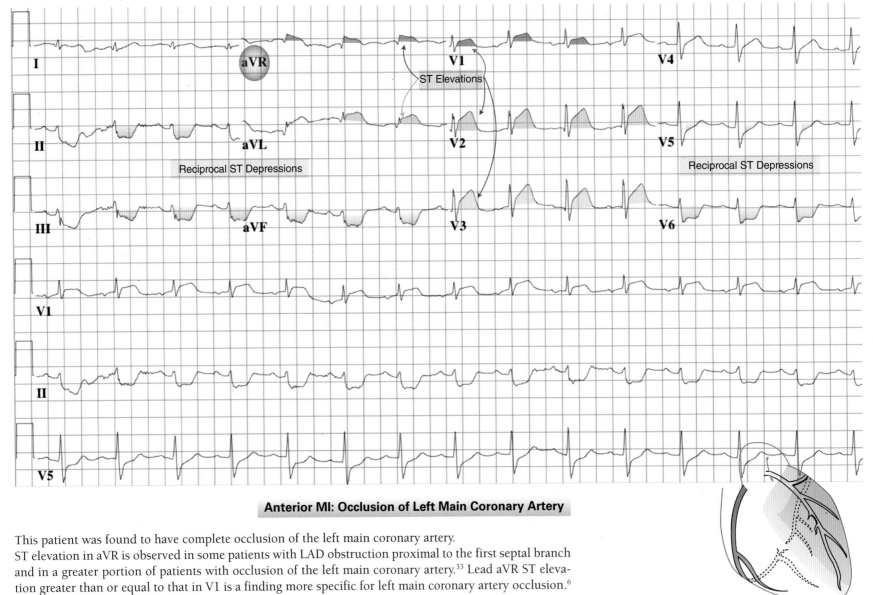

Anterior MI: Occlusion of Left Main Coronary Artery

This patient was found to have complete occlusion of the left main coronary artery.
ST elevation in aVR is observed in some patients with LAD obstruction proximal to the first septal branch and in a greater portion of patients with occlusion of the left main coronary artery.[33] Lead aVR ST elevation greater than or equal to that in V1 is a finding more specific for left main coronary artery occlusion.[6]

FIGURE 12.34 Territory infarcted by occlusion of the left main coronary artery.

Reference

1. Popma J. Coronary arteriography. In: Bonow RM, Zipes D, Libby P, eds. *Braunwald's Heart Disease: A Textbook of Cardiovascular Medicine*. Philadelphia,. PA: Elsevier; 2011.
2. Wagner GaL, T. Increased myocardial demand. In: *Marriott's Practical Electrocardiography*. 11th ed. Philadelphia, PA: Lippincott Williams & Wilkins; 2008: 154–162.
3. van 't Hof AW, Liem A, de Boer MJ, et al. Clinical value of 12-lead electrocardiogram after successful reperfusion therapy for acute myocardial infarction. Zwolle Myocardial infarction Study Group. *Lancet* 1997;350:615–619.
4. Schroder R, Dissmann R, Bruggemann T, et al. Extent of early ST segment elevation resolution: a simple but strong predictor of outcome in patients with acute myocardial infarction. *J Am Coll Cardiol* 1994;24:384–391.
5. Sgarbossa EaWG. Electrocardiography. In: Topol E, ed. *Cardiovascular Medicine*. 3rd ed. Philadelphia, PA: Lippincott Williams & Wilkins; 2007.
6. Yamaji H, Iwasaki K, Kusachi S, et al. Prediction of acute left main coronary artery obstruction by 12-lead electrocardiography. ST segment elevation in lead aVR with less ST segment elevation in lead V(1). *J Am Coll Cardiol* 2001;38:1348–1354.
7. Oraii S, Maleki M, Tavakolian AA, et al. Prevalence and outcome of ST-segment elevation in posterior electrocardiographic leads during acute myocardial infarction. *J Electrocardiol* 1999;32:275–278.
8. Melendez LJ, Jones DT, Salcedo JR. Usefulness of three additional electrocardiographic chest leads (V7, V8, and V9) in the diagnosis of acute myocardial infarction. *Can Med Assoc J* 1978;119:745–748.
9. Saw J, Davies C, Fung A, et al. Value of ST elevation in lead III greater than lead II in inferior wall acute myocardial infarction for predicting in-hospital mortality and diagnosing right ventricular infarction. *Am J Cardiol* 2001;87:448–450, A6.
10. O'Rourke RA, Dell'Italia LJ. Diagnosis and management of right ventricular myocardial infarction. *Curr Probl Cardiol* 2004;29:6–47.
11. Cohn JN, Guiha NH, Broder MI, et al. Right ventricular infarction. Clinical and hemodynamic features. *Am J Cardiol* 1974;33:209–214.
12. Baltazar R. Acute coronary syndrome: ST elevation myocardial infarction. In: *Basic and Bedside Electrocardiography*. Philadelphia, PA: Wolters Kluwer/Lippincott Williams & Wilkins; 2009:331–377.
13. LeWinter MaT. Pericardial diseases. In: Bonow RM, Zipes D, Libby P, eds. *Braunwald's Heart Disease: A Textbook of Cardiovascular Medicine*. 9th ed. Philadelphia, PA: Elsevier; 2011:1651–1671.
14. Spodick DH. Differential characteristics of the electrocardiogram in early repolarization and acute pericarditis. *N Engl J Med* 1976;295:523–526.
15. Baljepally R, Spodick DH. PR-segment deviation as the initial electrocardiographic response in acute pericarditis. *Am J Cardiol* 1998;81:1505–1506.
16. Napodano M, Tarantini G, Ramondo A, et al. Myocardial abnormalities underlying persistent ST-segment elevation after anterior myocardial infarction. *J Cardiovasc Med (Hagerstown)* 2009;10:44–50.
17. Mehta MC, Jain AC. Early repolarization on scalar electrocardiogram. *Am J Med Sci* 1995;309:305–311.
18. Ginzton LE, Laks MM. The differential diagnosis of acute pericarditis from the normal variant: new electrocardiographic criteria. *Circulation* 1982;65:1004–1009.
19. Mehta M, Jain AC, Mehta A. Early repolarization. *Clin Cardiol* 1999;22:59–65.
20. Sgarbossa EB, Pinski SL, Barbagelata A, et al. Electrocardiographic diagnosis of evolving acute myocardial infarction in the presence of left bundle-branch block. GUSTO-1 (Global Utilization of Streptokinase and Tissue Plasminogen Activator for Occluded Coronary Arteries) Investigators. *N Engl J Med* 1996;334:481–487.
21. Tabas JA, Rodriguez RM, Seligman HK, et al. Electrocardiographic criteria for detecting acute myocardial infarction in patients with left bundle branch block: a meta-analysis. *Ann Emerg Med* 2008;52:329–336 e1.
22. Falterman TJ, Martinez JA, Daberkow D, et al. Pulmonary embolism with ST segment elevation in leads V1 to V4: case report and review of the literature regarding electrocardiographic changes in acute pulmonary embolism. *J Emerg Med* 2001;21:255–261.
23. Lin JF, Li YC, Yang PL. A case of massive pulmonary embolism with ST elevation in leads V1–4. *Circ J* 2009;73:1157–1159.
24. Yeh KH, Chang HC. Massive pulmonary embolism with anterolateral ST-segment elevation: electrocardiogram limitations and the role of echocardiogram. *Am J Emerg Med* 2008;26:632 e1–633.
25. Simon BC. Pseudomyocardial infarction and hyperkalemia: a case report and subject review. *J Emerg Med* 1988;6:511–515.
26. Turhan S, Kilickap M, Kilinc S. ST segment elevation mimicking acute myocardial infarction in hypercalcaemia. *Heart* 2005;91:999.
27. Ashizawa N, Arakawa S, Koide Y, et al. Hypercalcemia due to vitamin D intoxication with clinical features mimicking acute myocardial infarction. *Intern Med* 2003;42:340–344.

28. Wesson LC, Suresh V, Parry RG. Severe hypercalcaemia mimicking acute myocardial infarction. *Clin Med* 2009;9:186–187.

29. Gurevitz O, Fogel RI, Herner ME, et al. Patients with an ICD can safely resume work in industrial facilities following simple screening for electromagnetic interference. *Pacing Clin Electrophysiol* 2003;26:1675–1678.

30. Reddy RK, Gleva MJ, Gliner BE, et al. Biphasic transthoracic defibrillation causes fewer ECG ST-segment changes after shock. *Ann Emerg Med* 1997;30:127–134.

31. Finn AV, Antman EM. Images in clinical medicine. Isolated right ventricular infarction. *N Engl J Med* 2003;349:1636.

32. Barold SS, Hayes DL. Second-degree atrioventricular block: a reappraisal. *Mayo Clin Proc* 2001;76:44–57.

33. Gorgels AP, Engelen DJ, Wellens HJ. Lead aVR, a mostly ignored but very valuable lead in clinical electrocardiography. *J Am Coll Cardiol* 2001;38:1355–1356.

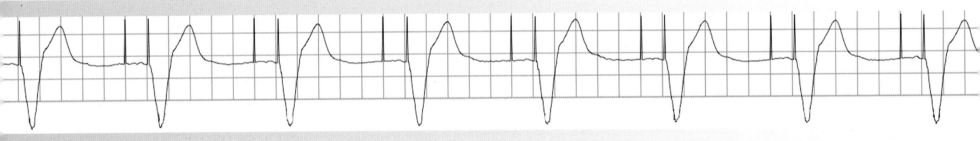

The Pacemaker

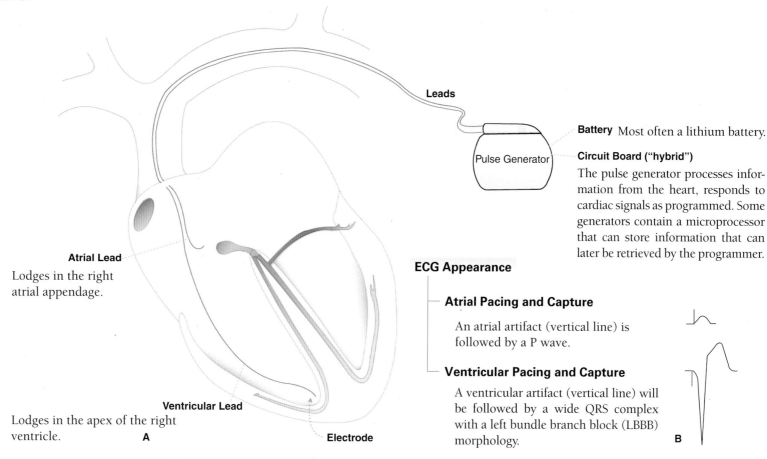

Leads

Battery Most often a lithium battery.

Circuit Board ("hybrid")
The pulse generator processes information from the heart, responds to cardiac signals as programmed. Some generators contain a microprocessor that can store information that can later be retrieved by the programmer.

Pulse Generator

Atrial Lead
Lodges in the right atrial appendage.

ECG Appearance

Atrial Pacing and Capture

An atrial artifact (vertical line) is followed by a P wave.

Ventricular Pacing and Capture

A ventricular artifact (vertical line) will be followed by a wide QRS complex with a left bundle branch block (LBBB) morphology.

Ventricular Lead
Lodges in the apex of the right ventricle.   **A**

Electrode

B

FIGURE 13.1 A. Anatomy of a dual chamber pacemaker.
B. ECG appearance of atrial and ventricular pacing.

Electrode Types

Unipolar

Cathode is on the lead tip; anode is located proximally within the pulse generator.

Pacemaker artifacts are generally more conspicuous.

Bipolar

Cathode and anode are located 1 cm apart at the distal end of the lead.

Pacemaker artifacts are smaller and may be difficult to appreciate.

Pacemaker Nomenclature

A five-letter code has been adopted to identify different types of pacemakers.[1] The first letter identifies the number and location of leads (single versus dual and atrial versus ventricular). The second letter corresponds to the presence or absence of sensing capability (the ability to sense a chamber's native impulse conduction). The third letter indicates the pacemaker's response to a sensed impulse. The fourth letter indicates the pacemaker's programmability and capacity for rate modulation. The fifth letter indicates the anti-tachydysrhythmia functions of the pacemaker.

Table 13.1 North American Society of Pacing and Electrophysiology/British Pacing and Electrophysiology Group (NBG Code) System of Categorizing Pacemakers.

I Chamber(s) Paced	II Chamber(s) Sensed	III Response to Sensing	IV Programmability and Rate Modulation	V Anti-tachydysrhythmia Functions
0	0	0	0	0
A	A	T	P	P
V	V	I	M	S
D	D	D	C	D
			R	

0: None	0: None	0: None	0: None	0: None
A: Atrial	A: Atrial	T: Triggered	P: Simple Programmable	P: Simple Programmable
V: Ventricular	V: Ventricular	I: Inhibited	M: Multiprogrammable	S: Shock
D: Dual (Atrial + Ventricular)	D: Dual (Atrial + Ventricular)	D: Dual (Triggered and Inhibited)	C: Communicating	D: Dual pacing and shock
			R: Rate Modulation	

Pacemakers are typically referred to by the first three letters of the NBG code. Common pacemaker modes are VVI and DDD.

Single Chamber Pacing

Atrial Pacemakers

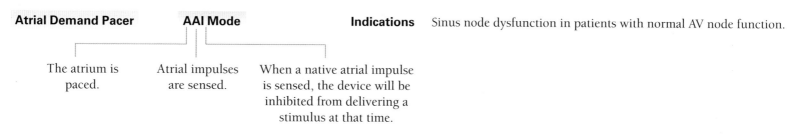

| Atrial Demand Pacer | AAI Mode | | Indications | Sinus node dysfunction in patients with normal AV node function. |

The atrium is paced.

Atrial impulses are sensed.

When a native atrial impulse is sensed, the device will be inhibited from delivering a stimulus at that time.

Ventricular Pacemakers

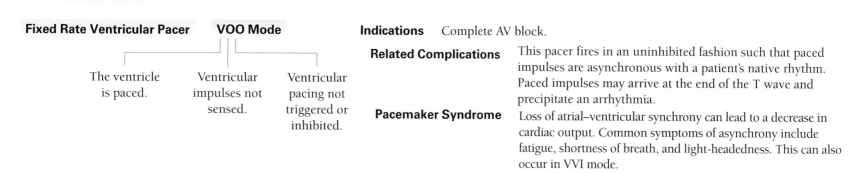

Fixed Rate Ventricular Pacer   **VOO Mode**

Indications   Complete AV block.

The ventricle is paced.

Ventricular impulses not sensed.

Ventricular pacing not triggered or inhibited.

Related Complications   This pacer fires in an uninhibited fashion such that paced impulses are asynchronous with a patient's native rhythm. Paced impulses may arrive at the end of the T wave and precipitate an arrhythmia.

Pacemaker Syndrome   Loss of atrial–ventricular synchrony can lead to a decrease in cardiac output. Common symptoms of asynchrony include fatigue, shortness of breath, and light-headedness. This can also occur in VVI mode.

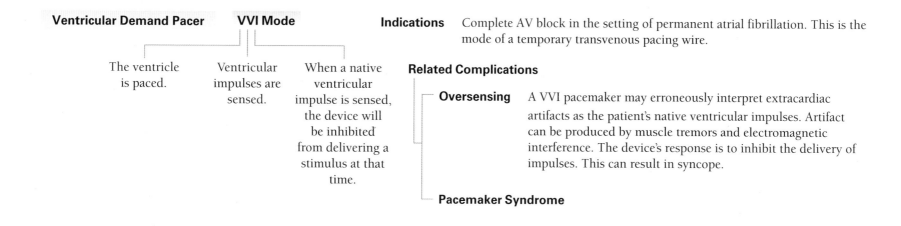

Ventricular Demand Pacer   **VVI Mode**

Indications   Complete AV block in the setting of permanent atrial fibrillation. This is the mode of a temporary transvenous pacing wire.

The ventricle is paced.

Ventricular impulses are sensed.

When a native ventricular impulse is sensed, the device will be inhibited from delivering a stimulus at that time.

Related Complications

Oversensing   A VVI pacemaker may erroneously interpret extracardiac artifacts as the patient's native ventricular impulses. Artifact can be produced by muscle tremors and electromagnetic interference. The device's response is to inhibit the delivery of impulses. This can result in syncope.

Pacemaker Syndrome

Dual Chamber Pacing

Dual chamber pacemakers consist of both atrial and ventricular leads capable of pacing and sensing. The principal advantage of DDD pacers is preservation of atrial–ventricular synchrony.

Table 13.2 Different Patterns of Sensing and Pacing Seen in Dual Chamber Pacemakers

Atrial Complex	Ventricular Complex	Description	ECG Appearance
Native	Native	The atrial channel senses a native atrial impulse and is inhibited from firing. This atrial impulse may successfully conduct to the ventricle (sensed by the ventricular channel) and result in a native QRS complex.	Absent Pacer Spikes
Native	Paced	The atrial impulse is inhibited by sensing a native atrial impulse. The atrial impulse fails to conduct to the ventricles. The atrial channel triggers the ventricular channel to fire, resulting in a paced ventricular complex.	Ventricular Pacer Spike
Paced	Native	Atrial conduction depends on the firing of the atrial channel resulting in a paced atrial complex. This paced atrial impulse can conduct successfully to the ventricles and result in a native QRS complex.	Atrial Pacer Spike
Paced	Paced	Both atrial and ventricular conduction depend on the pacemaker. A paced ventricular impulse is delivered after a programmed interval following the paced atrial impulse.	Atrial Pacer Spike / Ventricular Pacer Spike

Biventricular Pacing (Cardiac Resynchronization Therapy)

Desynchrony in Heart Failure

Ventricular conduction delay is a common abnormality in patients with heart failure. Delay in ventricular activation renders the mechanics of ventricular contraction suboptimal.

Synchronizing left and right ventricular contraction through left and right ventricular pacemaker leads has been shown to improve clinical outcomes in randomized controlled trials.[2,3]

Indications[4]

Ejection Fraction ≤ 35%

QRS ≥ 120 msec

Sinus Rhythm

NYHA Class III or IV Heart Failure

CRT is also considered for patients with the above criteria who have atrial fibrillation.

Anatomy

The left ventricular lead enters the ostium of the coronary sinus after passing through the right atrium. The lead passes through the coronary sinus and enters a cardiac vein and a tributary that leads to the ventricular wall. The electrode is often passively fixed in the midlateral aspect of the left ventricular wall.

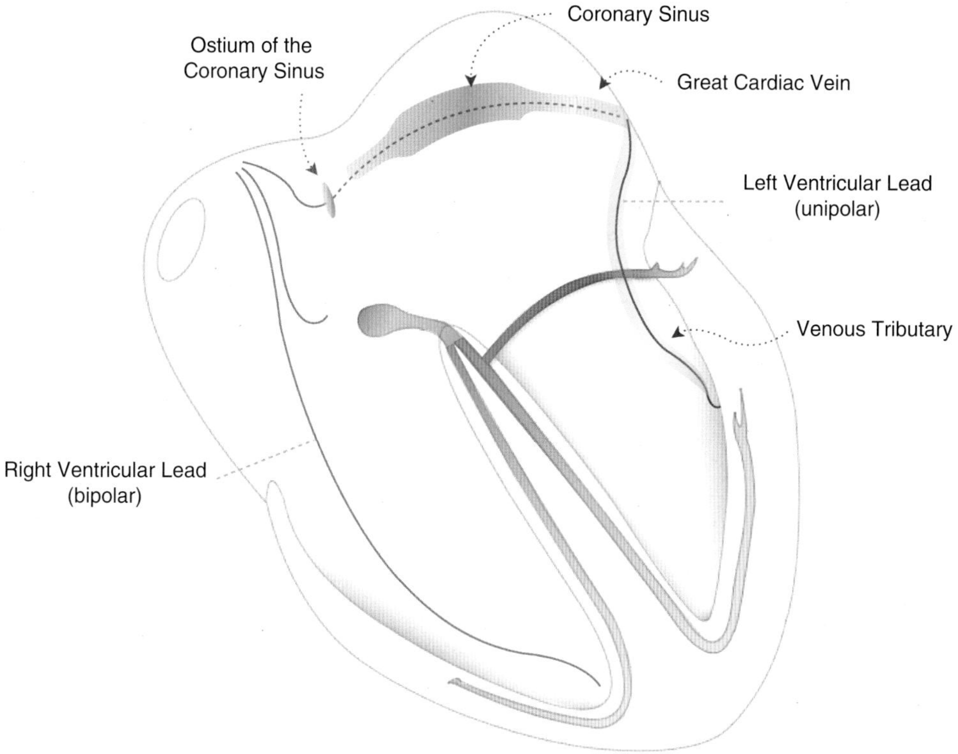

ECG Appearance

Relative Narrowing of QRS

Right bundle branch block (RBBB) Morphology

FIGURE 13.2 Anatomical positioning of the leads in a biventricular pacer.

Often the morphology of the QRS complex changes to that of a RBBB.

Pacemaker-Mediated Tachycardia

Pacemaker-mediated tachycardia (PMT) is a form of tachycardia that involves the pacemaker itself as a part of the conduction pathway. Endless loop tachycardia is a form of PMT in which retrograde ventricular–atrial conduction results in repetitive atrial sensing and triggering of a ventricular impulse.

Mechanism

A premature ventricular contraction occurring after the atrial refractory period may be conducted in retrograde fashion past the AV node and result in atrial depolarization. Atrial depolarization then triggers ventricular pacing.

After a pacer-stimulus is delivered to the ventricle, conduction can travel in a retrograde fashion to the atria through the normal conduction system.

The atrial electrode senses the retrograde atrial conduction. This triggers the ventricular electrode to pace the ventricle and the cycle repeats until the retrograde ventricular–atrial conduction is interrupted.

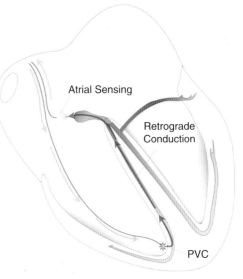

FIGURE 13.3 Conduction pathway of PMT.

ECG Appearance

Inverted P Waves Retrograde conduction from ventricle to atria will result in inverted P waves in II, III, and aVF.

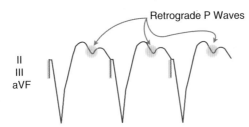

FIGURE 13.4 ECG appearance of PMT in an inferior limb lead.

Rate The ventricular rate should approximate the programmed upper limit of the pacemaker.

Mistaken for

Sinus tachycardia

Ventricular tachycardia
(if pacer artifacts from bipolar leads are barely visible)

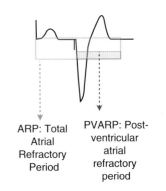

FIGURE 13.5 Atrial refractory periods in a dual chamber pacemaker.

Treatment

PMT can be broken by disabling the sensing capability of the atrial electrode. This can be accomplished in several ways.

Magnet A magnet placed over the pacemaker generator will render a DDD system incapable of sensing atrial and ventricular impulses. It will function as a fixed rate pacer (DOO mode).

Mode Switch Programming the pacemaker to DVI or VVI mode will also prevent the atrial electrode from sensing.

Postventricular Atrial Refractory Period The pacemaker can be programmed to have a longer postventricular atrial refractory period (PVARP) during which the atrial channel is incapable of sensing.

Pacemaker Failures

Failure to Capture

ECG Appearance Pacing artifacts are present, but not followed by an atrial or ventricular complex.

Causes[5]

Elevated Capture Threshold

Metabolic disturbance (hyperkalemia, acidosis, alkalosis)
Myocardial fibrosis near the electrode
Myocardial infarction (MI) near the electrode
Class IC Drugs (flecainide, propafenone)

Lead Failure

Conductor coil fracture
Insulation defect
Lead dislodgment

FIGURE 13.6 ECG appearance of a pacemaker failing to capture.

Failure to Pace

ECG Appearance Pacing artifacts are absent where there is an indication for pacing.

Causes

Output Failure

Battery depletion
Conductor coil fracture
Insulation defect

Oversensing

Electromagnetic interference (MRI, electrocautery, lithotripsy, arc welding, cellular telephones)
Crosstalk: The ventricular channel inappropriately senses atrial pacing and inhibits ventricular output
Sensing myopotentials (diaphragm, rectus abdominal muscles, pectoralis muscles)
Oversensing T waves

FIGURE 13.7 ECG appearance of a pacemaker failing to pace.

Failure to Sense

Undersensing occurs when the pacemaker fails to detect intrinsic depolarizations and inappropriately fires.

ECG Appearance Pacemaker artifact will appear at inappropriate times.

Causes
Metabolic disturbance
Myocardial fibrosis
Myocardial infarction
Pulse generator failure
Lead dislodgment/insulation failure
Conductor coil fracture

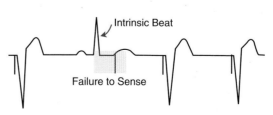

FIGURE 13.8 ECG appearance of a pacemaker failing to sense

The Magnet

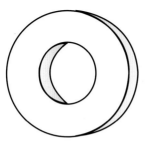

FIGURE 13.9 Appearance of a magnet.

Mechanism

Placing a magnet over the pulse generator of a pacer reprograms the pacemaker to an asynchronous mode (VOO or DOO), which renders it incapable of sensing.

Indications for a Magnet

Failure to Pace

An ECG may fail to show pacer artifacts in a patient with symptomatic bradycardia. Placement of a magnet can help differentiate output failure from oversensing as causes of failure to pace.

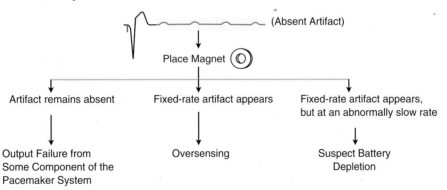

FIGURE 13.10 Role of magnet in evaluating failure to pace.

Pacemaker-Mediated Tachycardia

The atrial sensing of retrograde ventricular-atrial conduction can be halted by a magnet. This is a temporary therapeutic maneuver.

Inappropriate Firing of an ICD

Placement of a magnet over an ICD device will inhibit the device's ability to defibrillate.

ECG 13.1a

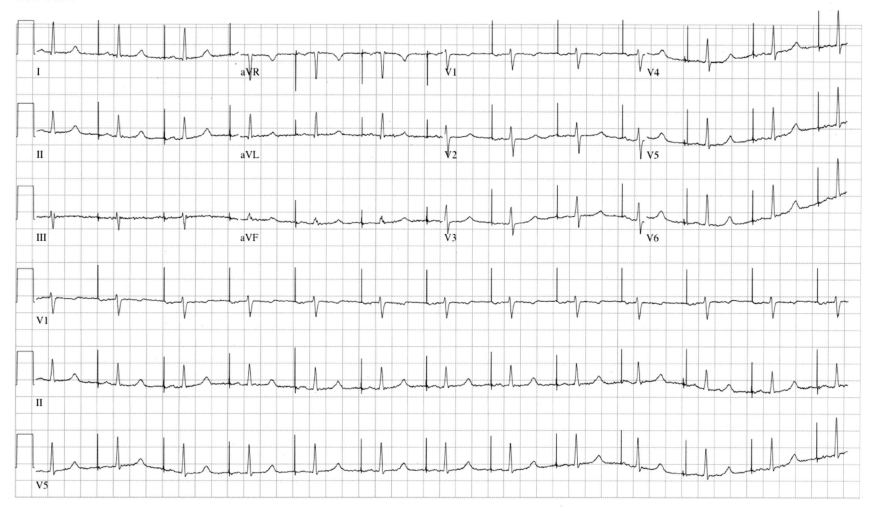

ECG 13.1b

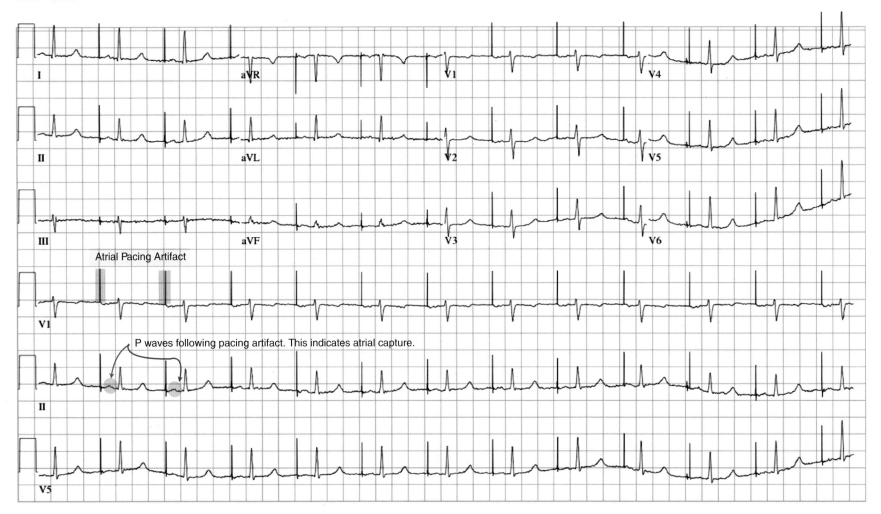

Atrial Pacing Artifact

P waves following pacing artifact. This indicates atrial capture.

Atrial Pacing

ECG 13.2a

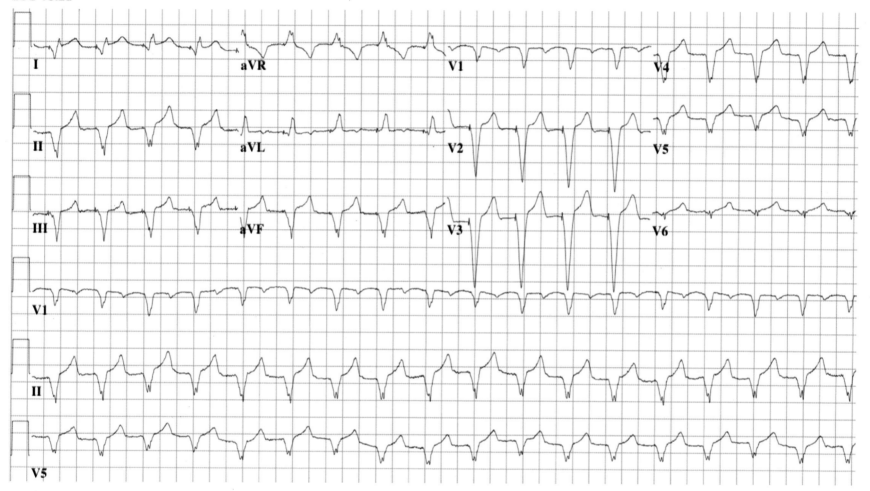

ECG 13.2b

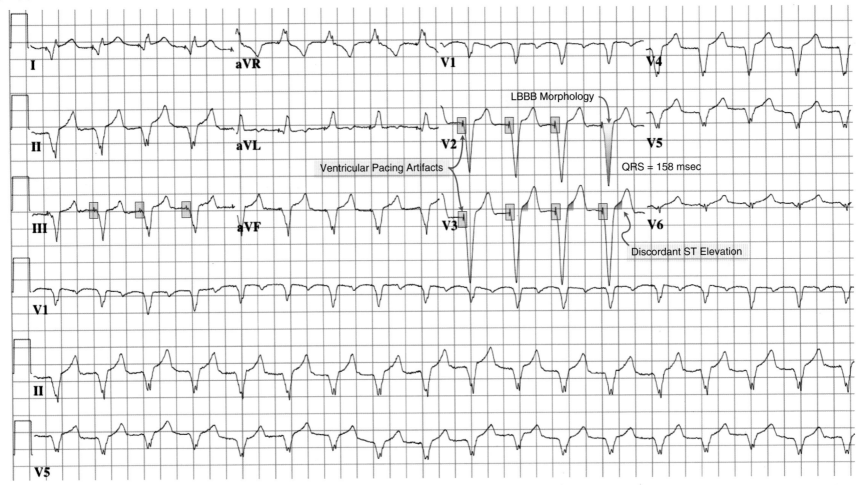

Ventricular Pacing

ECG 13.3a

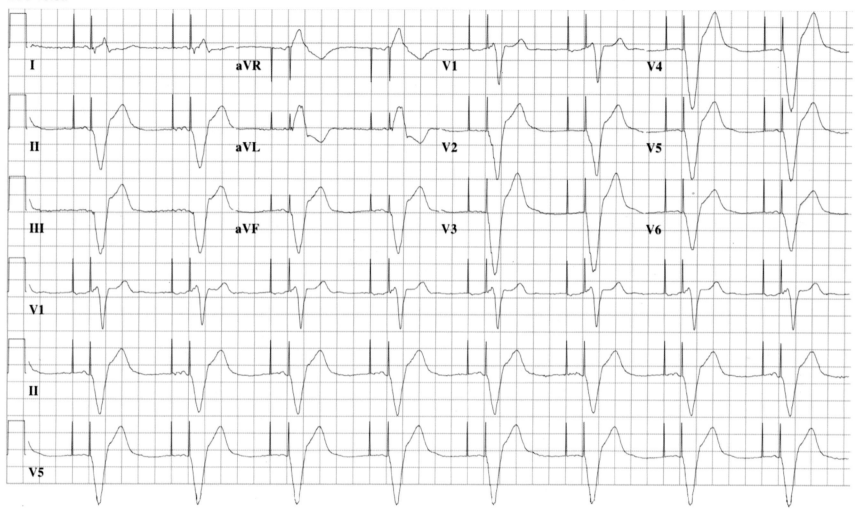

ECG 13.3b

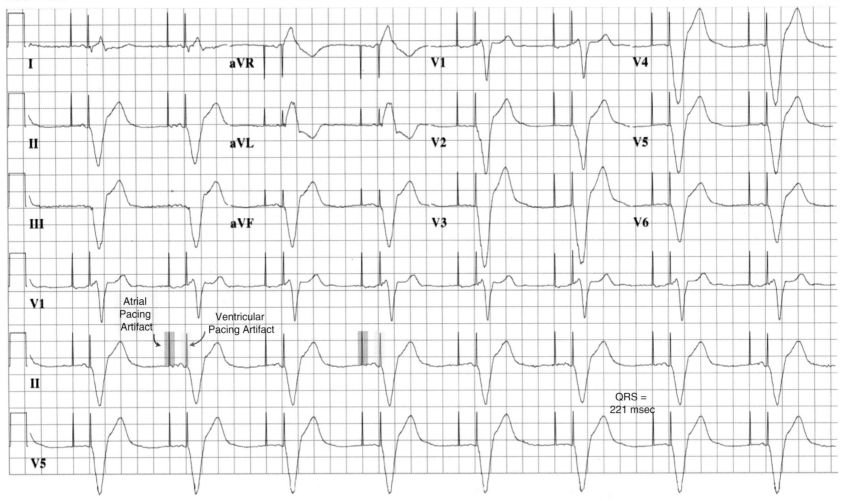

Atrial Pacing Artifact

Ventricular Pacing Artifact

QRS = 221 msec

AV Paced Rhythm

ECG 13.4a A 69-year-old male with a dual-chamber pacemaker.

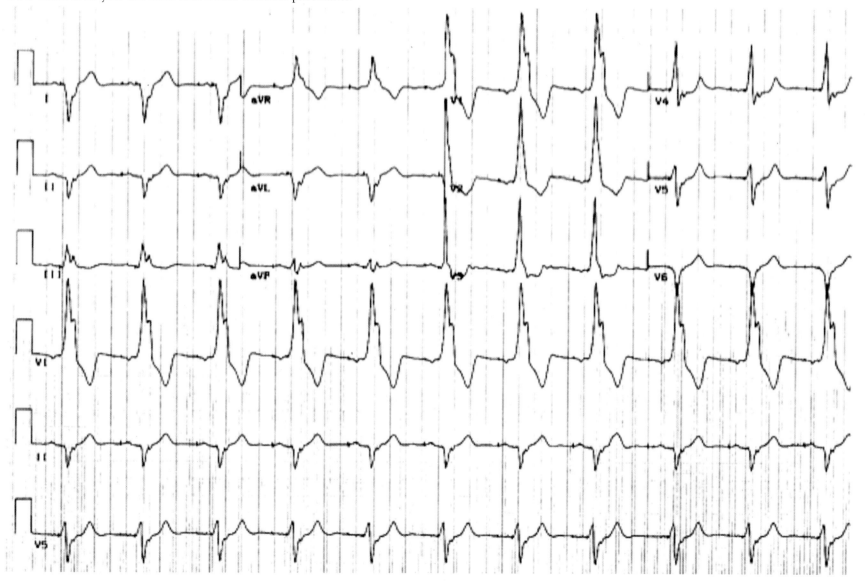

ECG 13.4b A 69-year-old male with a dual-chamber pacemaker.

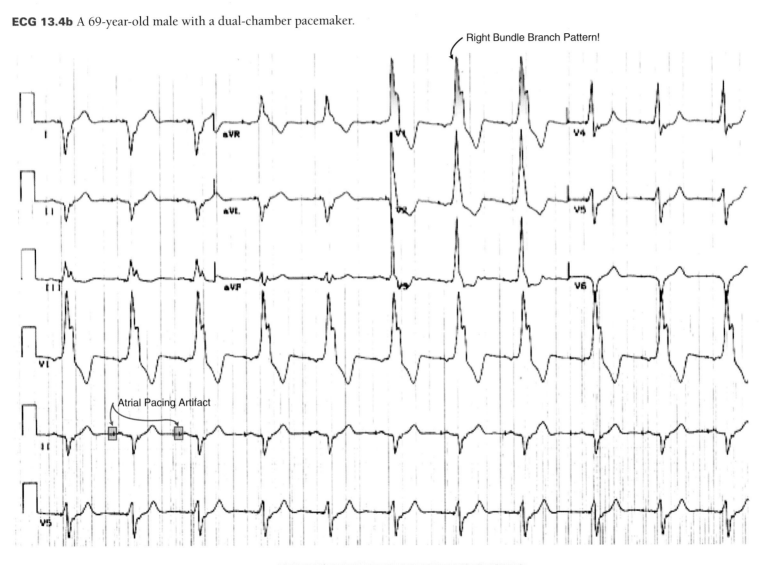

Right Bundle Branch Pattern!

Atrial Pacing Artifact

Septal Perforation by the Ventricular Lead

RBBB morphology in a patient with a dual-chamber pacer should raise suspicion of lead migration into the left ventricle. The RBBB pattern results from ventricular depolarization spreading through myocardial cells from a site in the left ventricle. Lead migration from right to left ventricle can occur during pacemaker placement through an atrial septal defect,[6] a patent foramen ovale,[7] or a sinus venosus defect.[8] A lead may also perforate the interventricular septum and migrate to the left ventricle, as occurred in this patient.

A pattern of RBBB can also occur when the right ventricular lead is appropriately positioned in the right ventricular apex.

ECG 13.5a

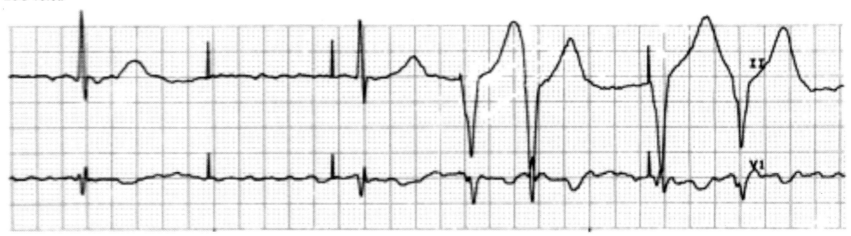

Image courtesy of Theofanie Mela, MD.

ECG 13.5b

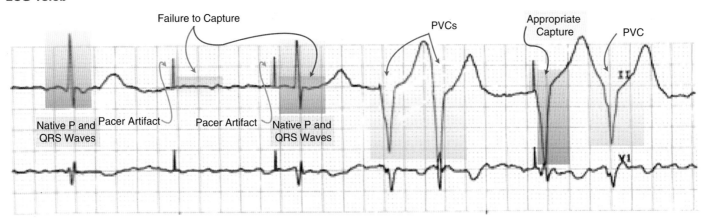

Failure to Capture

Loss of ventricular capture in this case was secondary to dislodgment of the pacer lead in this VVI pacer. The dislodged lead may be responsible for inducing the ventricular ectopy seen in the latter half of this strip.

ECG 13.6a

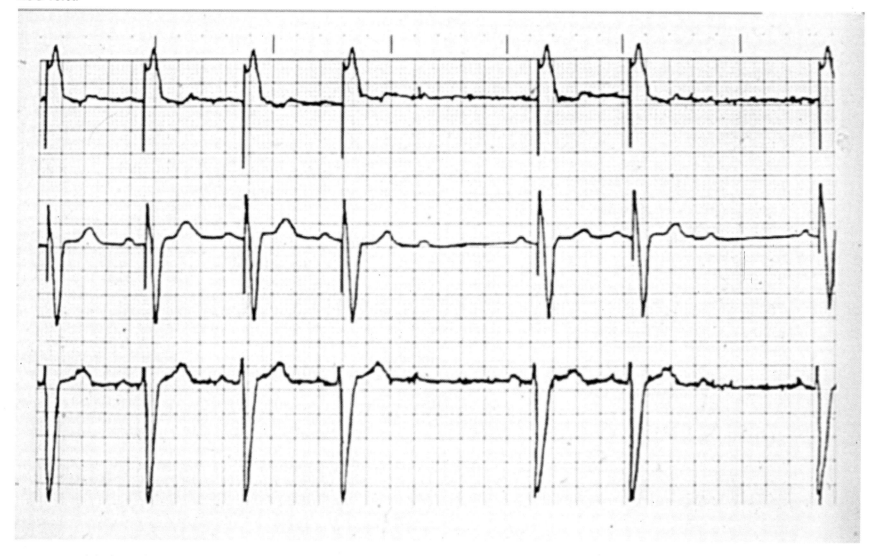

Image courtesy of Theofanie Mela, MD.

ECG 13.6b

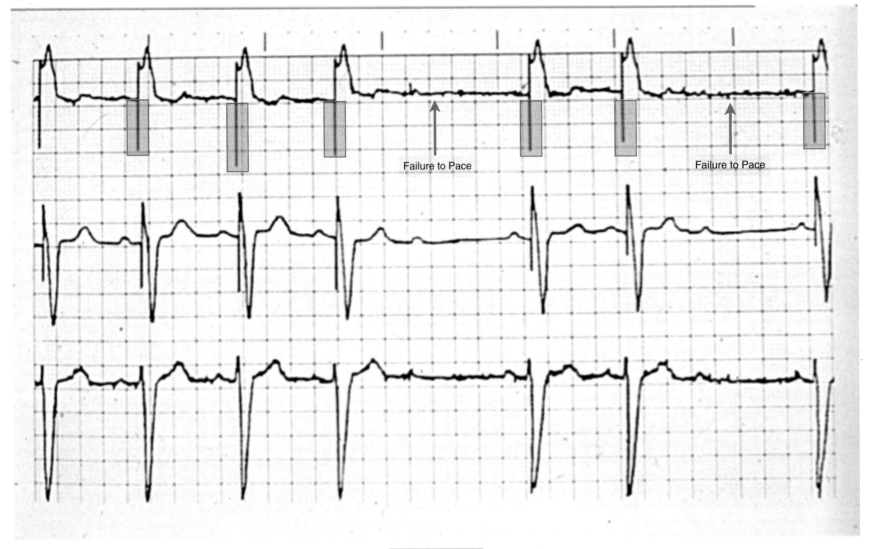

Failure to Pace

Failure to Pace

Failure to Pace

Failure to pace could result from output failure (battery depletion) or oversensing.

ECG 13.7a

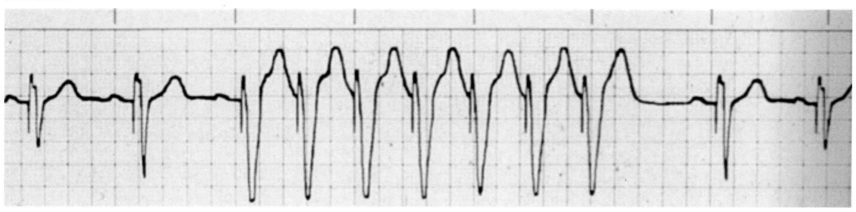

Image courtesy of Theofanie Mela, MD.

ECG 13.7b

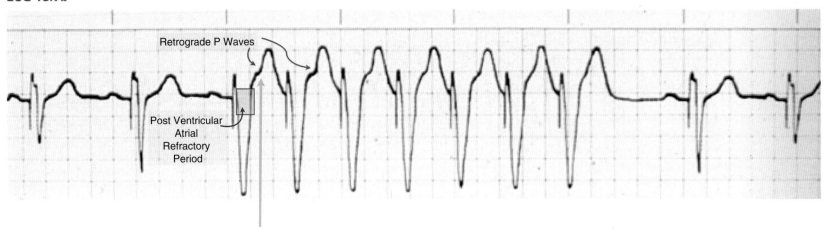

Retrograde P Waves

Post Ventricular
Atrial
Refractory
Period

The retrograde P wave occurs outside of the post-ventricular atrial
refractory period (PVARP).

Pacemaker-Mediated Tachycardia

ECG 13.8a A 74-year-old female with COPD and severe CHF.

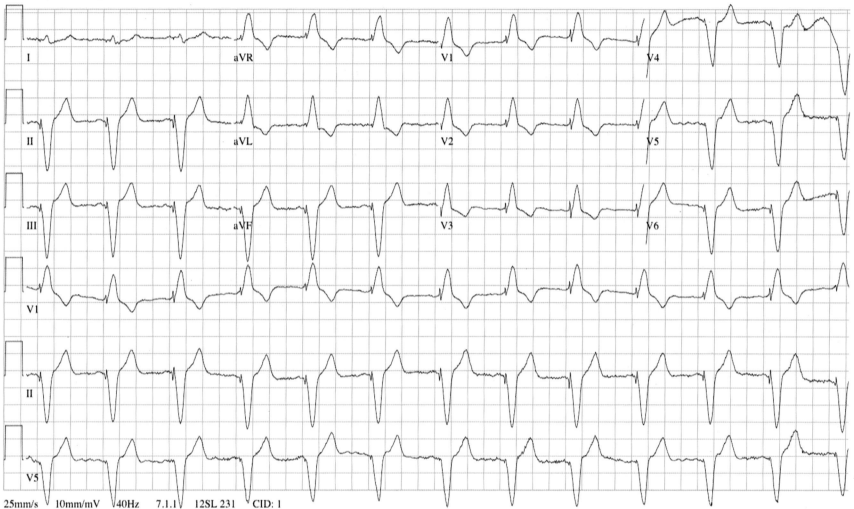

25mm/s   10mm/mV   40Hz   7.1.1   12SL 231   CID: 1

ECG 13.8b A 74-year-old female with COPD and severe CHF.

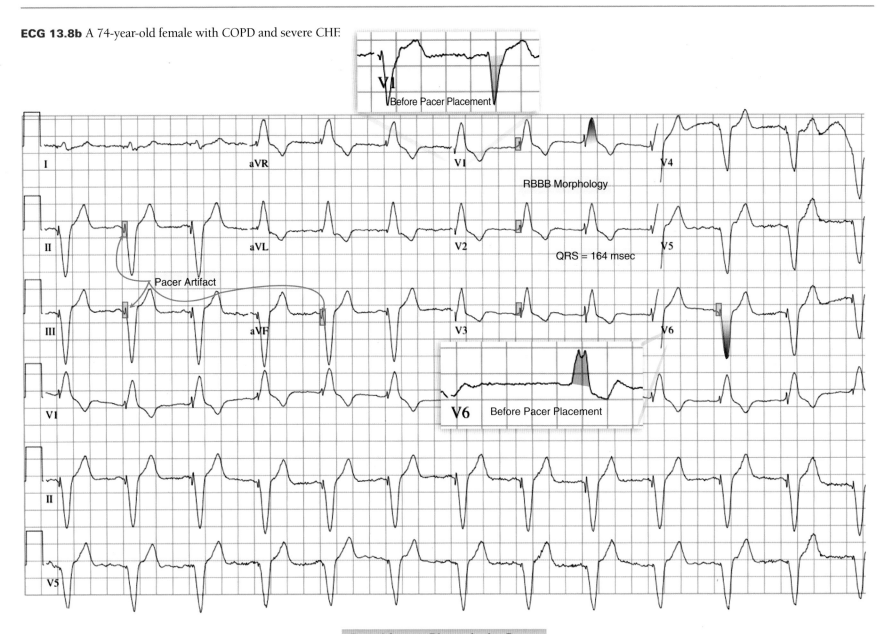

Paced from a Biventricular Pacer

This patient has severe adriamycin-induced cardiomyopathy. Despite biventricular pacing, the QRS complex remains wide.

ECG 13.9a

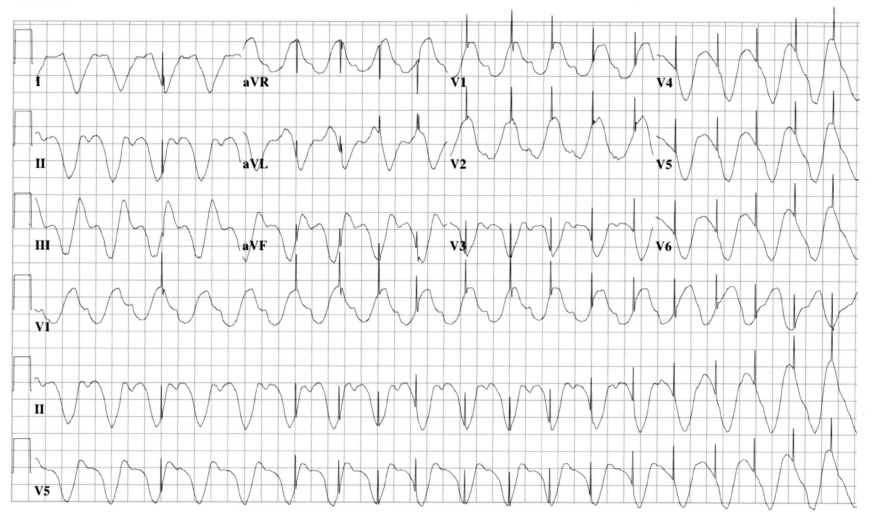

ECG 13.9b

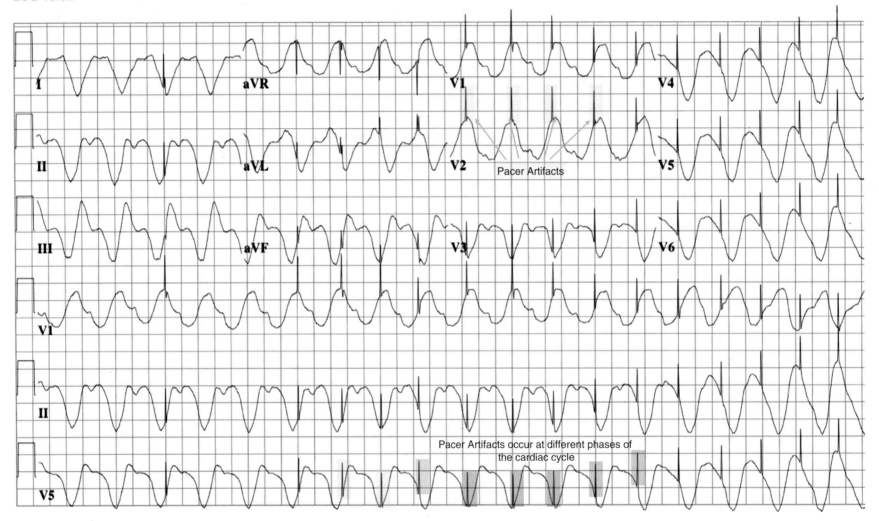

Pacemaker Malfunction Secondary to Severe Hyperkalemia

This patient's potassium level was 7.8 mg/dL. Note the extremely wide QRS complexes. Pacing spikes appear intermittently and at different phases of the cardiac cycle. Hyperkalemia can cause failure to capture.

ECG 13.10a A 95-year-old with sick sinus syndrome and coronary artery disease is found unresponsive in a nursing home.

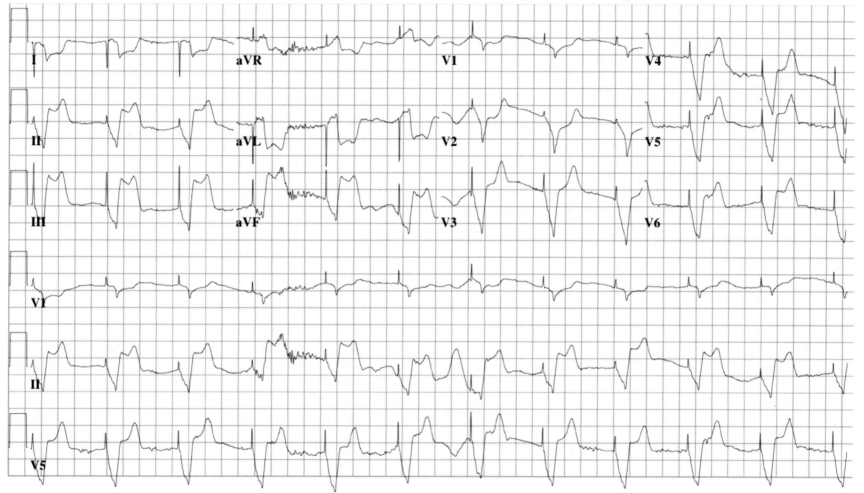

ECG 13.10b A 95-year-old with sick sinus syndrome and coronary artery disease is found unresponsive in a nursing home.

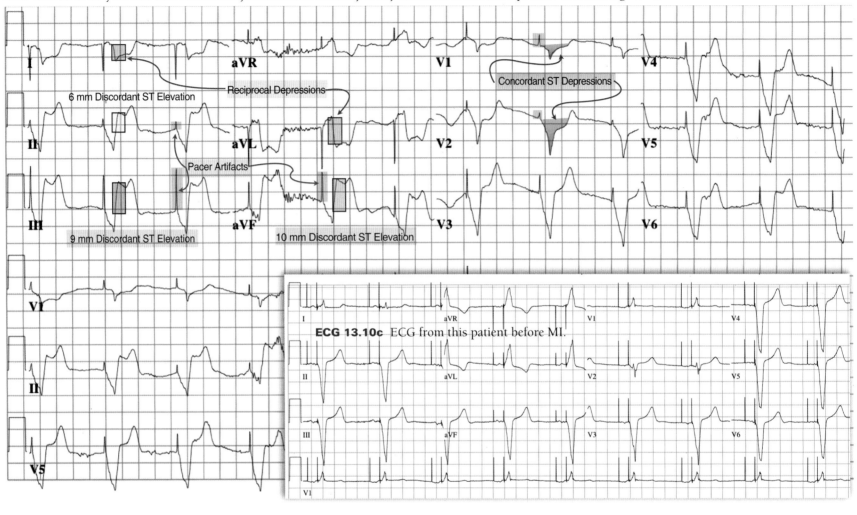

Inferior STEMI: Ventricular Paced

Ruling out acute MI in a ventricular-paced ECG is difficult because there are no findings that are sensitive for this diagnosis. However, Sgarbossa found that the same abnormalities specific for MI in the presence of a LBBB (ST depression in leads V1–V3, exaggerated discordance, and concordant ST elevation) were also specific for the diagnosis of MI in ventricular paced rhythms. The finding of discordant ST elevation of ≥ 5 mm has demonstrated the highest specificity.[9,10] This ECG demonstrates inappropriate concordance and exaggerated discordance in a ventricular paced rhythm. The ST segments are markedly elevated in the inferior limb leads with reciprocal ST depressions in I and aVL. Concordant ST depressions could represent posterior extension of the area of infarction or reciprocal changes.

Cardiac markers in this patient were significantly elevated. The patient suffered cardiac arrest and expired shortly after this ECG was obtained.

References

1. Bernstein AD, Daubert JC, Fletcher RD, et al. The revised NASPE/BPEG generic code for antibradycardia, adaptive-rate, and multisite pacing. North American Society of Pacing and Electrophysiology/British Pacing and Electrophysiology Group. *Pacing Clin Electrophysiol* 2002;25:260–264.
2. Abraham WT. Cardiac resynchronization therapy for heart failure: biventricular pacing and beyond. *Curr Opin Cardiol* 2002;17:346–352.
3. Cazeau S, Leclercq C, Lavergne T, et al. Effects of multisite biventricular pacing in patients with heart failure and intraventricular conduction delay. *N Engl J Med* 2001;344:873–880.
4. Vardas PE, Auricchio A, Blanc JJ, et al. Guidelines for cardiac pacing and cardiac resynchronization therapy: The Task Force for Cardiac Pacing and Cardiac Resynchronization Therapy of the European Society of Cardiology. Developed in collaboration with the European Heart Rhythm Association. *Eur Heart J* 2007; 28:2256–2295.
5. Mahoney TaT, P. Cardiac Pacing. In: Griffin BaT, E, ed. *Manual of Cardiovascular Medicine.* 3rd ed. Philadelphia, PA: Wolters Kluwer/Lippincott Williams & Wilkins; 2009.
6. Huang WM, Xin ZP, Tung CL. An unusual electrocardiographic pattern of left ventricular endocardial pacing. *Pacing Clin Electrophysiol* 1980;3:597–599.
7. Shmuely H, Erdman S, Strasberg B, et al. Seven years of left ventricular pacing due to malposition of pacing electrode. *Pacing Clin Electrophysiol* 1992;15:369–372.
8. Van Erckelens F, Sigmund M, Lambertz H, et al. Asymptomatic left ventricular malposition of a transvenous pacemaker lead through a sinus venosus defect: follow-up over 17 years. *Pacing Clin Electrophysiol* 1991;14:989–993.
9. Sgarbossa EB, Pinski SL, Gates KB, et al. Early electrocardiographic diagnosis of acute myocardial infarction in the presence of ventricular paced rhythm. GUSTO-I investigators. *Am J Cardiol* 1996;77:423–424.
10. Maloy KR, Bhat R, Davis J, et al. Sgarbossa criteria are highly specific for acute myocardial infarction with pacemakers. *West J Emerg Med* 2010;11:354–357.

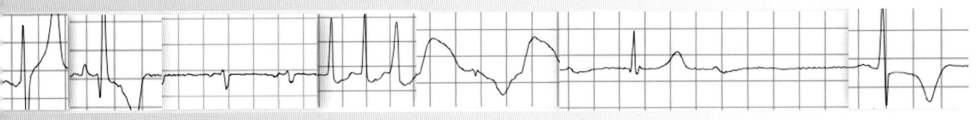

Repetition helps with pattern recognition. The following ECG excerpts represent classic ECG patterns and morphologies. Try to identify the ECG abnormality and clinical correlate.

Table 14.1a

Image	ECG Abnormality	Clinical Significance

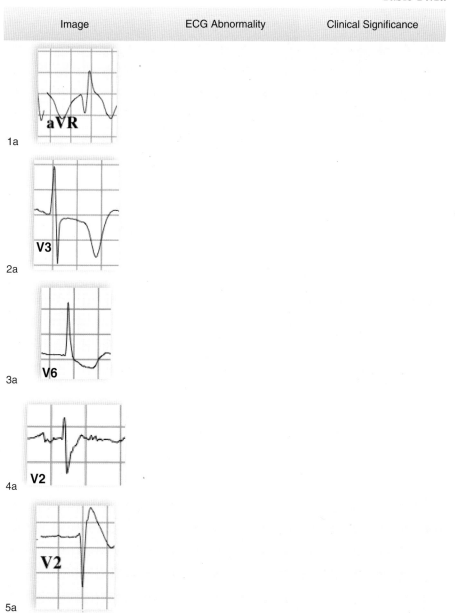

1a

2a

3a

4a

5a

Table 14.1b

Image	ECG Abnormality	Clinical Significance
1b	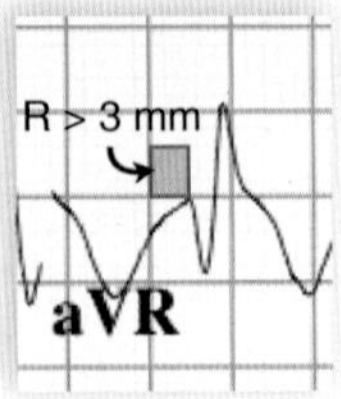 R in aVR QRS Widening	Na$^+$ Channel Blocker Toxicity (Cocaine, TCA)
2b	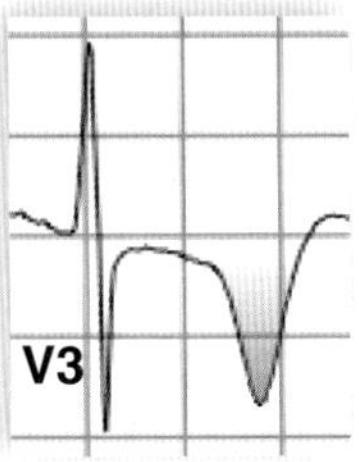 Deep Symmetric TWI	Wellens Syndrome (Proximal LAD Occlusion)
3b	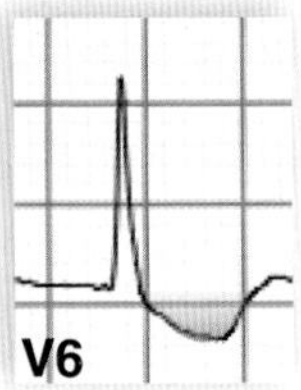 ST Depression and Scooped T Wave Inversion	Digoxin Effect (not toxicity)
4b	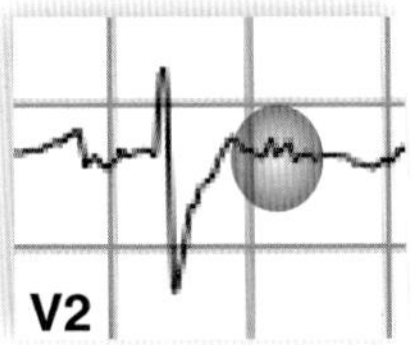 Epsilon Wave	Arrhythmogenic Right Ventricular Dysplasia
5b	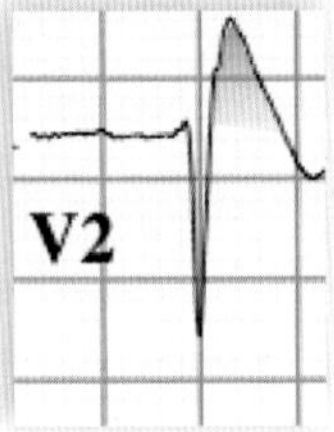 Coved ST Elevation in Right Precordial Lead	Brugada Syndrome (Type 1)

Table 14.2a

Image	ECG Abnormality	Clinical Significance

6a

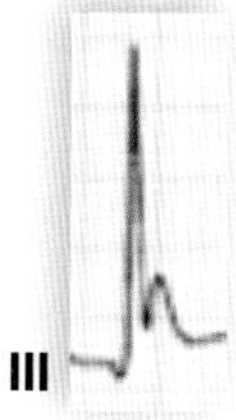

7a

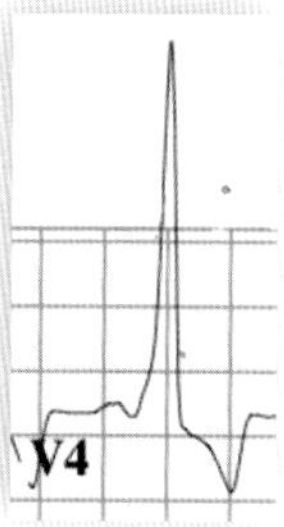

8a

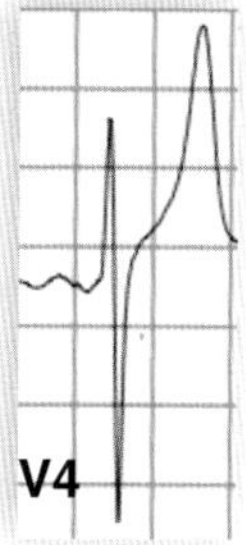

9a

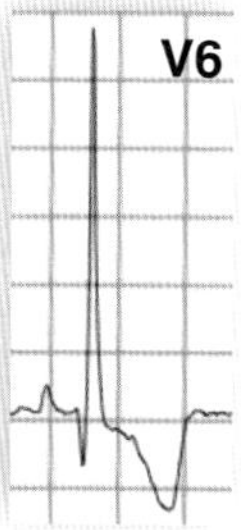

Table 14.2b

Image	ECG Abnormality	Clinical Significance
 III 6b	Osborn Wave (J wave)	Hypothermia (less likely subarachnoid hemorrhage, hypercalcemia)
 V4 7b	Short PR Interval Delta Wave QRS Widening	WPW Pattern
 V4 8b	Peaked T Wave	Hyperkalemia
 V6 9b	Deep and Narrow Q Wave Alongside High-Amplitude QRS	Hypertrophic Cardiomyopathy

Table 14.3a

Image	ECG Abnormality	Clinical Significance

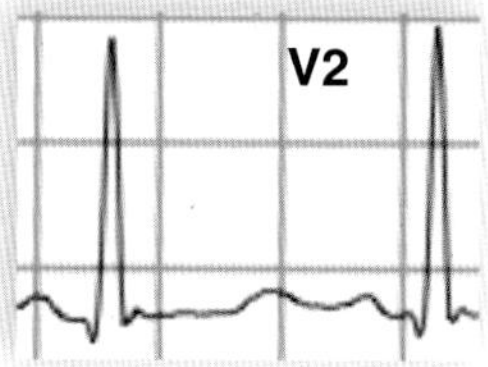

10a

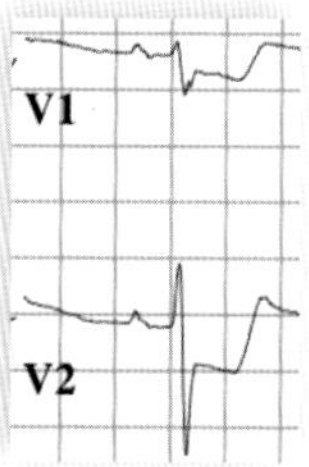

11a

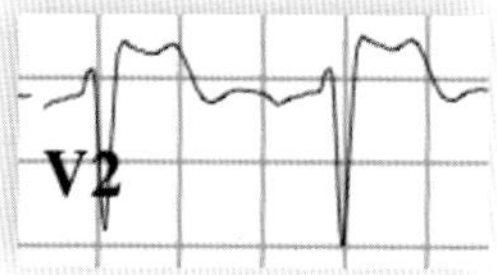

12a

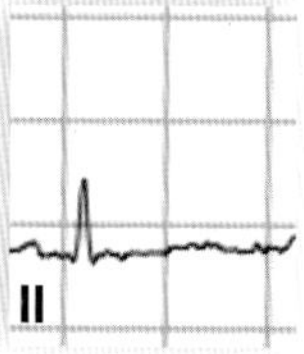

13a

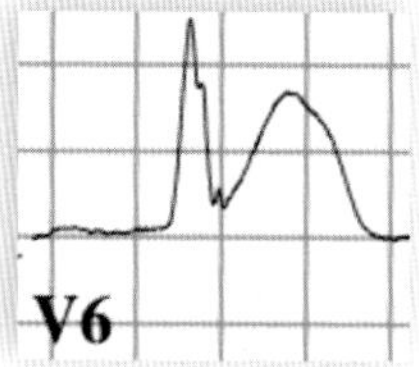

14a

Table 14.3b

Image	ECG Abnormality	Clinical Significance
 10b	QT Prolongation	Increased Risk for Torsades Look for correctable causes
 11b	ST Depression in V1 and V2	Possible Posterior STEMI Consider reciprocal ST depression or anterior subendocardial ischemia as other causes
 12b	Incomplete RBBB ST Elevation with Saddleback Morphology	Type 2 Brugada
 13b	Low Voltage	Consider pericardial effusion Go through low voltage differential
 14b	Concordant ST Elevation with LBBB Morphology	Consider ST Elevation MI

Table 14.4a

Image	ECG Abnormality	Clinical Significance

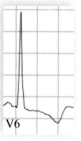

15a

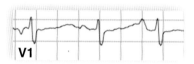

16a

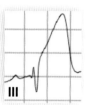

17a

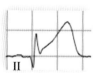

18a

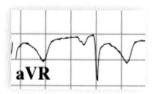

19a

Table 14.4b

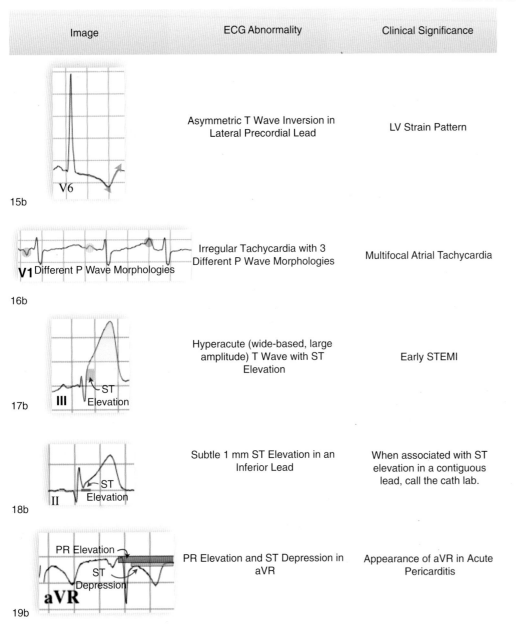

Image	ECG Abnormality	Clinical Significance
15b	Asymmetric T Wave Inversion in Lateral Precordial Lead	LV Strain Pattern
16b	Irregular Tachycardia with 3 Different P Wave Morphologies	Multifocal Atrial Tachycardia
17b	Hyperacute (wide-based, large amplitude) T Wave with ST Elevation	Early STEMI
18b	Subtle 1 mm ST Elevation in an Inferior Lead	When associated with ST elevation in a contiguous lead, call the cath lab.
19b	PR Elevation and ST Depression in aVR	Appearance of aVR in Acute Pericarditis

Table 14.5a

Image	ECG Abnormality

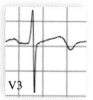

20a

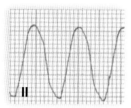

21a

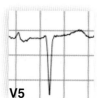

22a

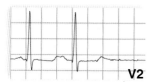

23a

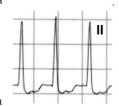

24a

Table 14.5b

Image	ECG Abnormality	Clinicial Significance
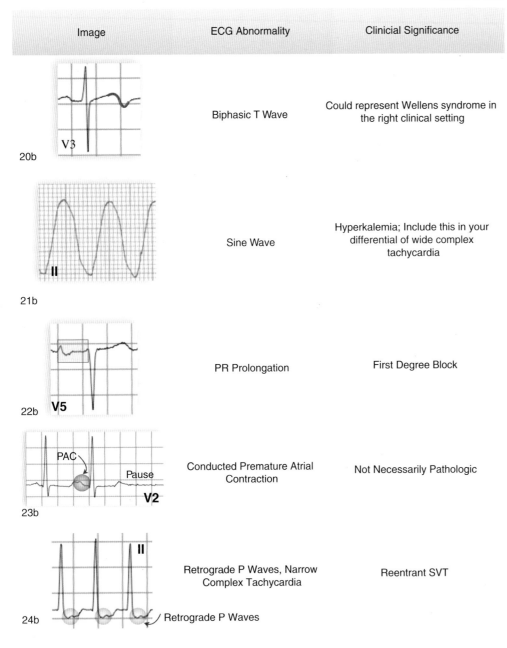		

20b — Biphasic T Wave — Could represent Wellens syndrome in the right clinical setting

21b — Sine Wave — Hyperkalemia; Include this in your differential of wide complex tachycardia

22b — PR Prolongation — First Degree Block

23b — Conducted Premature Atrial Contraction — Not Necessarily Pathologic

24b — Retrograde P Waves, Narrow Complex Tachycardia — Reentrant SVT

APPENDIX
COMMON ABBREVIATIONS

AF	Atrial Fibrillation
AICD	Automatic Implantable Cardioverter-Defibrillator
ARVD	Arrhythmogenic Right Ventricular Dysplasia
AVNRT	Atrioventricular Nodal Reentrant Tachycardia
AVRT	Atrioventricular Reciprocating Tachycardia
BBB	Bundle Branch Block
BER	Benign Early Repolarization
CHB	Complete Heart Block
ICD	Implantable Cardioverter-Defibrillator
IMI	Inferior Myocardial Infarction
LAD	Left Anterior Descending Artery
LAFB	Left Anterior Fascicular Block
LBBB	Left Bundle Branch Block
LPFB	Left Posterior Fascicular Block
LV	Left Ventricle
LVH	Left Ventricular Hypertrophy
LVOT	Left Ventricular Outflow Tract Tachycardia
MAT	Multifocal Atrial Tachycardia
MI	Myocardial Infarction
NSR	Normal Sinus Rhythm
NSTEMI	Non-ST Elevation MI
OM	Obtuse Marginal

PAC	Premature Atrial Contraction
PDA	Posterior Descending Artery
PJC	Premature Junctional Complex
PMT	Pacemaker Mediated Tachycardia
PRWP	Poor R-Wave Progression
PVC	Premature Ventricular Contraction
QTc	Corrected QT interval
RBBB	Right Bundle Branch Block
RCA	Right Coronary Artery
RV	Right Ventricle
RVH	Right Ventricular Hypertrophy
RVMI	Right Ventricular Myocardial Infarction
RVOT	Right Ventricular Outflow Tract Tachycardia
STD	ST Depression
STE	ST Elevation
STEMI	ST Elevation MI
SVT	Supraventricular Tachycardia
TWF	T Wave Flattening
TWI	T Wave Inversion
VF	Ventricular Fibrillation
VT	Ventricular Tachycardia
WPW	Wolff-Parkinson-White

INDEX

(Note: Page number in *italics* indicates figures and page numbers followed by "t" indicates tables)

A

Aberrancy, 319
Accelerated idioventricular rhythm, 24
Accelerated junctional rhythm, 111–112,
    291–292
    AV dissociation, 70, *70*, 91–92
    premature junctional contraction, 97, *97*
Action potential
    myocardial cell, 2, *2*
    pacemaker cell, 3, *3*
Adrenergic ventricular tachycardia, 312
Annular ventricular tachycardia, 312
Anterior myocardial infarction,
    169–170, 361
    acute complications, 362
    atrial fibrillation with, 379–380
    atrioventricular block with, 393–394
    evolution of ECG appearance, 417–418
    LAD
        lesions location, 364, *364*
        proximal occlusion of, 413–414
    left main coronary artery occlusion,
        429–430
    mistaken for VT, ECG, 409–410
    with right bundle branch block, 381–382
    subtypes, 362t
Arrhythmogenic right ventricular dysplasia
    (ARVD)
    arrhythmias, 119
    clinical course, 119
    diagnosis, 119
    ECG, 119, 125–126, 155–156
    management, 119
    pathogenesis, 119
Ashman phenomenon, 29, *29*, 319
Atrial demand pacer, 433
Atrial fibrillation, 265
    with aberrancy, 325–326, 341–342

with complete heart block, 69, *69*
with digoxin toxicity, 91–92
with left bundle branch block, 343–344
mechanism of, 265
with rapid ventricular response, 24,
    281–282, 301–302
with right ventricular MI, 366
with 3-second sinus pause, 24
types of, 265
Wolff–Parkinson–White pattern, 120,
    325–326, 341–342
Atrial flutter, 266
    aberrancy, 333–334
    with 2:1 conduction, 285–286
    mimics, 266
    reverse typical atrial flutter, 266
    typical atrial flutter, 266
    with variable block, 295–296
Atrial infarction, 363
Atrial pacemakers, 433
Atrial pacing and capture, 431, 439–440
Atrial tachycardia, 270
    with 2:1 AV block, 297–298
    with 4:1 AV block, 283–284
    ECG, 303–304
    multifocal (*see* Multifocal atrial tachy-
        cardia)
    premature atrial contractions, 96–97
Atrioventricular block, 363
    in chronic atrial fibrillation, 90
    first degree, 64, *64*
    right ventricular MI, 366
    second degree (*see* Second degree AV
        block)
    third degree (*see* Third degree AV block;
        Complete heart block)
Atrioventricular (AV) dissociation, 70, *70*
    accelerated junctional rhythm, 91, 92

isorhythmic dissociation, 89, 90
ventricular tachycardia, 313
Atrioventricular nodal reentrant tachycardia
    (AVNRT), 267
    atypical, 268, *268*
    ECGs 277–280, 289–290, 305–306
Atrioventricular paced rhythm, 443–444
Atrioventricular reciprocating tachycardia,
    269
    antidromic AVRT, 269
    ECG, 287–288
    orthodromic AVRT, 269
Arrhythmias (*see also* Supraventricular
    tachyarrhythmias)
    sinus arrhythmia
        ECG appearance, 17, *17*, 21
        nonrespiratory, 17
        respiratory, 17
    uniform P wave morphology, 22
Axis deviation, 7, *7*

B

Benign early repolarization (BER)
    ECG, 369, 377–378
Bifascicular block
    LAFB + LPFB, 35, *35*
    LAFB + RBBB, 47–56
    RBBB + LAFB, 35, *35*
Bigeminy
    atrial, 96, 103–106
    ventricular, 98
Bipolar electrode, 435
Biventricular pacing, 435, *435*
Bradycardia
    in hyperkalemia, 223–224
    in hypothermia, 139
    inappropriate, 20

junctional, 21, 22
in myxedema coma, 249–250
pacemaker therapy, 192
right ventricular MI, 366
sinus bradycardia
    first degree AV block, 22, 24
    2.4-second sinus pause, 22
Brugada pattern and syndrome
    clinical course, 118
    differential diagnosis, 118
    ECG features, 118, *118*
    pathogenesis, 118
    treatment, 118
    type I pattern, 137–138, 141–142,
        151–152
    type 2 pattern, 145–146, 465t, 466t

C

Capture beats, 313, *313*
Cardiac glycosides, 273
Cardiac resynchronization therapy, 435,
    435, 453–454
    biventricular pacing (*see* Biventricular
        pacing)
Cardiac tamponade
    ECG, 253–254, 257–258
Catecholaminergic polymorphic VT, 315
Cerebral T waves
    ECG, 166, 177–178, 183–184
Chronic obstructive pulmonary disease
    (COPD)
    ECG findings, 231, 245–246
    Lead I sign, 231
    RVH in, 231
Circumflex artery, 357, *357*
Class IA antiarrhythmics, 4
Class III antiarrhythmics, 4

Cocaine overdose
  action potential, *147*
  Brugada pattern, 118
  ECG appearance, 147–148
  Na⁺ channel–blocking drugs, 122
Complete heart block, 69, *69*
  atrial fibrillation with, 69, *69*, 91, 92
  AV dissociation, 70
  ECG, 70–76, 79–80, 89–92
Concealed retrograde conduction, 6, *6*
Conducted premature atrial contractions,
    469t, 470t
  normal sinus rhythm with, 107–108
Conduction
  anatomy, 5, *5*
  retrograde conduction patterns, 6, *6*
Congenital long QT syndrome
  ECG features, 192, *192*, 205–206
  mutations and channels, 192, *192*
  treatment, 192
Coronary anatomy, 357, *357*

D

DDD pacing, 434, 436
Delta wave, 120, 127–128, 131–134
Diastolic dysfunction, 366
Digitalis effect, 165, *165*, 179–180,
    461t, 462t
Digitalis toxicity
  electrophysiology of, 273
  ECG, 274, 283–284, 297–298
Dual chamber pacemaker, 434
  ECG, 445–446

E

Early repolarization (*see* Benign early
    repolarization)
ECG interpretation
  axis, 13
  clinical history, 13
  general approach to, 15
  intervals, 14
  ischemia, 14
  QRS voltage and width, 13
  rate, 13
  rhythm, 13
  wave morphologies, 14
Ectopic atrial impulse, 319, *319*

Effective refractory periods, 4, *4*
Electrical alternans
  ECG, 233–234, 239–240
Epsilon wave, 461t, 462t
Escape rhythm (*see* Junctional escape
    rhythm; Ventricular escape
    rhythm)

F

Fascicular ventricular tachycardia, 312,
    345–346
First degree AV block
  causes, 64
  ECG features, 64, *64*, 67, 71, 72
  extreme first degree block, 73–78
  pitfalls in diagnosis, 64, *64*
  PR prolongation, 469t, 470t
First degree SA block, 19, *19*
Fixed rate ventricular pacer, 433
Flecainide toxicity
  ECG appearance, 157–158
Friedreich's ataxia, 235–236
Frontal leads, 7, *7*
Fusion beats, 313

H

Hexaxial method, 7
Hyperacute T waves, 181–182
  in anterior STEMI, 169–170, 395–396,
    418–419
  ischemic T-wave changes, 162
Hypercalcemia
  ECG, 201–202
  QT abnormalities, 194, *194*
  ST segment, 12
Hyperkalemia, 195, *195*, 199–200,
    203–204, 207–208
  pacemaker failure in, 211–212, 455–456
  PR prolongation in, 207–208
  peaked T Wave, 173–174, 463t, 464t
  progressive dyspnea, 337–338
  sine wave, 203–204, 337–338, 353–354,
    469t, 470t
Hypertrophic cardiomyopathy, 229
  clinical complications, 229
  clinical presentations, 229
  ECG, 229, 235–236, 255–256, 463t,
    464t

Hypocalcemia
  ECG, 97–98
  QT abnormalities
    action potential, *194*
    QT prolongation secondary to,
      197–198
    ST segment, 12
Hypokalemia
  ECG, 195, *196*, 210, 213–214, 219–220
Hypotension
  right ventricular MI, 366
Hypothermia, 243–244
  ECG, 249–250
  J waves, 121, *121*, 135–136, 139–140,
    153–154, 463t, 464t

I

Idiopathic ventricular tachycardia, 312
Inappropriate bradycardia, 20
Incomplete left bundle branch block,
    32, *32*
Inferior myocardial infarction, 361
  anatomy, 363, *363*
  complications, 363
  extending to right ventricle, 374–375,
    383–384
  mistaken for VT, 403–406
  second degree AV block, 393–394,
    423–424
  subtle ST elevation in, 388–389,
    411–412
  subtypes, 363
Inferolateral myocardial infarction, 363
Inferoposterior myocardial infarction, 363
  ECG, 403–404
Ischemic T-wave changes
  hyperacute T waves, 162
  pseudonormalization, 162, *162*
  T waves inversions, 162, *162*, 162t
Isorhythmic AV dissociation, 89–90

J

J waves, 121, *121*, 135–136, 139–140, 463t,
    464t
Junctional escape rhythm
  sinus node dysfunction, 18, *18*, 24
Junctional tachycardia
  AV dissociation, 70

digoxin toxicity, 274
nonparoxysmal, 97, 264
supraventricular tachyarrhythmia
  ECG features, 271
  increased automaticity, 271t
  mechanism, 271
  misdiagnosis, 271
  retrograde conduction, *271*
Juvenile T-wave pattern, 165, *165*

L

Lateral myocardial infarction, 421–422
Left anterior fascicular (LAF) block
  causes, 33, *33*
  criteria for, 33t
  ECG, 33, 43–46
Left bundle branch block (LBBB), 37–38,
    41–42, 371, *371*
  aberrant septal depolarization, 30
  cardiac resynchronization therapy, 32
  clinical significance, 32
  criteria for, 32
  discordance, 32
  ECG appearance, 37–38, 41–42
  incomplete, 32, *32*
  inferoposterior MI with, 401–402
  location, 32
  right ventricular outflow tachycardia,
    31, *31*
  right-sided bypass tract, 31, *31*
  ventricular depolarization, 30, *30*
  ventricular pacing, 31, *31*
Left main coronary artery occlusion
  anterolateral MI, 361
  territory infarction, 429–430
Left posterior fascicular (LPF) block, 34,
    34, 34t
Left ventricular aneurysm
  anatomy, 368, *368*
  clinical course, 368
  ECG, 368, *368*, 391–392
  pathology, 368
Left ventricular strain, 164, 167–168,
    185–186
Left ventricular hypertrophy
  causes, 228
  ECG, 228, *228*, 247–248
Left ventricular outflow tract tachycardia,
    312

Lenegre disease, 68
Lev disease, 68
Long QT syndrome, (see Congenital long
    QT syndrome)
Low voltage ECG, 232, 251–252, 465t, 466t
LV strain pattern, 167–168, 186–187
    asymmetric T wave inversion, 467t, 468t
    digitalis effect, 165, *165*, 179–180
    ECG features, 164, *164*
    mechanism, 164, *164*
    ST depression, 164
    T-wave morphology, 164
Lyme carditis, 76

M
Magnet, 438
Mitral annulus ventricular tachycardia, 312
Mobitz I block
    causes, 65, *65*
    ECG features, 89–92
        grouped beating, 65
        PR interval lengthening, 65, *65*
        R-R interval variable, 65, *65*
        shortest PR interval, 65
    location, 65
    mechanism, 65
Mobitz II block
    causes, 66
    ECG features
        constant PR length, 66
        variable conduction, 81–82
        wide QRS Complexes, 66
    location, 66
    mechanism, 66
    vs. Mobitz I block, 66t
Monomorphic ventricular tachycardia
    causes, 311
    ECG features, 313, *313*
    location, 311
    mechanism, 311
    origins of, 312
    V1 and V6 morphologies, 314, *314*
Multifocal atrial tachycardia (MAT),
    293–294, 467t, 468t
    causes and clinical course, 272
    ECG, 272, *272*, 293–294, 299–300,
        307–308
    mechanism, 272
    misdiagnosis, 272

Myocardial infarction (see also ST elevation
    myocardial infarction)
    anterior (see Anterior myocardial infarction)
    hyperkalemia, 354
    inferior (see Inferior myocardial infarc-
        tion)
    inferior ventricular, 373–374
    inferolateral, 363
    inferoposterior, 363
    lateral, 421–422
    ventricular tachycardia
        acute dyspnea, treadmill, 327–328
        and congestive heart failure, 351–352
        shortness of breath, 351–352
Myocarditis, 340, 372, 419–420
Myxedema coma
    ECG, 243–244, 249–250

N
Nonconducted premature atrial contrac-
    tions, 101, 102
Normal sinus rhythm, 24
Normal T wave, 162

O
Obtuse marginal (OM) arteries, 357, *357*
Orthodromic atrioventricular reciprocating
    tachycardia, 269, *269*
Osborn wave (see J wave)
Outflow tract tachycardia, 312

P
P wave, 12
Pacemaker
    anatomy of, *435*
    atrial demand pacemaker, 433
    biventricular pacing, 435, *435*
    dual chamber pacing, 434, 434t
    ECG appearance, 431, *431*
    electrode types, 431
    failures, 437, *437*
        failure to capture, 447–449,
        455–456
        failure to pace, 449–450
        failure to sense, 449–450
    fixed rate ventricular pacer, 433
    magnet, 438, *438*

    malfunction, hyperkalemia
        ECG, 455–456
    nomenclature, 432, 432t
    oversensing, 433
    pacemaker-mediated tachycardia,
        436, *436*
    septal perforation by pacer lead, 446
    single chamber pacing, 433
    ST elevation MI in, 457–458
    ventricular demand pacer, 433
Pacemaker syndrome, 433
Pacemaker-mediated tachycardia (PMT)
    conduction pathway, *436*
    ECG appearance, 436, *436*, 451–452
    mechanism, 436
    misdiagnosis, 436
    treatment, 436
Papillary muscle rupture, 363
Paroxysmal atrial tachycardia, 270, 297–298
Pericarditis
    clinical characteristics, 367
    ECG, 367, *367*, 367t, 385–386, 407–408
    after penetrating trauma, 415–416
    persistent juvenile T-wave pattern, 165
    PR elevation and ST depression in avR,
        467t, 468t
Polymorphic ventricular tachycardia, 315, *315*
    ECG, 324, *324*, 349–350
    Torsades de Pointes (see Torsades de
        Pointes)
Posterior descending artery (PDA), 357, *357*
Posterior myocardial infarction
    anatomy, 364
    ECG features, 364, *364*, 364t
    mid circumflex occlusion, 375–376
    with posterior leads shown, 389–390
    resulting in VT, 397–398
Postinfarction T waves, 187–188
Postventricular atrial refractory period
    (PVARP), 436
PR interval, 12
PR segment, 12
Precordial leads, 8, *8*
Premature atrial contractions (PACs)
    with aberrant ventricular conduction,
        99–100
    atrial tachycardia, 96
    conducted PAC, 96, *96*, 105–108
    grouped beats, *101*, 102
    noncompensatory pause, 99, 100

    nonconducted PAC, 96, *96*, 101, 103
Premature junctional contractions (PJCs)
    accelerated junctional rhythm, 97,
        97, 112
    anterograde and retrograde conduction,
        97, *97*
    different appearances of, *97*
    ECG features, 97
Premature ventricular contraction (PVC)
    bigeminy pattern, 98, *98*, 99, 100
    couplet, 98, *98*, 109–110
    coupling intervals, 98, *98*
    ECG appearance, 98, *98*
    multifocal, 113–114
    polymorphic, 98, *98*
    recurring, 98, *98*
    trigeminy pattern, 98, 99, 100
Prinzmetal angina, 359
Pulmonary embolism, 231
    ECG, 237–238
Pulse generator, 431

Q
QRS morphology, abnormal
    ARVD (see Arrhythmogenic right ven-
        tricular dysplasia (ARVD))
    Brugada pattern and syndrome (see
        Brugada pattern and syndrome)
    hypothermia, 121, *121*, 135, 136,
        139, 140
    Na$^+$ channel blockade, 122, *122*
    Wolff–Parkinson–White pattern (see
        Wolff–Parkinson–White pattern)
QRS wave, 12
    morphology, 9
    septal depolarization, 9
    ventricular depolarization, 9, *9*
QRS widening
    ECG abnormality, 461t, 462t
QT abnormalities
    congenital long QT syndrome (see
        Congenital long QT syndrome)
    hypercalcemia (see Hypercalcemia)
    hyperkalemia (see Hyperkalemia)
    hypocalcemia, 194, *194*, 197–198
    hypokalemia (see Hypokalemia)
    QT interval, 191, *191*
    short QT syndrome (see Short QT
        syndrome)

QT interval, 12, 191, *191*
QT prolongation, 217–218, *218*
  ECG, 217, 218, 324
  hypocalcemia, 197–198
  intraparenchymal hemorrhage, 221–222

R
R in aVR 122, 131, 145, 149, 151, 159
Reentrant circuit, 4, *4*
Reentrant SVT
  AVNRT *vs.* AVRT, 275–276
  dyspnea and heart racing, 279–280
  retrograde P waves, 469t, 470t
Refractory periods, 4, *4*
Relative refractory periods, 4, *4*
Respiratory sinus arrhythmia, 17
Rhythm nomenclature, 11, *11*, 11t
Right bundle branch block (RBBB),
    39–40
  anterior MI, with 381–382
  criteria for, 29
  depolarization pattern, 28, *28*
  discordance, 29
  ECG appearance, 39, 40
  incomplete, 29
  left ventricular activation, 28
  QRS morphologies in V1, 29
  septal depolarization, 28
Right bundle branch block pattern
  Ashman phenomenon, 29, *29*
  VT from left ventricular focus,
    29, *29*
Right coronary artery (RCA), 357, *357*
Right coronary dominance, 357
Right ventricular hypertrophy
  causes, 230
  ECG, 241–242
Right ventricular MI, 363, 373–374
  anatomy, 365, *365*
  complications of, 366
  ECG features, 365, *365*
  with second degree AV block,
    373–374
  with ST elevation in V1, 383–384
Right ventricular outflow tract tachycardia,
    31, *31*, 312, 331–332
R-on-T phenomenon, 98
RR interval, 12

S
Second degree AV block
  advanced, 67, *67*, 85, 86
    3:1 conduction, 87–88
  2:1 conduction
    ECG appearance, 73–76, 83, 84
  high-grade, 85–86
  Mobitz I block
    causes, 65, *65*
    ECG appearance, 65, *65*, 71, 72,
      89–90, 101, 393–394
    location, 65
    mechanism, 65
    pitfalls, 65
    variable conduction 80, 81
  Mobitz II block
    causes, 66
    ECG features, 66, 71
    in setting of MI, 425
    location, 66
    mechanism, 66
    pitfalls, 66, 66t
Second degree SA block, 19, *19*
Septal depolarization
  aberrant, 30
  left bundle branch block, 30
  QRS wave, 9
  right bundle branch block, 28
Septal perforation, 446
Short QT syndrome
  arrhythmias, 193
  differential diagnosis, 193
  ECG appearance, 193, *193*
  management, 193
  mutations, 193
Sick sinus syndrome, 20, 457–458
Sine wave, 195, *204*, 354, 470t
Single chamber pacemaker, 433
Sinoatrial exit block
  causes, 19
  subtypes, 19, *19*
Sinus arrest, 18, *18*, 24
Sinus arrhythmia
  ECG appearance, 17, *17*, 21, 22
Sinus bradycardia
  first degree AV block, 22, 24
  2.4-second sinus pause, 22
Sinus dysfunction
  inappropriate bradycardia, 20

junctional escape rhythm, 18, *18*
  sick sinus syndrome, 20
  sinoatrial exit block, 19, *19*
  sinus arrest, 18, *18*
  sinus arrhythmia, 17, *17*
  tachycardia-bradycardia syndrome, 20
  ventricular escape rhythm, 18, *18*
  wandering atrial pacemaker, 17, *17*
Sinus node dysfunction, 18, *18*
Sinus tachycardia
  Na+ channel–blocking drugs, 122
  tricyclic antidepressant overdose,
    129–130
  wide-complex tachycardia, 316
Sodium channel blockade, 122, *122*
  cocaine overdose 147, 148
  tricyclic antidepressant overdose
    129–130, 143–144, 149–150
ST depression, 358, *358*
ST elevation
  in lead aVR, 425–426
ST elevation myocardial infarction (STEMI)
  (*see also* Anterior ST elevation myo-
    cardial infarction)
  acute ischemia, 359, *359*
  coronary artery occlusion sites, 361, *361*
  evolution of ECG changes, 359, *359*
  LBBB morphology, 314, 401–402, 465t,
    466t
  mimics of, 372
  morphologies of, *360*
  pathophysiology, 359
  reperfusion, 359
  ST vector, 359, *359*
ST segment, 12
Subarachnoid hemorrhage 178–179,
    183–184
Subendocardial ischemia
  ECG features, 358, *358*
  pathophysiology, 358, *358*
Supraventricular tachyarrhythmia
  atrial fibrillation (*see* Atrial fibrillation)
  atrial flutter (*see* Atrial flutter)
  AVNRT (*see* AV nodal reentrant tachy-
    cardia)
  AVRT (*see* Atrioventricular reciprocating
    tachycardia)
  focal atrial tachycardia, 270, *270*
  junctional tachycardia, 271, *271*, 271t

mechanisms
  increased automaticity, 263, *263*
  reentry, 263, *263*, 263t, 275–276
  triggered activity, 263, *263*
multifocal atrial tachycardia (*see* Multifocal atrial tachycardia)
narrow complex tachycardias, 264, *264*
Systolic dysfunction, 366

T
T wave, 12
  cerebral T waves, 166, 177–178,
    183–184
  inversions (TWI), 163
    in digitalis effect, 165, 179–180
    ischemic, 187–188
    in LV strain 164, 185–186
    in Wellens syndrome, 163
  peaked (*see* hyperkalemia)
  pseudonormalization, 162
T waves, abnormal
  anterior MI, 169–170
  cerebral T waves (*see* Cerebral T waves)
  hyperkalemia, 165, *165*, 173–174
  ischemic T-wave changes, 162,
    162, 162t
  LV strain pattern (*see* LV strain pattern)
  persistent juvenile T-wave pattern,
    165, *165*
  Wellens syndrome (*see* Wellens
    syndrome)
Tachycardia–bradycardia syndrome, 20
Takotsubo cardiomyopathy
  angiographic appearance, 370, *370*
  ECG appearance, 370, *370*
  ECG progression, 399–400
  clinical presentation, 370
  ECG appearance, 370, *370*
  prognosis, 370
Tamponade (*see* Cardiac tamponade)
Third degree AV block
  causes, 68
  clinical significance, 68
  location, 68
Third degree SA block, 19, *19*
Torsades de Pointes, 315, 324, 329–330,
    465t, 466t
Tricuspid annulus VT, 312

Tricyclic antidepressant overdose
ECG, 129–130, 143–144, 149–150
Trifascicular block, 36, *36*
RBBB + LAFB + second degree AV block, 59–60
RBBB + LPFB + first degree AV block, 53–54
Trigeminy (*see* Premature ventricular contractions)

U

U wave, 12
Unipolar electrode, 431

V

Vagal stimulation, 366
Ventricular demand pacer, 433
Ventricular depolarization, 324
action potential, 2
left bundle branch block, 30, *30*

QRS wave, 9, 12
QT interval, 191
RBBB morphology, 446
Ventricular escape rhythm, 18, *18*
Ventricular fibrillation, 315, *315*
ECG, 323–324
Ventricular flutter
ECG appearance of, 315, *315*
ECG, 339–340
Ventricular pacemakers, 433
Ventricular pacing and capture, 431
ECG, 441–442
Ventricular pre-excitation, 31
Ventricular rate, 10, *10*
Ventricular tachycardia (VT)
ECG, 335–336, 347–348, 351–352
fascicular, 312, 345–346
left ventricular outflow tract, 321–322
right ventricular outflow tract, 331–332
monomorphic VT (*see* Monomorphic VT)
polymorphic VT, 315, *315*(*see also* Polymorphic VT)

Ventriculoatrial conduction, 6, *6*
VVI pacing, 433, *448*

W

Wandering atrial pacemaker, 17, *17*, 21
Wellens syndrome
biphasic T wave, 469t, 470t
criteria, 163
ECG appearance, 175–176
ECG features, 163, *163*
management, 163
prognosis, 163
symmetric T wave inversion 163
Wenckebach block (*see also* Second degree AV block; Mobitz I block)
causes, 65, *65*
ECG features, 65, *65*
location, 65
mechanism, 65
Wide-complex tachycardia

acute MI with extreme ST elevation, 320, *320*
hyperkalemia, 320, *320*
mechanisms, 316
Na⁺ channel blockade, 320, *320*
supraventricular causes
antidromic AVRT, 317, *317*
atrial fibrillation, 318, *318*
ECG features, 316, *316*
preexisting BBB, 319, *319*
rate-related BBB, 319, *319*
Wolff–Parkinson–White pattern
arrhythmias, 120
with atrial fibrillation, 325–326, 341–342
delta wave and QRS widening, 463t, 464t
direction of conduction, 120, *120*
ECG appearance, 120, 123, 124, 134, 135
left-sided bypass tract, 127–128, *128*
right-sided bypass tract, 131–132
location, 120, *120*
pathogenesis, 120

DATE DUE

RRS1202